Firesetting and Mental Health

Theory, Research and Practice

Edited by Geoffrey L. Dickens,
Philip A. Sugarman and Theresa A. Gannon

D1423831

RCPsych Publications

© The Royal College of Psychiatrists 2012

RCPsych Publications is an imprint of the Royal College of Psychiatrists,
17 Belgrave Square, London SW1X 8PG
http://www.rcpsych.ac.uk

British Library Cataloguing-in-Publication Data.
A catalogue record for this book is available from the British Library.

ISBN 978-1-908020-37-6

Distributed in North America by Publishers Storage and Shipping Company.

Printed in the UK by Bell & Bain Limited, Glasgow.

Contents

Part II: Practice and law

Figures, tables and boxes

Figures

Tables

Boxes

Contributors

Sally Averill, Barrister, Senior Policy Advisor, Crown Prosecution Service, London, UK

Magali Barnoux, PhD Candidate, CORE-FP, School of Psychology, University of Kent, UK

Sabyasachi Bhaumik, Medical Director and Consultant Psychiatrist, Learning Disability Service, Leicestershire Partnership NHS Trust, UK

John Devapriam, Consultant Psychiatrist, Learning Disability Service, Leicestershire Partnership NHS Trust, UK

Geoff Dickens, Head of Nursing Research, St Andrew's Healthcare, Northampton; Visiting Lecturer in Forensic Mental Health, King's College London Institute of Psychiatry; Senior Lecturer, University of Northampton, UK

Rebekah M. Doley, Assistant Professor and Director, Clinical and Forensic Psychology Programmes, School of Psychology, Bond University, Queensland, Australia

Mairead Dolan, Professor of Forensic Psychiatry, Monash University, and Assistant Clinical Director (Research), Centre for Forensic Behavioural Science, Victorian Institute for Forensic Mental Health, Victoria, Australia

Kenneth R. Fineman, Associate Clinical Professor of Medical Psychology, Department of Psychiatry and Human Behavior, University of California, Irvine, USA

Katarina Fritzon, Associate Professor, Bond University, Queensland, Australia

Theresa A. Gannon, Reader in Forensic Psychology and Chartered Forensic Psychologist, CORE-FP, School of Psychology, University of Kent, UK

Allan Grice, Former Senior Fire Safety and Operations Officer, North East Area London Fire Brigade; Late Principal Fire Safety Officer, Devon Fire and Rescue Service; Visiting Lecturer, Applied Fire Safety Law, University of Leeds; Independent Fire Safety Advisor

Clive R. Hollin, Professor of Criminological Psychology, University of Leicester, UK

Troy E. McEwan, Australian Research Council Postdoctoral Fellow, Centre for Behavioural Science, Monash University, and Clinical and Forensic Psychologist, Victorian Institute of Forensic Mental Health, Victoria, Australia

Sherri MacKay, Assistant Professor, Department of Psychiatry, University of Toronto, and Psychologist, Provincial Director of The Arson Prevention Program for Children (TAPP-C), Centre for Addiction and Mental Health (CAMH), Toronto, Canada

Afroditi Pina, Lecturer in Forensic Psychology, CORE-FP, School of Psychology, University of Kent, UK

Tim Rogers, Consultant Forensic Psychiatrist, North London Forensic Service, UK

Erin M. Ruttle, PhD Candidate, Clinical Development Psychology, York University; Research Coordinator, The Arson Prevention Program for Children (TAPP-C), Centre for Addiction and Mental Health (CAMH), Toronto, Canada

Philip Sugarman, Chief Executive and Medical Director, St Andrew's Healthcare, Northampton; Visiting Senior Lecturer, King's College London Institute of Psychiatry; Visiting Professor, University of Northampton, UK

Nichola Tyler, PhD Candidate, CORE-FP, School of Psychology, University of Kent, UK

Ashley K. Ward, PhD Candidate, Clinical Development Psychology, York University Program Co-ordinator, The Arson Prevention Program for Children (TAPP-C), Centre for Addiction and Mental Health (CAMH), Toronto, Canada

Bruce D. Watt, Assistant Professor, School of Psychology, Bond University, Queensland, Australia

Preface

Geoff Dickens, Philip Sugarman and Theresa A. Gannon

Arson and other types of deliberate firesetting have major human and financial costs. People with mental disorder are disproportionately involved, and mental health and criminal justice practitioners are often required to assess, treat and manage this troubling group. The literature on juvenile firesetting is advanced relative to that on adult firesetting but around half of all deliberate fire-related damage is caused by adults, so it is surprising that professionals who want to learn more about adult firesetting have been so poorly served, with no specialist single-subject text until now. This volume aims to provide a fresh, focused look at firesetting, at its interface with mental health and mental disorder; and to bring together research evidence, theory and practitioner advice from multiple perspectives in one accessible volume.

Medico-legal interest in deliberate firesetting can be dated, at least in the United Kingdom, to 1829 when Jonathan Martin the York Minster arsonist was declared not guilty on the grounds of insanity (Balston, 1945). However, interest and research on the subject has been sporadic. Although this means that there are considerable opportunities for future research on the topic, it also means that the existing literature is limited. In the current volume we have taken a decision that individual chapter authors be allowed to develop their ideas using the whole of the available literature. This means that, inevitably, there is some repetition between chapters when referring to theories, definitions and so on. However, this approach has also facilitated a situation where individual chapters all stand on their own merits and without repeated reference to one another.

Terminology

Both *firesetting* and *arson* are commonly used terms in the literature. In brief, *firesetting* describes a particular behaviour (the deliberate setting of fires), while *arson* is a legal term that varies across jurisdictions in its precise meaning. Although we have preferred firesetting in our title, our approach in commissioning chapters has been to give authors the freedom to use their own preferred terminology, with the proviso that they specify and justify their own definitions.

The future

In the UK the number of deliberately set fires fell year on year from 2002 to 2007 (the most recent annual figure at the time of writing); and the frequency of fatalities and non-fatal casualties has also decreased in recent years (Department for Communities and Local Government, 2009). Indeed, 2007 saw the lowest number of fire-related deaths in the UK since 1950. This marked reduction in the UK reflects the success of a coordinated, government-supported strategic initiative to tackle the problem by the Arson Control Forum (ACF). Established in 2001 the ACF brought together wide-ranging groups with an interest in arson, including representatives from the police and fire services, the Home Office, local government, business leaders, the Crown Prosecution Service and the insurance industry. Refreshed in 2008, the ACF now aims to sustain the reduction in the numbers of deliberate fires and related deaths and injuries.

There are still too many deliberate fires and too many fatalities and casualties resulting from them. Firesetting remains a particularly visible issue for clinical mental health professionals, for a number of reasons. Reports by the ACF (Office of the Deputy Prime Minister 2004; Department for Communities and Local Government, 2006) have consistently highlighted the increased risk of both accidental and deliberate fires in poorer, socially excluded communities. People with mental health problems comprise one of the most socially excluded groups in terms of lack of employment and premature death. Mental health professionals focus on the assessment of risk and dangerousness, on treatment and intervention, and on advising the legal system about the role of mental disorder and intentionality in firesetting behaviour. We believe this mental health approach to firesetting will be key to the development of the new interventions of the future which will help further reduce the toll of casualties and damage.

References

Balston, T. (1945) The Life of Jonathan Martin Incendiary of York Minster. Macmillan.

Department for Communities and Local Government (2006) *Learning Lessons from Real Fires: Findings from Fatal Fire Investigation Reports*. Research bulletin no. 9. Arson Control Forum (http://www.arsoncontrolforum.gov.uk/download/628).

Department for Communities and Local Government (2009) *Fire Statistics United Kingdom 2007*. Department for Communities and Local Government (http://www.communities.gov.uk/documents/statistics/pdf/1320522.pdf).

Office of the Deputy Prime Minister (2004) *Social Exclusion and the Risk of Fire*. Research bulletin no. 4. Arson Control Forum (http://www.communities.gov.uk/documents/fire/pdf/130697.pdf).

Part I: Theory and research

CHAPTER 1

Adult firesetters: prevalence, characteristics and psychopathology

Geoff Dickens and Philip Sugarman

Introduction

In the USA, one in 100 adults has a self-reported lifetime history of deliberate firesetting and, for 38% of these firesetting persisted beyond the age of 15 years (Blanco *et al*, 2010; Vaughn *et al*, 2010). These statistics, findings from the National Epidemiologic Survey on Alcohol and Related Conditions (NESARC), represent the first attempt worldwide to gauge the extent of intentional firesetting in a general adult population. If it is accurate, then, based on US population figures (US Census Bureau, 2010), there are roughly 1 million US adults who have deliberately set fires since age 15. In the UK the figure would approach 200 000 (Office for National Statistics, 2005). This chapter critically explores the current evidence base on the prevalence of firesetting behaviour and examines these new findings in the light of previous research on arson and firesetting among more highly selected offending and clinical populations. The key questions addressed relate first to the credibility of this new evidence, and the extent to which it supports the current knowledge base about the correlates, characteristics and psychopathology of arsonists and firesetters. Second, the chapter synthesises the current knowledge of the characteristics of those who deliberately set fires, and addresses the sociodemographic factors, psychopathological features, co-offending behaviours and developmental characteristics associated with deliberate firesetting (see Table 1.1). The chapter provides practitioners with state-of-the-art information on which to base clinical decision-making in this difficult and sometimes misunderstood area, and highlights gaps in knowledge, where future research is needed.

'Arson' is a legal term which defines the specific criminal act of intentionally or recklessly setting fire to property or wildland areas; an arsonist has, by definition, been convicted of the crime of arson. A firesetter displays a behavioural phenotype, the deliberate setting of fires, which may not have been prosecuted, for a number of reasons: the fire has been insufficiently severe to cause damage or has not been detected as a deliberate fire; it has not been possible to identify who set the fire; there is insufficient evidence to gain a conviction; or the young age of the firesetter. 'Firesetting' is therefore applicable to a wider range of people who deliberately set fires than the narrow legal definition represented by the term 'arson'. In this chapter firesetting is the preferred term; however, arson is used when it is accurate to do so in the context of individual studies that have been conducted with that subgroup of firesetters who hold a conviction for arson.

Prevalence

Adults

The NESARC study recruited a representative sample in excess of 40 000 non-institutionalised adults resident across the USA. Vaughn *et al* (2010) describe the diligence with which representativeness was ensured both by over-sampling hard-to-reach groups (including young adults and minority ethnic groups) and by weighting results to adjust for over-sampling and non-response. Data for the study were collected using standardised instrumentation by trained US census workers during face-to-face interviews. In total, 407 participants answered 'Yes' to the following item embedded in the Antisocial Personality Disorder (ASPD) interview module of the survey:

In your entire life, did you ever start a fire on purpose to destroy someone else's property or just to see it burn?

On the basis of the one study, it was separately reported that, after weighting the data, the lifetime prevalence rate of firesetting was 1.0% (Vaughn *et al*, 2010) or 1.13% (Blanco *et al*, 2010). The disparity between reported results appears to reflect different approaches to data analysis. Firesetters, defined as those affirming the above statement, were compared with non-firesetting population controls ($n=$ 41 552) across a range of sociodemographic and psychopathological variables, and to antisocial and offending behaviours. Blanco *et al* (2010) reported that 38% of firesetters affirmed a subsequent questionnaire statement that this behaviour had persisted beyond the age of 15 years. Unfortunately, no further analysis of data for this subgroup was presented.

The size and representativeness of the NESARC study (Blanco *et al*, 2010; Vaughn *et al*, 2010) are its key strengths. The sample recruited can confidently be expected to reflect the 'true' population response to the firesetting question within a fraction of a percentage point. The question item used to define firesetting, however, imposes a limitation on the study. Firesetting behaviour that is indicative of arson ('to destroy someone else's property') and other firesetting behaviour for imputed thrill- or pleasure-seeking ('just to see it burn') are conflated. It is possible, and is stated by the researchers, that non-pathological behaviour such as safely lighting bonfires could be defined as firesetting under the latter part of the definition, as could childhood fire play or experimentation. The potential effect of this conflation is an overestimation of the prevalence of deliberate firesetting. A second limitation, common to all survey studies, is the potential for response bias. In the NESARC study, underestimation of the true prevalence of lifetime firesetting is suggested by the relatively low rate reported compared with studies of children and adolescents (for figures see 'Children and adolescents' below). This may simply reflect the fact that respondents fail to remember their own childhood behaviour accurately. A likely candidate cause of under-reporting of lifetime firesetting among adults, however, was the mode of data collection employed in the NESARC study. That is, the face-to-face interview may be more prone to social desirability bias than are, for example, anonymous self-interviewing techniques (Clark Newman *et al*, 2002), reflecting that respondents simply may not wish to admit to undesirable behaviours.

A subsequent UK study of the prevalence of self-reported deliberate firesetting behaviour among adults (Gannon & Barrowcliffe, 2011) approached the problem from a different and enlightening perspective. The potential for pro-social response bias was reduced by requesting participants ($n = 158$) to complete a questionnaire booklet anonymously. More detailed information about the respondent's firesetting history, where reported, was elicited by items that enquired about each individual's reasons for setting fires. Additionally, more precise operational definitions were given to respondents to exclude reporting of firesetting prior to age 10 years and non-problematical or non-deliberate firesetting, including bonfires or accidental fires. In total, 11% of participants reported that they had intentionally set fires. Two (1.3%) respondents reported setting fires during adulthood, and the remainder reported this behaviour during adolescence only. Gannon & Barrowcliffe's sample is, inevitably, less representative of the general adult population than that recruited for the NESARC study. In particular, there was an over-preponderance of female participants, and almost certainly of more highly educated respondents, which could have led to an underestimation of the population prevalence for firesetting. Their study does suggest, however, that increased rigour in the design of research questions about adult firesetting, and the use of data collection modes that act to minimise response bias, may lead to more accurate estimations of firesetting prevalence during adulthood. If anything, the true prevalence of adult firesetting is likely to be higher than current estimates suggest. However, on the current evidence, this is little more than informed guesswork.

Despite their limitations, the studies discussed above are the first serious attempts to measure the prevalence of firesetting in the general adult population. While estimations of the number of firesetters in the population are almost certainly imprecise due to the methodological limitations outlined, they hint at the scale of this potentially problematical and harmful behaviour. Alternative methods of estimating the prevalence of firesetting are also limited. For example, we know that around 323 900 intentionally set fires were recorded by US fire departments in 2005, and that these fires caused 490 deaths, 9100 injuries and created $1 billion worth of costs related to property damage (Hall, 2007). However, the number of fires thought to be deliberate tells us little about the number of people responsible for those fires.

Children and adolescents

An interesting aspect of the NESARC firesetting study (Blanco *et al*, 2010; Vaughn *et al*, 2010) is its failure to reflect findings from the far more numerous epidemiological surveys of firesetting among children and adolescents. Different samples, definitions and measurements have been used by various researchers and therefore it is worth briefly describing a selection of studies. Dadds & Fraser (2006) collected data from the parent-reported Fire History Screen (Kolko & Kazdin, 1988) on 1359 Australian children aged 4–9 years. Fire play, as opposed to fire interest or match play, was reported by parents of 2% of 4- to 6-year-olds and over 5% of 7- to 9-year-olds. Del Bove *et al* (2008) reported that 29% of 567 Italian 11- to 18-year-olds self-reported 'yes' to the item 'I have set fires' on the Youth Self-Report form (YSR; Achenbach, 1991). Mackay *et al* (2009) collected self-report data from 396 Canadian pupils aged 11–19 years from 137 schools in 42 school boards. Firesetting was measured by response to the question 'In the last 12 months, how many times have you set something on fire that you weren't supposed to?' Only 32% selected the response 'Never in lifetime'. In contrast, 41% of respondents said they had set fires in their lifetime but not in the past 12 months, and the remaining 27% self-reported at least one incident of firesetting in the past year. Chen *et al* (2003) presented self-report data from a representative US national sample of 4595 adolescent respondents to the 1995 National Household Survey on Drug Abuse. Interestingly, this study examined the recent incidence of firesetting behaviour as opposed to the lifetime prevalence. An adapted form of the YSR employed in the study included an item about setting fires in the 6 months before interview. The self-reported 6-month incidence of firesetting was 6%. The study authors give the caveat that this YSR item may not discriminate between firesetting and experimentation.

The above studies indicate that firesetting behaviour is common in both children and adolescents. Indeed, Mackay *et al*'s (2009) survey results suggest that, for adolescents, some lifetime firesetting behaviour is the norm. The inescapable conclusion is that reported *lifetime* firesetting behaviour should, or certainly could, be equally prevalent among adults. The reasons for the discrepancy between self-reported lifetime prevalence of firesetting in adults (1%) and self-reported prevalence in children and adolescents (as high as 68% in Mackay *et al*, 2009) are not entirely clear, but to varying extents will include inconsistency between reporting measures and definitions, modes of data collection, pro-social bias and increased inability with advancing age to recall incidents of firesetting in youth. It is also possible that some people simply regard their own childhood firesetting as fairly unimportant or trivial and therefore do not report it.

In summary, fire interest appears to be common in children and adolescents in the general population and some firesetting behaviour, particularly during adolescence, is widespread. While the new information about adult self-reported firesetting from the NESARC study is welcome, current knowledge about the epidemiology of adult firesetting does not approach that of juvenile firesetting.

Characteristics of firesetters

Knowledge about the characteristics of those who deliberately set fires has traditionally been limited to the subset of those who come to the attention of the criminal justice and mental health services, chiefly convicted arsonists. The new epidemiological evidence from the NESARC study (Blanco *et al*, 2010; Vaughn *et al*, 2010), despite its limitations, together with the most recent studies of criminal and clinical samples, offers the opportunity to take a fresh look at the issue (Box 1.1). In this section, findings from the NESARC study regarding the characteristics of firesetters are discussed alongside those from studies of criminal justice and psychiatric samples in order to assess the extent to which new epidemiological information supports or challenges our knowledge of firesetting gained from less representative samples.

Sociodemographic factors

Gender

Results from the NESARC study (Blanco *et al*, 2010; Vaughn *et al*, 2010) highlighted that in excess of 80% of self-reported firesetters were men, a male:female gender ratio approximating 5:1. Gender ratios approaching or, in certain cases, exceeding this are common in various selected samples. Lewis & Yarnell (1951) identified 1346 adult arsonists from underwriting and insurance records and reported a male:female ratio of 6:1. Soothill *et al* (2004) reported a 9:1 ratio among 10 271 people convicted of arson in England and Wales between 1963 and 2001. Interestingly, the proportion of females convicted of arson increased from 4% (25 males to 1 female) in 1963–65 to 12% (8 males to 1 female) in 1980–81 and again to 14% (6 males for every female) in 2000–01, suggesting that the gender imbalance is not static across time. Anwar *et al* (2011) reported a ratio of nearly 4 males to 1 female based on the national database records of convictions for arson in Sweden from 1988 to 2000 (*n* = 1340). The lower male:female ratio in their study may reflect that, in Sweden, individuals are found guilty irrespective of mental illness and therefore any bias whereby women are diverted from the criminal justice system is removed.

Box 1.1 Common characteristics of firesetters

Sociodemographic features

- Predominantly male, white and young
- Unskilled employment or unemployment, low socioeconomic status
- Single, living alone, never married
- Low educational achievement

Psychopathology

- High rates of antisocial personality disorder and other personality disorders
- High levels of substance misuse as principal or comorbid disorder
- Most frequent other diagnoses include schizophrenia and affective disorders; the risk for firesetting is increased in those with schizophrenia
- Low numbers of those meeting full criteria for pyromania but emerging evidence (from relatively small populations) suggests a prevalence rate of 3–10% among those with depression or impulse control disorders
- No evidence for a link between firesetting and sexual pathology or fetishism
- Lack of assertiveness and communication skills, and presence of inwardly directed hostility and punitiveness
- Poor self-esteem, high levels of anxiety, guilt and low mood

Neurodevelopmental, developmental features and family history

- Intellectual disability may be a feature of about 10% of firesetters and there is some evidence of neurodevelopmental disorders in males (7% may have Asperger syndrome)
- Low IQ levels relative to general population
- Family history of offending is frequent
- Common reports of childhood behavioural disturbance, truancy, reading difficulties
- Childhood institutionalisation is common

History of offending and antisocial behaviour

- Firesetters have often been involved in an array of other offending and antisocial behaviours
- Offending behaviours are mostly non-violent offending but some firesetters are also violent

---

A similar gender imbalance, although slightly less pronounced, is also a feature of psychiatric samples. Enayati *et al* (2008) examined the Swedish national database, which held records of all 214 people convicted of arson between 1997 and 2001 who were subsequently referred for forensic psychiatric assessment, and reported a ratio of about 3:1. This supports the suggestion above that women are more likely than men to be referred to psychiatric services following arson or firesetting. Other studies, largely with samples referred for pre-trial or pre-sentencing reports, have reported male:female ratios of between 3:1 and 6:1 (Fleszar-Szumigajowa, 1969; Bradford, 1982; Bourget & Bradford, 1989; Leong, 1992; Rix, 1994; Puri *et al*, 1995; Ritchie & Huff, 1999; Jayaraman & Frazer, 2006; Dickens *et al*, 2009), most lying towards the lower end of this range. One study, by Swinton & Ahmed (2001), reported a male:female ratio of just over 1.5:1 among their sample of 79 arsonists detained in a high-security psychiatric hospital. This suggests that women who deliberately set fires are disproportionately over-represented in high-security settings.

In summary, the pronounced over-representation of males suggested by the epidemiological evidence on firesetting is largely replicated in arson conviction data and in findings from highly selected psychiatric samples. Deliberate firesetting is, therefore, largely a male activity. Where research results are not presented separately by gender then study findings will largely reflect the over-preponderance of men in research samples, and care should be taken before generalising them to women. In the current chapter the reader should generally assume that quoted results, unless specifically stated otherwise, refer to male samples or to samples which are predominantly male. For an in-depth discussion of the characteristics of female arsonists, see Chapter 7 (also Gannon, 2010).

Age

The NESARC study (Blanco *et al*, 2010; Vaughn *et al*, 2010) reported that more than half (51%) of self-reported firesetters were aged 18–35 years, compared with 31% of non-firesetter population controls. Older firesetters were relatively rare: just 4% were aged 65 years and above, compared with 16% of population controls. Gannon & Barrowcliffe (2011) reported a non-statistically significant trend for firesetters to be younger (mean age 27 years) than non-firesetters (mean age 30 years) in a self-selected general population sample.

The tendency towards youth as a risk factor is common across studies of various samples. Lewis & Yarnell (1951) demonstrated a highly positively skewed age distribution among those arrested for arson. Soothill & Pope (1973) reported a mean age of 30 years for all 83 arsonists convicted at high court in England and Wales in 1951. Subsequently, Soothill *et al* (2004) studied convictions from all court cases including those aged from as young as 10. The mean age they reported is inevitably significantly lower in this later study: 23 years for men and 27 years for women in 2000, a statistically significant gender difference. Convicted arsonists in Sweden were significantly younger than general-population controls, irrespective of gender (Anwar *et al*, 2011). The mean age of firesetters and arsonists in psychiatric samples ranges from the mid-20s (Bourget & Bradford, 1989; Puri *et al*, 1995) to the mid-30s (Repo, 1998; Enayati *et al*, 2008). Males are generally found to be significantly younger than females (Bourget & Bradford, 1989; Dickens *et al*, 2007a; Enayati *et al*, 2008).

Firesetters are, therefore, generally young, but there is mixed evidence as to whether this differentiates them from other offenders. Use of a control group of non-firesetting offenders is a key strength of a number of studies. Hurley & Monahan (1969) examined 50 male arsonists in prison and compared them with a control group of 100 randomly selected inmates. Arsonists (mean age 25 years 10 months, range 15–57 years) were generally younger than controls, with only 14% older than 35 years at conviction, compared with 33% of controls. Jackson et al (1986) reported that male arsonists detained in a maximum-security hospital were younger (mean age 27 years) than non-arsonists (28 years), but this was not statistically significant, possibly due to the small sample size ($n = 18$ per group). Rice & Harris (1991) reported mean ages of 29 years and 32 years respectively for firesetters ($n = 243$) and controls ($n = 100$) detained in a maximum-security hospital, a statistically significant difference. More recently, Labree et al (2010) examined 25 arsonists detained in a maximum-security forensic hospital in the Netherlands and found no significant age difference between them and a control group of non-arsonist violent and sexual offenders. Furthermore, they did not differ on age at admission, first conviction or age at first psychiatric treatment. Conversely, Bradford (1982) reported that arsonists were significantly older than controls, although this result was from one of the smaller samples reported in the literature. Soothill et al (2004) found that all convictions for arson involving those aged over 62 years involved men only and this suggested that 'geriatric arson', a rare thing in itself, is solely a male phenomenon.

In summary, arsonists and firesetters are usually reported to be young. On the whole, the evidence suggests *statistically* significant age differences between firesetters and non-firesetting control offenders, but the clinical utility of this information is questionable given the small differences involved. There are clear gender differences, however, with female firesetters generally being older than males.

Ethnicity and immigration

People of Hispanic or African American origin were under-represented among self-reported firesetters (7% and 9%, respectively) compared with population controls (12% and 11%) in the NESARC study (Blanco et al, 2010; Vaughn et al, 2010). White firesetters (81%) were over-represented compared with population controls (70%). Self-reported firesetters were more likely to be US natives (94%) when compared with controls (85%). In contrast, Anwar et al (2011) found that, in Sweden, immigrant status among convicted arsonists, at around 20% for both men and women, was about double that in the general population. This was also reflected in a sample of arsonists convicted in Sweden and subsequently referred for forensic psychiatric examination (Enayati et al, 2008). The reasons for relatively low self-reported firesetting among non-nationals in a US general population sample and the relatively high immigrant status of convicted Swedish arsonists are not known, but may simply reflect the fact that convicted arsonists are a subset of firesetters as a whole and the two sets of information are not directly comparable. The ethnicity of clinical samples of arsonists has been reported to be largely White or Caucasian and broadly reflective of the countries and regions from which samples are drawn (Rix, 1994; Dickens *et al*, 2009). Lewis & Yarnell (1951) reported that 6% of their sample were foreign-born and that 'practically every nationality' was represented. Ritchie & Huff (1999) presented contradictory evidence: that 54% of their sample of 283 arsonists from US prisons and hospitals were White. However, this figure was based on data from incomplete medical and other records from a highly selected sample. There is therefore little strong evidence for any particular association between ethnicity and firesetting.

Environment, education, employment and social class

The NESARC general population study found no difference in terms of education, income or marital status between self-reported firesetters and general population controls. Neither was urban or rural dwelling a risk factor for firesetting (Blanco *et al*, 2010; Vaughn *et al*, 2010). Respondents from the west of the USA were more likely to report firesetting than those from the north-east, mid-west or south. Vaughn *et al* (2010) suggest this explanation: the number of campfires that are set in the west as opposed to other areas could fit the study description (see above) of starting a fire 'just to see it burn' and thus may represent false positive reporting of firesetting behaviour in these populations.

Lewis & Yarnell (1951) believed there was insufficient evidence to confirm or refute the hypothesis (Aschaffenberg, 1913) that rural location would be associated with increased firesetting, but felt that different geographical areas could well be associated with differently motivated types of firesetting.

Among more highly selected samples there is evidence that arsonists are more likely to be unemployed or unskilled than other non-firesetting offenders (Bradford, 1982; Harris & Rice, 1991) and more likely to be disadvantaged in terms of social class (Hurley & Monahan, 1969). Compared with population controls, convicted arsonists in Sweden were clearly disadvantaged in terms of individual income, unemployment and receipt of social welfare benefits (Anwar *et al*, 2011). Firesetters in psychiatric samples have been reported to be likely to be living alone and never to have married (Bourget & Bradford, 1989; Puri *et al*, 1995; Ritchie & Huff, 1999; Dickens *et al*, 2009) and this appears to differentiate them from non-firesetting control offenders (Harris & Rice, 1991) and from the general population (Anwar *et al*, 2011). Arsonists appear to be low achievers educationally, as evidenced by completion of elementary school only among both males (63%) and females (62%) compared with population controls (39% and 41%, respectively) (Anwar *et al*, 2011). However, Labree *et al* (2010) reported no difference between arsonists and a control group of violent and sexual offenders in terms of high-school completion.

In summary, there is some good evidence that firesetters may tend to be low achievers educationally, may have difficulties forming lasting relationships, and are likely to be unemployed, unskilled or disadvantaged on other social measures, including class and receipt of welfare benefits. However, this may not reliably distinguish them from other serious offenders.

Psychopathology

General psychopathology

Results from the NESARC study (Blanco *et al*, 2010; Vaughn *et al*, 2010) were based on a fully structured diagnostic interview conducted by trained US census workers using the valid and reliable Alcohol Use Disorder and Associated Disability Interview Schedule DSM-IV version (AUDADIS-IV) (Grant *et al*, 1995; Hasin *et al*, 1997) to assess substance use disorder, including alcohol and drug dependence, mood and anxiety disorders. Antisocial personality disorder (ASPD) and other personality disorder symptom sets were assessed. Possible psychotic disorder was assessed through self-report. Among self-reported firesetters any Axis I diagnosis was present in 91% of respondents but only 51% of population controls. Any Axis II diagnosis was recorded in 69% of firesetters and in 15% of controls. Alcohol use disorder was the most prevalent diagnosis and was present in significantly more self-reported firesetters (72%) than population controls (30%). Mood, specifically bipolar disorder, and anxiety disorders were more prevalent in firesetters than in controls after adjustment for sociodemographic characteristics (Blanco *et al*, 2010). The most prominent association was between firesetting and ASPD (52% of firesetters versus 3% of population controls). After adjusting for sociodemographic characteristics, ASPD was 22 times more likely in the firesetting population than in controls. ASPD remained strongly associated with firesetting even after controlling for substance use disorder and this suggested an independent relationship between the two variables. Conduct disorder and other personality disorders were also relatively common in firesetters following adjustment for sociodemographic variables. An increased prevalence of pathological gambling, substance use disorder and bipolar disorder in firesetters after adjustment was interpreted as suggestive of an underlying deficit in impulse control (Blanco *et al*, 2010). Interestingly, significantly more firesetters (46%) reported lifetime mental health treatment than did controls (19%). This supports studies of convicted arsonists in prison in which previous psychiatric treatment was found to be common (Sapsford *et al*, 1978); and studies of maximum-security psychiatric patients, among whom 84% of arsonists had previously received psychiatric treatment, compared with 60% of control non-arson offenders (Labree *et al*, 2010). This suggests that, in line with research findings presented above, firesetting may be common in clinical samples and should be screened for during psychiatric assessment. In brief, the large general population sample suggests that the lifetime prevalence rates of ASPD and other personality disorders and substance use disorder were higher among a sample of self-reporting firesetters compared with the general population.

In both prison and psychiatric samples, personality disorder has been found to be common. For example, in a study of 266 jailed arsonists 61% of those sentenced to life imprisonment and 25% of other arsonists were reported to be psychopathic by Sapsford *et al* (1978). Ritchie & Huff (1999) reported that 20% of their sample of arsonists had a primary or secondary diagnosis of personality disorder. Among samples referred for psychiatric assessment, the prevalence of personality disorder has been reported to be 54% among 153 arsonists (Rix, 1994) and 41% among 92 arsonists (Bourget & Bradford, 1989). Among 79 arsonists resident in a UK high-security psychiatric hospital, the prevalence of personality disorder was 44% (Swinton & Ahmed, 2001). However, when compared with non-arsonist offender controls, psychopathy is no more prevalent: for example, 48% of 155 male and 41% of 59 female arsonists were diagnosed with personality disorder in Sweden (Enayati *et al*, 2008), but this was not significantly higher than among controls referred for non-arson offences. Labree *et al* (2010) reported that scores on the Psychopathy Checklist Revised (PCL-R; Hare, 2003) indicated no significant differences between arsonists and violent and sexual offending controls. Duggan & Shine (2001) examined data taken from a routinely recorded measure of ten personality disorder traits (Personality Diagnostic Questionnaire, fourth version; Hyler, 1994) for 68 male arsonists and 380 male offender control inmates of a UK prison. The only significant difference was in levels of borderline personality traits and the authors rejected their hypothesis that more personality disturbance would be present in arsonists than in controls. These findings are confirmed by results from a high-security psychiatric setting reported by Rice & Harris (1991), where 50% of arsonists and offender controls had a personality disorder, and by Jackson *et al* (1987), who found that 66% of arsonists and 78% of controls had a personality disorder (a statistically non-significant difference). Repo (1998) categorised male firesetters in three groups: those who had committed only one offence, that being arson ($n = 59$); those who had committed other non-violent crimes alongside arson ($n = 110$); and those who had committed other violent crimes in addition to arson ($n = 113$). ASPD was more common in the violent firesetting group (27%) than in the non-violent (9%) and one-time firesetting groups (3%). This may suggest that ASPD is associated with the most dangerous firesetters. Personality disorder appears to be a common feature of people referred to forensic psychiatric services, including firesetters. However, it has been reported at much lower rates in those with firesetting behaviour in general psychiatric settings (e.g., 4% with a primary diagnosis of personality disorder; Geller *et al*, 1992).

The prevalence of lifetime substance misuse, particularly alcohol misuse, in general population research on firesetters is mirrored to a large extent in prison and clinical samples. Again, however, this is not generally found to distinguish firesetters from control samples of other offenders. Enayati *et al* (2008) reported that 47% of males and 48% of females had a principal or comorbid substance disorder, but this was not significantly higher than among control offenders. Hurley & Monahan (1969) reported higher, but not significantly higher, levels of alcoholism (44%) compared with non-arson offending controls (32%). Other samples have reported a common history of alcohol or substance misuse if not an actual disorder (Bourget & Bradford, 1989; Puri *et al*, 1995; Ritchie & Huff, 1999; Jayaraman & Frazer, 2006; Dickens *et al*, 2009). Alcohol intoxication at the time of the index offence may be especially common (Jayaraman & Frazer, 2006; Repo, 1998) particularly among men (Fleszar-Szumigajowa, 1969; Ritchie & Huff, 1999; Dickens *et al*, 2009).

Psychosis (not including bipolar disorder) was present in 25% of males and 48% of females among Swedish arsonists referred for forensic psychiatric examination (Enayati *et al*, 2008) and schizophrenia was diagnosed in 37% of Puri *et al*'s (1995) similarly referred, but smaller, sample ($n = 36$). Geller *et al* (1992) examined the hospital records of all 279 patients resident in a US psychiatric hospital. Of those with a history of firesetting behaviour ($n = 76$; 27%) 65% were diagnosed with schizophrenia, compared with 55% of controls with no firesetting history. This was not a statistically significant difference. When interpreting results from this study, consideration should be given to its wide definition of 'firesetting', which included 'careless smoking' and false activation of fire alarms. Anwar *et al*'s (2011) study of convicted arsonists in Sweden found that both men and women arson offenders were significantly more likely than controls to be diagnosed with schizophrenia or other psychoses than were population controls. The increased risks for arson among those with schizophrenia were very high: a 20-fold increase in men and a near 40-fold increase in women compared with non-arson offenders after adjusting for sociodemographic factors. This is reported as being equivalent to the increased risk for homicide in this group. Arsonists with schizophrenia or psychosis were responsible for 8% of arson in Sweden over a 12-year period. Relative risk was highest among those individuals with comorbid personality disorder, substance use disorder or both.

Psychological traits

Only a few studies of arsonists have reported data from valid psychometric assessment tools. Jackson *et al* (1987) found arsonists detained in a maximum-security hospital to be considerably less assertive and to have poorer communication skills than violent offender controls and population controls (hospital staff). Both arsonists and violent offenders were found to be more depressed than population controls. Koson & Dvoskin (1982) administered the Minnesota Multiphasic Personality Inventory (Hathaway & McKinley, 1940) to 26 pre-trial arsonists in a maximum-security hospital and reported that scores indicated a great level of inwardly directed hostility or aggressiveness. This was supported by Duggan & Shine (2001), who reported that male arsonists ($n = 83$) in prison scored more highly on a measure of inwardly directed hostility (Hostility and Direction of Hostility Questionnaire, HDHQ; Caine et al, 1967) than offender controls ($n = 498$). Day (2001) conducted case-file reviews of 20 male arsonists, 20 male sex offenders and 20 male violent offenders in an English prison, which included routinely recorded psychometric data, but found no difference between arsonists and the other offenders on measures of self-esteem, social desirability, impulsivity, rumination, assertiveness or emotional loneliness. Duggan & Shine (2001) reported that arsonists had lower self-esteem as measured on all scales of the Culture Free Self-Esteem Inventory (Battle, 1992) than control prisoners, a finding consistent with those of Smith & Short (1995) and Swaffer et al (2001). Results from the revised Eysenck Personality Questionnaire (Eysenck & Eysenck, 1991) also indicated that arsonists had an increased tendency to suffer anxiety, guilt and low mood. Hurley & Monahan (1969) similarly reported a high incidence of neurotic features among imprisoned arsonists based on scores from the Eysenck Personality Inventory (Eysenck & Eysenck, 1964) and the Maudsley Personality Inventory (Eysenck, 1959), but no difference from offending, non-arsonist controls. The most robust data here suggest associations between firesetting and arson and self-esteem, inwardly directed hostility, lack of assertiveness and anxiety.

Pyromania

Pyromania is classified within DSM-IV-TR (American Psychiatric Association, 2000) as a psychiatric impulse control disorder not otherwise specified (312:33). Other impulse control disorders are pathological gambling, trichotillomania, intermittent explosive disorder, kleptomania, compulsive buying and compulsive sexual behaviour. Impulsivity, in a psychiatric context, has been defined by Moeller et al (2001, p. 1784) as a 'predisposition toward rapid unplanned reactions to internal or external stimuli without regard to the negative consequences of these actions to the impulsive individual or others', a definition which these authors believe to be ideologically neutral and to encapsulate biological, psychological and social aetiology. In addition to specific impulse control disorders, impulsivity is a feature of a range of mental disorders, including personality disorder, substance misuse, bipolar disorder, attention-deficit hyperactivity disorder and conduct disorder, but firesetting in the context of other mental disorders or impaired judgement should not, under current criteria, attract the diagnosis of pyromania. Pyromania is defined in DSM-IV-TR as deliberate and purposeful firesetting on multiple occasions. The diagnosis applies only to those for whom firesetting is accompanied by tension or affective arousal prior to the act. Additionally, the individual will display fascination with, interest in, curiosity about, or attraction to fire and its situational contexts, and will gain pleasure, gratification or relief when setting fires, or when witnessing or participating in their aftermath. Additionally, the firesetting will not have been undertaken for monetary gain, as an expression of sociopolitical ideology, to conceal criminal activity, to express anger or vengeance, to improve living circumstances, in response to a delusion or hallucination, or as a result of impaired judgement (e.g., in dementia, mental retardation or substance intoxication). Finally, for pyromania to be diagnosed, the firesetting must not be better accounted for by conduct disorder, a manic episode or ASPD.

Pyromania was not addressed by the NESARC study and evidence for its prevalence must be drawn from other literature. In Lewis & Yarnell's (1951) classic work *Pathological Firesetting (Pyromania)*, 60% of their sample of 1145 male firesetters were classified as 'pyromaniacs', defined as 'offenders who said they set their fires for no practical reason and received no material profit from the act, their only motive being to gain some sensual satisfaction' (p. 86). This figure is far in excess of almost all other prevalence estimates and it is important to understand the historical context in which the research was conducted. Geller *et al* (1986) describe the wax and wane in the use of the term 'pyromania' in US psychiatry over a 150-year period up to 1985. A parallel is drawn between the use of the term and the ongoing wider debate in US psychiatry about issues of individual agency and responsibility. The growth in the use of the term, and the use of pyromania as a legal defence, in the period 1840–90 accompanied the development of the concepts of moral insanity and moral treatment. In this period, consensus viewed pyromania as a 'moral mania' or monomania, largely outside of the control of the individual: 'a morbid propensity to incendiarism, where the mind though otherwise sound, is borne on by an invisible power to the commission of this crime that has been so frequently observed, that it is now generally recognized as a distinct form of insanity' (Ray, 1838, p. 195). Present throughout this period, but usurping the notion of pyromania as an irresistible impulse towards its end, were arguments that emphasised the agency and culpability of offenders and railed against the idea of moral insanity:

symptoms of moral insanity … are all striking delineations of what common sense … would call *depravity*. Yet we are asked to believe that these signs constitute evidence of a form of insanity destroying human responsibility. They [the defenders of moral insanity] make it appear that the decalogue and all human laws are unjust because they visit penalties on disease. (Ordroneaux (1873: p. 321)

Between 1880 and 1917, interest in pyromania dwindled, but it re-emerged in the period 1924–57, spurred on by the development of psychoanalytic theory, which again endorsed the condition as a disease entity characterised as an irresistible impulse (Magee, 1933), a urethra-erotic character trait (Hinsie & Shatzky, 1940) or a psychosexually based impulse neurosis (Henderson & Gillespie, 1944). However, while pyromania was included in DSM-I (American Psychiatric Association, 1952), as an obsessive–compulsive reaction, it gained little support as a distinct psychiatric diagnosis and was not included in DSM-II (American Psychiatric Association,

1968). By the time it re-emerged as a nosological classification in DSM-III (American Psychiatric Association, 1980), the language had been inverted and instead of an 'irresistible impulse', pyromania was described as a 'recurrent failure to resist impulses to set fires'. The tight exclusion criteria, outlined above, may exclude many deliberate firesetters from the diagnosis.

In this context, it becomes clear that Lewis & Yarnell's (1951) study occurred during a period when, on balance, US psychiatrists were disposed to view firesetting for non-profit motives as pathological. Furthermore, their study pre-dated publication of DSM-I and their definition of pyromania was less exclusive. Indeed, Geller *et al* (1986) remarked that the use of the term 'pyromania' in parentheses in the title of their book indicated Lewis & Yarnell's own uncertainty about this diagnostic entity (see also Lewis & Yarnell, 1951, p. 86). It is notable that, while 60% of their sample were classified as 'pyromaniacs', Lewis & Yarnell identified a small subset of about 50 (4%) of the group as having 'true pyromania'. Of this subsample they wrote:

These are the mysterious 'firebugs' who terrorize neighborhoods by going on solitary firesetting sprees, often nocturnal, during which they touch off trash fires in rapid succession without regard to whose property is endangered. These offenders are able to give a classical description of the irresistible impulse. They describe the mounting tension, the restlessness, the urge for motion. (Lewis & Yarnell, 1951, pp. 86–87)

Subsequent studies of the prevalence of pyromania in clinical and criminal samples have been conducted largely with reference to the tighter operational definition detailed in DSM-III, DSM-III-R and DSM-IV and DSM-IV-TR (American Psychiatric Association, 1980, 1987, 1994, 2000). Doley (2003) reviewed the evidence base and found that most published studies at that time reported very low rates (less than 0.5%), or indeed the non-existence, of pyromania in criminal and clinical samples (Koson & Dvoskin, 1982; Harmon *et al*, 1985; Prins *et al*, 1985; O'Sullivan & Kelleher, 1987; Rice & Harris, 1991; Leong, 1992; Ritchie & Huff, 1999).

More recently, Lindberg *et al* (2005) reviewed the medical and psychiatric records of 90 males with a history of recidivist arson and found that just 3% met DSM-IV-TR criteria for pyromania, and suggested that a further 10% met all criteria except for absence of alcohol intoxication during the index arson. The authors appear to suggest that for these individuals alcohol consumption typically magnified the affective arousal that they were experiencing *in any event*, the implication being that they were likely to fit criteria for pyromania and that alcohol did not necessarily impair their judgement. Lindberg *et al* (2005) recommended that there should be reconsideration of the use of alcohol intoxication as an exclusion criterion for pyromania.

Two studies of non-offenders have used structured tools to assess pyromania and other impulse control disorders, in a sample of 107 people with major depressive disorder (Lejoyeux *et al*, 2002) and in a sample of

204 consecutively admitted patients to a private psychiatric hospital and a university hospital in the USA (Grant *et al*, 2005). Both reported a prevalence of 3%. Two smaller studies, each comprising reports of 20 individuals with the impulse control disorders kleptomania (McElroy *et al*, 1991) and compulsive buying (McElroy *et al*, 1994), found comorbidity rates of lifetime pyromania of 15% and 10%, respectively. Subsequently, Grant & Kim (2007) reported results from semi-structured interviews conducted with 21 adults and adolescents who met DSM-IV criteria for lifetime pyromania, 16 of whom also met criteria for current (defined as past 12 months) pyromania. Much of the firesetting reported by respondents did not meet the legal definition of 'arson'; for example, fires were small and controlled. However, firesetting was reported to be frequent and, on average, respondents reported setting a fire every 6 weeks. Psychiatric comorbidity was common, particularly for mood and substance use disorders. Grant & Kim (2007) raised the question of whether pyromania shares a neurobiology with other impulse control disorders, and suggested that undetected pyromania may mean that it is more prevalent than is currently conceded. This is an interesting development which may presage a change in the way pyromania is viewed by psychiatry, a new era in which a limited group of firesetters are again viewed as 'diseased', as were larger groups in the past (Geller *et al*, 1986).

In summary, the understanding of firesetting as a pathological behaviour and as a distinct mental disorder has changed over time. When the influence of psychoanalytical approaches was dominant, and firesetting was seen as a disease, Lewis & Yarnell (1951) reported high levels (60%) of pyromania but modified this to around 4% for those with 'true pyromania'. Increasingly tight operational definitions of pyromania in subsequent editions of the DSM, particularly the use of alcohol intoxication at index as an exclusion criterion, appear to have contributed to research findings of zero or near-zero prevalence of the disorder. Recent US studies have indicated a small but non-trivial prevalence of criteria for lifetime pyromania in clinical, non-offending samples. It is worth noting that the diagnosis of pyromania does not require that firesetting behaviour meets the legal definition of arson. Rather, the fires set by those meeting the criteria for pyromania may be small and controllable. As a result, it may be suggested that samples of convicted arsonists, largely typified by the presence of ASPD, may be a group distinct from those meeting criteria for pyromania.

Neurodevelopmental, developmental features and family history

Intellectual disability and neurodevelopmental disorders

Few researchers have formally assessed intellectual disability among firesetters and the picture is clouded by the differing definitions employed between studies. Lewis & Yarnell (1951) reported 70% of their sample to be at least below average intelligence, 48% of whom were classified as 'morons or imbeciles', suggesting an IQ between 20 and 70 for nearly half their sample (Reber, 1995). Fleszar-Szumigajowa (1969) reported 'mental deficiency' in 19% of incendiarists. Dickens et al (2007b) reported IQ to be below 85 in 44% of arsonists. Rix (1994) reported 11% to be 'learning disabled' and Puri et al (1995) just 3%. More recently, Enayati et al (2008) have reported learning disability to be a feature in 10% of males and 9% of female convicted arsonists referred for forensic psychiatric examination, significantly greater levels than among offending controls (3% for both males and females). However, among a group of arsonists detained under maximum security, Labree et al (2010) found 8% of arsonists and violent offender controls had 'mental retardation', as indicated by scores below 70 on the WAIS-R or WAIS-III (Wechsler, 1981, 1997). Räsänen et al (1994) found the full-scale IQ on the Wechsler Adult Intelligence Scale test (Wechsler, 1965) of both arsonists and control offenders charged with homicide to be in the 'dull normal' range, with no significant difference between them. Among arsonists referred for psychiatric assessment, Dickens et al (2007b) reported that those with low normal and below intelligence were characterised by a pattern of lifelong temperamental problems. While intellectual disability may not be as prevalent among those who deliberately set fires as perhaps once thought, it may increase the risk for arson more than for other offences, although perhaps this is not the case among the most serious offenders. See Chapter 6 for a wider-reaching discussion of firesetting and intellectual disability.

There is little evidence relating to neurodevelopmental disorders and firesetting. Enayati et al (2008) reported that autism (excluding Asperger syndrome) was rare in both arsonists and control offenders referred for forensic psychiatric assessment. However, there was a significantly higher prevalence of Asperger syndrome among convicted arsonists (7%) relative to other offender controls (3%). There are several published case studies of firesetting or arson conducted by males with Asperger syndrome (Everall & LeCouter, 1990; Tantam, 1991; Murrie et al, 2002).

Other family and developmental factors

The developmental features of adult, as opposed to child and adolescent, firesetters have been insufficiently studied; moreover, as noted above, no longitudinal study has followed juvenile firesetters through to adulthood. In the general population there is a high prevalence of family history of antisocial behaviour among self-reported firesetters (60%) relative to population controls (23%) (Vaughn et al, 2010). From studies of more highly selected samples there are few reports of the family or developmental features of adult arsonists or firesetters compared with control groups. Hence, while apparently high rates of childhood disturbance are commonly reported, including behavioural disturbance, truancy and reading difficulties (Puri et al, 1995; Dickens et al, 2009), there is little control information to contextualise this. Evidence is largely from psychiatric populations and is indirect. For example, Harris & Rice (1991) compared 243 men admitted to a maximum-security psychiatric institution for firesetting and compared them with non-firesetting control patients. There was little significant difference in terms of childhood history, including childhood poverty, reported parental physical abuse, presence of the MacDonald triad (animal cruelty, enuresis and obsession with firesetting), or of childhood aggression. Significantly more firesetters had been institutionalised during childhood and about 10% had a family history of firesetting, lending support to a social learning component to their behaviour. More arsonists than controls came from 'broken homes' (Hurley & Monahan, 1969). Bradford (1982) compared arsonists referred for pre-trial forensic examination with offending, non-arsonist controls and found, similarly, that more arsonists had been reared outside of their natural birth family, but proportionately fewer reported parental childhood abuse. The evidence is mixed, however, and Labree *et al* (2010) found no difference between arsonists and control patients in a maximum-security hospital in terms of having been raised in their natural (biological) home. Hurley & Monahan (1969) reported that most arsonists came from large families (four or more children); however, they did not present control data for this variable and they noted that this may not distinguish the firesetters from other offenders. Dickens *et al* (2007a) found more evidence of childhood sexual abuse among female arsonists than among males.

Gannon & Pina (2010) reviewed the developmental features of adult arsonists and noted the preponderance of single men who are typified by loneliness and impoverished social support networks (Inciardi, 1970; Barracato, 1979; Bennett & Hess, 1984; Leong, 1992; Ritchie & Huff, 1999; Rice & Harris, 1991, 2008). Hurley & Monahan (1969) noted that a high proportion (62%) of arsonists were found to have difficulty forming social relationships with women. However, these features are also found among other non-firesetting criminals (Ward *et al*, 1996; Van Ijzendoorn *et al*, 1997; Frodi *et al*, 2001; Ross & Pfäfflin, 2007) and it is therefore questionable the extent to which conclusions can be drawn from these findings.

Offending and antisocial behaviour

Epidemiological research (Blanco *et al*, 2010; Vaughn *et al*, 2010) has suggested that, compared with controls, firesetters self-reported a wide range of antisocial or offending behaviours. This ranged from relatively trivial issues such as playing truant (61% of firesetters *v.* 21% of controls), repeated school or work absence (33% *v.* 7%), repeated lying (33% *v.* 5%), or loss of driving licence (26% *v.* 8%). More serious acquisitive offending behaviours among firesetters compared with controls included shoplifting (58% *v.* 11%) and illegal money-making (28% *v.* 3%); non-acquisitive property crimes were also more common among firesetters and included destruction of others' property (50% *v.* 3%). Finally, a self-reported history of violent offending was far more prevalent in firesetters, including 'hitting someone sufficiently hard to injure them' (35% *v.* 6%), using a weapon in a fight (21% *v.* 3%) and forcing someone to have sex (1.4% *v.* 0.1%). Blanco *et al* (2010) report that 76% of firesetters affirmed the statement that they had done 'anything that you could have been arrested for', compared with 15% of controls. The behaviours most associated with firesetters relative to controls were robbing, mugging or purse-snatching (5% *v.* 0%) and harassing, threatening or blackmailing someone (22% *v.* 2%). In short, in this large general population survey, self-reported lifetime firesetting was associated with a wide range of other self-reported antisocial or offending behaviours, including non-violent and serious violent crime. However, whether this pattern of offending differentiates firesetters from non-firesetting offenders is not known.

Soothill *et al* (2004) identified past convictions for a period of up to 37 years among 3335 arsonists convicted in England and Wales in 2000–01. More than two-fifths (43%) had at least one previous conviction; the most common were for theft (28%), criminal damage (23%), violence (20%) and motoring offences (18%). Sexual offending was relatively uncommon (1.6%) but it is not known whether arsonists are less likely than other non-sexual offenders to commit sexually offences. The proportion of those with previous convictions for violence had risen from 8% in 1951 to 12% in 1980–81 and to 20% in 2000–01. Soothill *et al* (2004) reflected that this probably indicated the increasing relevance of the prior offending record in any decision to prosecute. There was a small but increasing proportion of previous convictions for arson among convicted arsonists (1% in 1951 to 11% in 2000–01). This was argued to reflect the decreased probability of arson fires being detected in the war years, which formed a significant period of the pre-1951 conviction data-set. These data support the arguments that many arsonists are versatile in their offending behaviour and that some arsonists are also violent offenders: it is notable that in one study those with a conviction for arson were as likely subsequently to commit homicide as were those who had blackmailed and made threats to kill (Soothill *et al*, 2008).

On the whole, however, it would appear that most arsonists are not characterised by violent behaviour. Jackson *et al* (1986) compared arsonists without mental disorder or intellectual disability to controls with index offences involving interpersonal violence. Arsonists had significantly fewer recorded incidents of assaults both prior to and since admission than did violent offenders. This is supported by work among males referred for psychiatric assessment conducted by Hill *et al* (1982), who, interestingly, found that arsonists (*n* = 38) were less violent than violent offenders (*n* = 24) but more violent than property offenders (*n* = 30). Labree *et al* (2010) found no difference in the number of previous convictions between arsonists and non-arsonist offending controls, but did not report on the severity or type of previous offending. Hurley & Monahan (1969) reported lower rates of previous imprisonment (42%) among arsonists compared with offending controls (77%), and a smaller proportion of arsonists (15%)

had previous convictions for violence than did controls (32%). Arsonists had more previous convictions for property damage (26% v. 7%) but fewer convictions than controls for sex offences (15% v. 31%), larceny (37% v. 78%), breaking and entering (25% v. 63%) or deception (4% v. 33%). In psychiatric samples, aggression to others (53% v. 82%) and sexual offences (9% v. 82%) have been reported to be less common among arsonists than among controls (McKerracher & Dacre, 1966). However, there appear to be few hard-and-fast rules about offending and some arsonists do recidivate violently. For example, Rice & Harris (1996) reported a 57% rate of non-violent recidivism and a rate of 31% for violent recidivism in arsonists over an average follow-up of 7.8 years.

To summarise, it appears that firesetting is often part of a general array of offending behaviour. However, from the available evidence, firesetters and arsonists as a group are more like property offenders than violent offenders, but a minority of firesetters are also violent recidivists.

Summary and conclusions

This chapter has provided an overview of the emerging epidemiological evidence on firesetting in the general adult population. The NESARC study suggests a headline figure of 1% for lifetime prevalence of deliberate firesetting. Furthermore, 38% of firesetters reported this behaviour persisting after age 15 (Blanco et al, 2010; Vaughn et al, 2010). The extent to which this is a credible finding is offset by poor phrasing of survey questions and the potential for response bias in the original survey design. Nevertheless, this new epidemiological evidence largely supports previous empirical work on the sociodemographic characteristics of firesetters conducted with more highly selected samples of criminal and clinical populations. Those who deliberately set fires are predominantly young, White males. Low educational achievement is common and there is evidence that arsonists may experience difficulty in forming lasting relationships. However, studies of those convicted of arson suggest that many of these characteristics probably do not distinguish arsonists from other young men who offend. Firesetting does appear to be sufficiently prevalent among young men with mental disorder to warrant routine screening for evidence of the behaviour during psychiatric assessment. Early identification will inform risk assessment and any subsequent management plan.

In terms of psychopathology, the new population data also largely support what is known from clinical and criminal samples. Substance use disorders, ASPD and other personality disorders have been reported to be common in multiple studies. However, this is also true of many young men who offend. There is some evidence that firesetters may lack assertiveness and self-esteem, and be prone to inwardly directed hostility. It is noteworthy that risk for arson is particularly increased relative to population controls among those with schizophrenia and other psychoses. Questions pertinent to firesetting are certainly warranted when assessing this group. Pyromania, or at least firesetting that shares some of its characteristics (including intense pleasure and interest in fire and emotional arousal associated with lighting fires) may be present in a small proportion of individuals, but historical reports of pyromania appear to reflect shifting attitudes as much as fundamental shifts in firesetting behaviour in the population. The presence of pyromania among samples of people with other impulse control disorders (kleptomania and compulsive buying) and in other disorders associated with impulse control deficits (ASPD, substance misuse) may suggest a biological basis for a small subset of those who set fires. However, the potential biological basis of firesetting behaviour is outside the scope of the current chapter and readers are advised to consult Chapter 4 for a summary of this area.

Evidence from population studies suggests that firesetters have been frequently involved in a variety of antisocial and offending behaviours relative to the general population, and a small subset have been involved in very serious violent and sexual acts. Those who are convicted of arson are usually versatile in their offending behaviour and a proportion have convictions for grave crimes. On the whole, the evidence suggests that most of those who deliberately set fires share more in common with property offenders than with violent offenders. However, this is not true of all firesetters and practitioners should of course bear in mind that some arsonists deliberately set out to endanger life and thus more closely resemble violent offenders. Current classificatory systems for those who set fires are unsatisfactory (Gannon & Pina, 2010) and more work needs to be done to aid in the assessment of those who will go on to set the most dangerous fires (Dickens *et al*, 2009).

Finally, the emerging epidemiological data, though limited, provide a welcome advance from the position espoused by Barker (1994, p. 88), who suggested that such a comprehensive survey would be impracticable and cause 'at best, outright hostility' among respondents. Moving forwards, research is needed which combines the representativeness of the NESARC study with the detailed questioning and minimisation of response bias employed by Gannon & Barrowcliffe (2011) and the better epidemiological studies of firesetting in children and adolescents in order to improve the epidemiological picture. Epidemiological evidence for firesetting among juveniles is currently far more advanced than that for adults. However, it is claimed that only half of intentional firesetting brought to the attention of professionals is committed by juveniles (Cassel & Bernstein, 2007) and there is an urgent need to build the current evidence base on adult firesetting in order to inform assessment and treatment. In particular, there is a dearth of longitudinal studies that follow children into adulthood, meaning that we know very little about whether those who set fires as children go on to do so as adults. This issue can be addressed only by the initiation of a far-sighted project which aims to identify specific risk factors for adult firesetting.

References

Achenbach, T. M. (1991) *Manual for the Child Behavior Checklist (CBCL)/4–18 and 1991 Profile.* University of Vermont Department of Psychiatry.

American Psychiatric Association (1952) *Diagnostic and Statistical Manual of Mental Disorders* (1st edn) (DSM-I). APA.

American Psychiatric Association (1968) *Diagnostic and Statistical Manual of Mental Disorders* (2nd edn) (DSM-II). APA.

American Psychiatric Association (1980) *Diagnostic and Statistical Manual of Mental Disorders* (3rd edn) (DSM-III). APA.

American Psychiatric Association (1987) *Diagnostic and Statistical Manual of Mental Disorders* (3rd edn, revised) (DSM-III-R). APA.

American Psychiatric Association (1994) *Diagnostic and Statistical Manual of Mental Disorders* (4th edn) (DSM-IV). APA.

American Psychiatric Association (2000) *Diagnostic and Statistical Manual of Mental Disorders* (4th edn, text revision) (DSM-IV-TR). APA.

Anwar, S., Långström, N., Grann, M., et al (2011) Is arson the crime most strongly associated with psychosis? A national case–control study of arson risk in schizophrenia and other psychoses. *Schizophrenia Bulletin*, **37**, 580–586 .

Aschaffenburg, G. (1913) *Crime and Its Repression*. Patterson Smith.

Barker, A. F. (1994) *Arson: A Review of the Psychiatric Literature*. Oxford University Press.

Barracato, J. (1979) *Fire: Is It Arson?* Aetna Life and Casualty.

Battle, J. (1992) *Culture-Free Self-Esteem Inventory*. Pro-Ed.

Bennett, W. M. & Hess, K. M. (1984) *The Arsonist: A Closer Look*. Charles C. Thomas.

Blanco, C., Alegria, A. A., Petry, N. M., et al (2010) Prevalence and correlates of fire-setting in the United States: results from the National Epidemiologic Survey on Alcohol and Related Conditions (NESARC). *Journal of Clinical Psychiatry*, **71**, 1218–1225.

Bourget, D. & Bradford, J. M. (1989) Female arsonists: a clinical study. *Bulletin of the American Academy of Psychiatry and the Law*, **17**, 293–300.

Bradford, J. M. (1982) Arson: a clinical study. *Canadian Journal of Psychiatry*, **27**, 188–193.

Caine, T., Foulds, G. & Hope, K. (1967) *The Hostility and Direction of Hostility Questionnaire*. University of London Press.

Cassel, E. & Bernstein, D. A. (2007) *Criminal Behaviour* (2nd edn). Pearson.

Chen, Y. H., Arria, A. M. & Anthony, J. C. (2003) Firesetting in adolescence and being aggressive, shy and rejected by peers: new epidemiologic evidence from a national sample survey. *Journal of the American Academy of Psychiatry and the Law*, **31**, 44–52.

Clark Newman, J., Des Jarlais, D. C., Turner, C. F., et al (2002) The differential effects of face-to-face and computer interview modes. *American Journal of Public Health*, **93**, 294–297.

Dadds, M. R & Fraser, J. A. (2006) Fire interest, fire setting and psychopathology in Australian children: a normative study. *Australian and New Zealand Journal of Psychiatry*, **40**, 581–586.

Day, J. (2001) Understanding the characteristics of fire-setters. *Prison Service Journal*, **133**, 6–8.

Del Bove, G., Caprara, G. V., Pastorelli, C., et al (2008) Juvenile firesetting in Italy: relationship to aggression, psychopathology, personality, self-efficacy and school functioning. *European Child and Adolescent Psychiatry*, **17**, 235–244.

Dickens, G., Sugarman, P., Ahmad, F., et al (2007a) Gender differences amongst adult arsonists at psychiatric assessment. *Medicine, Science and the Law*, **47**, 233–238.

Dickens, G., Sugarman, P., Ahmad, F., et al (2007b) Characteristics of low IQ arsonists at psychiatric assessment. *Medicine, Science and the Law*, **48**, 217–220.

Dickens, G., Sugarman, P., Ahmad, F., et al (2009) Recidivism and dangerousness in arsonists. *Journal of Forensic Psychiatry and Psychology*, **20**, 621–639.

Doley, R. (2003) Pyromania: fact or fiction? *British Journal of Criminology*, **43**, 797–807.

Duggan, L. & Shine, J. (2001) An investigation of the relationship between arson, personality disorder, hostility, neuroticism and self-esteem amongst incarcerated fire-setters. *Prison Service Journal*, **133**, 18–21.

Enayati, J., Grann, M., Lubbs, S., *et al* (2008) Psychiatric morbidity in arsonists referred for forensic psychiatric assessment in Sweden. *Journal of Forensic Psychiatry and Psychology*, **19**, 139–147.

Everall, L. P. & LeCouter, A. (1990) Firesetting in an adolescent boy with Asperger's syndrome. *British Journal of Psychiatry*, **157**, 284–287.

Eysenck, H. J. (1959) *The Maudsley Personality Inventory*. University of London Press.

Eysenck, H. J. & Eysenck, S. B. G. (1964) *Manual of the Eysenck Personality Inventory*. University of London Press.

Eysenck, H. J. & Eysenck, S. B. G. (1991) The Eysenck Personality Questionnaire. The revised version of the psychoticism scale. *Personality and Individual Differences*, **6**, 21–29.

Fleszar-Szumigajowa, J. (1969) The perpetrators of arson in forensic-psychiatric material. *Polish Medical Journal*, **9**, 212–219.

Frodi, A., Dernevik, M., Sepa, A. *et al* (2001) Current attachment representations of incarcerated offenders varying in degree of psychopathy. *Attachment and Human Development*, **3**, 269–283.

Gannon, T. A. (2010) Female arsonists: key features, psychopathologies and treatment needs. *Psychiatry*, **73**, 173–189.

Gannon, T. A. & Barrowcliffe, E. (2011) Firesetting in the general population: the development and validation of the Fire Setting and Fire Proclivity Scales. *Legal and Criminological Psychology*. DOI: 10.1348/135532510X523203.

Gannon, T. A. & Pina, A. (2010) Firesetting: psychopathology, theory and treatment. *Aggression and Violent Behaviour*, **15**, 224–238.

Geller, J. L., Erien, J. & Pinkus, R.L. (1986) A historical appraisal of America's experience with 'pyromania' – a diagnosis in search of a disorder. *International Journal of Law and Psychiatry*, **9**, 201–229.

Geller, J. L., Fisher, W. H. & Moynihan, K. (1992) Adult lifetime prevalence of firesetting behaviors in a state hospital population. *Psychiatric Quarterly*, **63**, 129–142.

Grant, B. F., Harford, T., Dawson, D. A., *et al* (1995) The Alcohol Use Disorder and Associated Disabilities Interview Schedule (AUDADIS): reliability of alcohol and drug modules in a general population sample. *Drug and Alcohol Dependence*, **39**, 37–44.

Grant, J. E. & Kim, S. W. (2007) Clinical characteristics and psychiatric comorbidity of pyromania. *Journal of Clinical Psychiatry*, **68**, 1717–1722.

Grant, J. E., Levine, L., Kim, D., *et al* (2005) Impulse control disorders in adult psychiatric inpatients. *American Journal of Psychiatry*, **162**, 2184–2188.

Hall, J. R. Jr. (2007) *Intentional Fires and Arson*. Fire Analysis and Research Division, National Fire Protection Association (http://www.nfpa.org/assets/files/pdf/arsonsummary.pdf).

Hare, R. D. (2003) *Hare Psychopathy Checklist Revised (PCL-R)* (2nd edn). Multi Health Systems.

Harmon, R. B., Rosner, R. & Wiederlight, M. (1985) Women and arson: a demographic study. *Journal of Forensic Sciences*, **30**, 467–477.

Harris, M. E. & Rice, G. (1991) Firesetters admitted to a maximum security psychiatric institution: offenders and offenses. *Journal of Interpersonal Violence*, **6**, 461–475.

Hasin, D., Carpenter, K. M., McCloud, S., *et al* (1997) The Alcohol Use Disorders and Associated Disabilities Interview Schedule (AUDADIS): reliability of alcohol and drug modules in a clinical sample. *Drug and Alcohol Dependence*, **44**, 133–141.

Hathaway, S. R. & McKinley, J. C. (1940) A multiphasic personality schedule (Minnesota): I. Construction of the schedule. *Journal of Psychology*, **10**, 249–254.

Henderson, D. K. & Gillespie, R. D. (1944) *A Textbook of Psychiatry for Students and Practitioners*. Oxford University Press.

Hill, R. W., Langevin, R., Paitich, D., *et al* (1982) Is arson an aggressive act or a property offense? A controlled study of psychiatric referrals. *Canadian Journal of Psychiatry*, **27**, 648–654.

Hinsie, L. E. & Shatzky, J. (1940) *Psychiatric Dictionary with Encyclopaedic Treatment of Modern Terms.* Oxford University Press.

Hurley, W. & Monahan, T. M. (1969) Arson: the criminal and the crime. *British Journal of Criminology,* **9,** 4–21.

Hyler, S. E. (1994) *Personality Diagnostic Questionnaire* (4th edn). New York State Psychiatric Institute.

Inciardi, J. (1970) The adult firesetter. *Criminology,* **8,** 145–155.

Jackson, H., Glass, C. & Hope, S. (1986) A functional analysis of recidivistic arson. *British Journal of Clinical Psychology,* **26,** 175–185.

Jackson, H., Glass, C. & Hope, S. (1987) Why are arsonists not violent offenders? *International Journal of Offender Therapy and Comparative Criminology,* **31,** 143–151.

Jayaraman, A. & Frazer, J. (2006) Arson: a growing inferno. *Medicine, Science and the Law,* **46,** 295–300.

Kolko, D. J. & Kazdin, A. E. (1988) Prevalence of firesetting and related behaviours among child psychiatric patients. *Journal of Consulting and Clinical Psychology,* **56,** 628–630.

Koson, D. F. & Dvoskin, J. (1982) Arson: a diagnostic study. *Bulletin of the American Academy of Psychiatry and the Law,* **10,** 39–40.

Labree, W., Nijman, H., van Marle, H., *et al* (2010) Backgrounds and characteristics of arsonists. *International Journal of Law and Psychiatry,* **33,** 149–153.

Lejoyeux, M., Arbaretaz, M., McLoughlin, M., *et al* (2002) Impulse control disorders and depression. *Journal of Nervous and Mental Disease,* **190,** 310–314.

Leong, G. B. (1992) A psychiatric study of persons charged with arson. *Journal of Forensic Science,* **37,** 1319–1326.

Lewis, N. O. C. & Yarnell, H. (1951) *Pathological Firesetting (Pyromania).* Nervous and Mental Disease Monographs no. 82. Coolidge Foundation.

Lindberg, N., Holi, M. M., Tani, P., *et al* (2005) Looking for pyromania: characteristics of a consecutive sample of Finnish male criminals with histories of recidivist fire-setting between 1973 and 1993. *BMC Psychiatry,* **5,** 1–5. At http://www.biomedcentral.com/content/pdf/1471-244x-5-47.pdf (accessed 17 December 2010).

Mackay, S., Paglia-Boak, A., MacKay, S., *et al* (2009) Epidemiology of firesetting in adolescents: mental health and substance use correlates. *Journal of Child Psychology and Psychiatry,* **50,** 1282–1290.

Magee, J. H. (1933) Pathological arson. *Scientific Monthly,* **37,** 358–361.

McElroy, S., Pope, H., Hudson, J., *et al* (1991) Kleptomania: a report on 20 cases. *American Journal of Psychiatry,* **148,** 652–657.

McElroy, S., Keck, P., Pope, H., *et al* (1994) Compulsive buying: a report of 20 cases. *Journal of Clinical Psychiatry,* **55,** 242–248.

McKerracher, D. & Dacre, A. (1966) A study of arsonists in a special security hospital. *British Journal of Psychiatry,* **112,** 1151–1154.

Moeller, F. G., Barratt, E. S., Dougherty, D. M., *et al* (2001) Psychiatric aspects of impulsivity. *American Journal of Psychiatry,* **158,** 1783–1793.

Murrie, D. C., Warren, J. I., Kristiansson, M., *et al* (2002) Asperger's syndrome in forensic settings. *International Journal of Forensic Mental Health,* **1,** 59–70.

Office for National Statistics (2005) *United Kingdom: Estimated Resident Population by Single Year of Age and Sex; Mid–2004 Population Estimates.* ONS. At http://www.statistics.gov.uk/cci/nugget.asp?id=6 (accessed 17 December 2010).

Ordroneaux, J. (1873) Moral insanity. *American Journal of Insanity,* **29,** 313–340.

O'Sullivan, G. H. & Kelleher, M. J. (1987) A study of firesetters in the south west of Ireland. *British Journal of Psychiatry,* **151,** 818–823.

Prins, H., Tennent, G. & Trick, K. (1985) Motives for arson (fire raising). *Medicine, Science and the Law,* **25,** 275–278.

Puri, B. K., Baxter, R. & Cordess, C. C. (1995) Characteristics of fire-setters. A study and proposed multiaxial psychiatric classification. *British Journal of Psychiatry,* **166,** 393–396.

Räsänen, P., Hirvenoja, R., Hakko, H., *et al* (1994) Cognitive functioning ability of arsonists. *Journal of Forensic Psychiatry,* **5,** 615–620.

Ray, I. (1838) *A Treatise on the Medical Jurisprudence of Insanity*. Charles C. Thomas & James Brown.

Reber, A. S. (1995) *The Penguin Dictionary of Psychology* (2nd edn). Penguin Books.

Repo, E. (1998) Finnish fire-setting offenders evaluated pre-trial. *Psychiatrica Fennica*, **29**, 175–189.

Rice, M. E. & Harris, G. (1991) Firesetters admitted to a maximum security psychiatric institution: offenders and offenses. *Journal of Interpersonal Violence*, **6**, 461–475.

Rice, M. E. & Harris, G. T. (1996) Predicting the recidivism of mentally disordered firesetters. *Journal of Interpersonal Violence*, **11**, 364–375.

Rice, M. E. & Harris, G. T. (2008) Arson. In *The Encyclopedia of Social Problems* (ed V. N. Parrillo). Sage.

Ritchie, E. C. & Huff, T. G. (1999) Psychiatric aspects of arsonists. *Journal of Forensic Science*, **44**, 733–740.

Rix, K. J. B. (1994) A psychiatric study of adult arsonists. *Medicine, Science and the Law*, **34**, 21–34.

Ross, T. & Pfäfflin, F. (2007) Attachment and interpersonal problems in a prison environment. *Journal of Forensic Psychiatry & Psychology*, **18**, 90–98.

Sapsford, R. J., Banks, C. & Smith, D. D. (1978) Arsonists in prison. *Medicine, Science and the Law*, **18**, 247–254.

Smith, J. & Short, J. (1995) Mentally disordered firesetters. *British Journal of Hospital Medicine*, **53**, 136–140.

Soothill, K. L. & Pope, P. J. (1973) Arson: a twenty-year cohort study. *Medicine, Science and the Law*, **13**, 127–138.

Soothill, K., Ackerley, E. & Francis, B. (2004) The criminal careers of arsonists. *Medicine, Science and the Law*, **44**, 27–40.

Soothill, K. Francis, B. & Liu, J. (2008) Does serious offending lead to homicide? Exploring the interrelationships and sequencing of serious crime. *British Journal of Criminology*, **48**, 522–537.

Swaffer, T., Haggett, M. & Oxley, T. (2001) Mentally disordered firesetters: a structured intervention programme. *Clinical Psychology and Psychotherapy*, **8**, 468–475.

Swinton, M. & Ahmed, A. (2001) Arsonists in maximum security: mental state at time of fire-setting and relationship between mental disorder and pattern of behaviour. *Medicine, Science and the Law*, **41**, 51–57.

Tantam, D. (1991) Asperger's syndrome in adulthood. In *Autism and Asperger Syndrome* (ed. U. Frith), pp. 147–183. Cambridge University Press.

US Census Bureau (2010) *US and World Population Clocks*. US Census Bureau. At http://www.census.gov/main/www/popclock.html (accessed 17 December 2010).

Van Ijzendoorn, M. H., Feldbrugge, J. T. T., Derks, F. C. H., *et al* (1997) Attachment representations of personality disordered criminal offenders. *American Journal of Orthopsychiatry*, **67**, 449–459.

Vaughn, M. G., Fu, Q., DeLisi, M., *et al* (2010) Prevalence and correlates of fire-setting in the United States: results from the National Epidemiological Survey on Alcohol and Related Conditions. *Comprehensive Psychiatry*, **51**, 217–223.

Ward, T., Hudson, S. M. & Marshal, W. L. (1996) Attachment style in sex offenders: a preliminary study. *Journal of Sex Research*, **33**, 17–26.

Wechsler, D. (1965) *Manual for the Wechsler Adult Intelligence Scale*. Psychological Corporation.

Wechsler, D. (1981) *Wechsler Adult Intelligence Scale – Revised (WAIS-R)*. Psychological Corporation.

Wechsler, D. (1997) *WAIS-III Administration and Scoring Manual*. Psychological Corporation.

CHAPTER 2

Theories on arson: the action systems model

Katarina Fritzon

This chapter develops an account of the utility of psychological models as an aid to understanding the crime of arson. A brief overview of some of the theories and typologies previously espoused is first presented. As its main focus the chapter then defines and provides an account of an 'action systems' model, which, in contrast to other arson typologies, produces empirically testable hypotheses. It goes on to describe how this model posits arson, and other crimes, as explicable along two axes relating to the arson target (object or person) and the arson objective (expressive or instrumental). The use of multidimensional scaling (MDS) analysis to map the characteristics of arson and arsonists onto these four modes is also described. The idea is developed of arsonists with psychiatric history as a distinct group, and the relationships between this distinct group of arsonists and the various arson modes are explored. The chapter lastly summarises how a typology based on arson mode and arsonist characteristics might affect clinical treatment.

Throughout the chapter the term 'arson' is used to denote adults who have set fires that in most cases would meet the legal criteria for arson. However, some studies are cited that include individuals who self-reported firesetting behaviour and were not necessarily convicted in court. Thus, these individuals are legally speaking not 'arsonists'; however, for simplicity the term 'arson' is used consistently throughout.

Arson and psychopathology

Much of what is known about adult arsonists is derived from studies of mentally disordered offenders. Studies based on these populations have informed ideas about what risk factors can predict arson recidivism (Dickens *et al*, 2009) as well as the primary treatment goals that might prevent reoffending (Swaffer *et al*, 2001). Whereas the literature on juvenile arson draws largely on community samples (Kolko & Kazdin, 1990; Kolko, 2002), adult arsonists mainly come to the attention of clinicians and researchers through the criminal justice system. Therefore research has relied on groups of incarcerated offenders – often in psychiatric institutions – to inform theories about motivations, characteristics and treatment needs. The current chapter summarises a number of theoretical perspectives on arson that are derived from this literature, while acknowledging that much of this existing knowledge may not apply to a broader sample of arsonists who either have no mental disorder or have not been convicted. Two recent studies have examined the prevalence of firesetting in the general community and found the self-reported rates to range from 1% (Vaughn et al, 2010) to 11.4% (Gannon & Barrowcliffe, 2011). Furthermore, a few studies have identified that the rate of past firesetting behaviour in individuals convicted for other index offences ranges from 25% (Lewis, 1999) to 54% (Doley, 2009). Clearly there are many individuals for whom firesetting has formed a part of their offending repertoire either historically or currently, but this may remain unidentified and unaddressed clinically.

This chapter also aims to draw on research on other types of crime to inform a broader theoretical perspective that is applicable to the general population of arsonists, including possibly those not convicted. The work of Tony Ward and colleagues in the area of sexual offending is particularly helpful, as parallels can be seen between his 'pathways' model (Ward & Siegert, 2002; Ward & Beech, 2006) and existing typologies of firesetting, especially the 'action systems framework' outlined by Fritzon and colleagues (e.g., Fritzon et al, 2001; Santtila et al, 2003a,b), but also other models of arson that have explicit practical relevance in terms of developing suitable treatment targets (e.g., Jackson et al, 1987; Jackson, 1994; Fineman, 1995).

Explanatory models of arson

As outlined by Gannon & Pina (2010) and Ward et al (2006), there are key criteria for evaluating competing theories relating to a phenomenon. These include: empirical adequacy, external consistency, unifying power, fertility and explanatory depth (Newton-Smith, 2002). *Empirical adequacy* refers to the evidential support for the theory; *external consistency* is the extent to which the theory is compatible with other accepted theories; *unifying power* is the extent to which a theory is able to account for all other theoretical perspectives and empirical findings; *fertility* refers to whether a theory gives rise to new lines of investigation; and *explanatory depth* refers to whether a theory is able to account sufficiently for all observed phenomena relating to the object of the theory. Multifactor theories are therefore preferred over single-factor theories, yet the literature on arson contains only two such theories, these being Jackson's functional analysis (Jackson et al, 1987; Jackson, 1994) and Fineman's (1995) dynamic behaviour models. Both frameworks view arson as a product of developmental experiences and reinforcement contingencies. While elements of these models can be seen to meet the criteria of empirical support and external consistency (in terms of clinical utility), they vary in relation to the criteria of explanatory depth and unifying power.

Jackson's functional analysis model proposes that recidivistic arson has a number of functions and motives, and argues that when the antecedents and consequences of arson are such that certain criteria are met, then the behaviour is likely to be repeated. According to the model, the key antecedents are: (1) psychosocial disadvantage (e.g., high incidence of mental illness and intellectual impairment leading to inadequacy in social situations); (2) dissatisfaction with life and the self (e.g., low self-esteem and depression); (3) social ineffectiveness (e.g., social isolation and poor social problem-solving skills); (4) specific psychosocial stimuli (e.g., previous exposure to fire); and (5) triggering stimuli (i.e., an undesired situation over which the arsonist is powerless, such as abuse). Jackson cites various research studies on the background characteristics of arsonists as support for these key factors. The consequences of arson are also hypothesised to function as positive or negative reinforcers; for example, the arsonist gains attention or is protected from further stressful situations. While this theory has received strong support from clinicians and is based on well-founded principles of social learning theory, there is relatively little empirical evidence for each of the key elements of the theory (Gannon & Pina, 2010). In addition, Gannon & Pina have argued that the theory is somewhat lacking in explanatory depth, as it fails to account explicitly for how cognitive or individual personality factors lead to a propensity to set fires.

Similarly, Fineman's model views arson as a product of: (1) historical factors that predispose to antisocial behaviour in general; (2) previous and existing reinforcement contingencies that reinforce firesetting behaviour specifically; and (3) environmental contingencies that encourage a specific instance of firesetting. The third aspect is further broken down into several factors, including triggering events (crisis or trauma), characteristics of the fire, cognitive distortions before, during and after the fire, feelings before during and after the fire, and internal and external reinforcements. The addition of cognitive factors is an improvement on Jackson's model, and each of the factors is developed in more detail as a sequence of events leading up to the fire. Thus Fineman's model arguably has greater explanatory depth than Jackson's functional analysis (Gannon & Pina, 2010).

Arson typologies

Typologies of arson, while useful as a way of potentially distinguishing between subgroups of offenders for the purpose of aiding treatment decisions, generally are neither comprehensive nor descriptive enough to be considered theories. Many of these typologies are essentially just lists of potential motives for arson and are not necessarily empirically derived, nor validated. Gannon & Pina's (2010) review and Dickens & Sugarman (see Chapter 3) should be consulted for a comprehensive overview of these typologies, including, in historical order: Lewis & Yarnell (1951), Inciardi (1970), Icove & Estepp (1987) and Prins (1994). Motives identified across such studies include: revenge/jealousy, excitement, vandalism, crime concealment, and a product of mental illness (e.g. delusional belief or command hallucination relating to fire). One of the very few empirically derived typologies of arsonists with a mental disorder was presented by Harris & Rice (1996), who studied a sample of 243 individuals held at the Penetanguishine forensic psychiatric institution in Canada, for each of whom there was at least one reported firesetting incident. Harris & Rice performed a cluster analysis on selected characteristics of both the crime scene and the offender and identified four subtypes of firesetters. These four groups were called 'psychotics', 'unassertives', 'multi-firesetters' and 'criminals'. The first of these groups made up a third ($n = 80$) of the sample. These individuals were usually diagnosed as schizophrenic, had set few fires in their lives, and did not have a history of criminal or aggressive behaviour. They were less likely than members of other clusters to have used accelerants while lighting the fire and their rate of recidivism was not particularly high for any further violent, non-violent or firesetting offences. No other fire-related characteristics were reported as significant for this group. The next largest group was the 'unassertives' ($n = 68$; 28%). They did not tend to have a history of aggression or criminal activity and were more intelligent and had better employment histories than the other groups. As the label suggests, these individuals were the least assertive of all the four types and were most likely to set fires out of anger or a desire for revenge. They were also most likely to report the fire themselves, to know the victim and to use accelerants. The 'multi-firesetters' accounted for 23% ($n = 56$) of the total sample. This group had the most adverse childhood histories and had high levels of aggression. Although they had little criminal history generally, they had previously set many fires. They were least intelligent, were most likely to have been institutionalised as children and had parents with psychiatric problems. They also were very unassertive, but were least likely to have been diagnosed as schizophrenic. In terms of the characteristics of their fires, they were most likely to have set fire to institutions and to have confessed. They were also most likely to have committed their offences during the day and exhibited a high rate of recidivism for all types of crime. Finally, the smallest subgroup was the 'criminals', making up 16% ($n = 39$) of the sample. These individuals had extensive criminal histories and poor childhood backgrounds marked by abusive parents. They were most likely to have been diagnosed as personality disordered. In terms of the fires they set, they were least likely to have known the victim of the fire, were most likely to set fire at night and were least likely to confess. These offenders were the most assertive and were most likely to commit further fire and violent offences when released.

Harris & Rice (1996) also attempted to develop a typology of the characteristics of the fires themselves and to relate this to the four subgroups of offender. A two-cluster solution was found, consisting of one large group

($n = 220$) of less serious fires and one small cluster ($n = 23$) of fires with high levels of injuries and property damage. This latter cluster was related to younger offenders with more extensive histories of firesetting. One possible reason for this inability to identify more substantial links between offence and offender characteristics is the absence of a theoretical framework underpinning the study. Without such a basis to guide hypotheses about expected differences in the characteristics of the fires set by each of the four groups of arsonists, it would be difficult to know what aspects of the fires to include in the analysis. Similarly, the labels given to describe the subgroups reflected concepts from a number of different domains, such as psychiatry and personality psychology. It is not clear why 'psychotics', for example, could not also be 'multi-firesetters', since one refers to a mental state and the other to behaviour.

It has been suggested that a useful offender classification should meet seven criteria: comprehensive coverage of the offender population; clear definitions of categories; sensitivity to changes; clinical relevance; economy of application; and both reliability and validity of distinctions (Megargee, 1977). Unfortunately, most existing classifications of arsonists fail to meet even the first of these criteria; in almost all of the typologies of motives, for example, there is included a 'motiveless/no apparent motive' category (e.g., Barker, 1994; Prins, 1994).

A further set of typologies, however, have used crime-scene data to classify subtypes of arsonists and are based on the assumption that the variations in arsonists' behaviour may reflect aspects of the arsonists' personal characteristics. These studies thus attempt to provide a more psychologically meaningful model of arson, with external validity and fertility in terms of providing guidance for mental health practitioners and agencies such as the police (e.g., Canter & Fritzon, 1998; Kocsis *et al*, 1998).

The action systems model (Canter & Fritzon, 1998; Fritzon *et al*, 2001; Almond *et al*, 2005) was created by investigative psychologists and holds some potential utility as a theory, given its potential to capture the behaviour and personal characteristics of the arsonist, and then to relate these to non-crime characteristics, such as response to therapy (Neville *et al*, 2007), and non-arson behaviours (Miller & Fritzon, 2007; Fritzon & Miller, 2010). The model has also been applied to other types of crime, such as school homicides (Fritzon & Brun, 2005), intra-familial homicide (Fritzon & Garbutt, 2001) and hostage-taking by terrorist groups (Fritzon *et al*, 2001).

The action systems framework

Systems theories of criminology arose from the work of von Bertalanffy (1968) and Parsons (1953) and have been applied to a diverse range of criminal activities, systems and networks. For example, following the terrorist attacks in the USA on 11 September 2001, ideas derived from systems theory were used to describe the actions and networks of Al-Qaeda terrorists (Lutes, 2001). The most common application of general systems theory today, however, is within family systems therapy, particularly around the theoretical orientation developed by Murray Bowen and colleagues (e.g., Kerr & Bowen, 1988).

Critics of Parsons' application of systemic models to criminology have pointed to the lack of acknowledgement of the role of human emotion, and have called for perspectives that take into account both the rational and the non-rational elements of human decision-making (Fish, 2004). However, within the more recent applications of Shye's (1985) behavioural action systems framework, the role of human emotion is acknowledged, both as an internal driver for behaviour and as a target for behavioural change, thus overcoming some of the criticisms of the original systems theories. More recent applications of the behavioural action systems framework integrate theory with methodology, utilising multidimensional scaling (MDS) procedures to show that, across various behavioural, social and cultural settings, four modes of functioning can be found to describe interactions that occur between the 'system' and the environment. A refinement incorporating elements of facet theory (Canter, 1985) has been labelled faceted action systems theory (FAST) by Canter, Fritzon and colleagues (e.g., Fritzon & Brun, 2005).

Shye (1985) defines a system as a collection of members that maintain interrelationships among themselves. To the extent that such a system is *active, open, organised* and *stable*, it can be regarded as an action system. The *active* nature of a behavioural action system is evidenced by the manifestations of both the sources of behaviours and the desired effect of these behaviours. To the extent that behaviours arise from person–environment interactions, they are considered *open*. The *organisation* and *stability* of criminal behaviour were challenges in applying Shye's (1985) model, which was essentially derived from a number of studies of high-functioning, pro-social systems, but a number of studies have now shown links between different forms of behaviour within the same individual across time (e.g., Miller & Fritzon, 2007; Neville *et al*, 2007; Fritzon & Miller, 2010).

The action systems model as originally developed by Shye (1985) was a way of modelling quality-of-life concerns (e.g., in adjusting to a new residential neighbourhood) and proposed that behaviour can be differentiated according to whether it derives from internal or external sources, and has as its desired locus of effect an internal or external target. In applying this model to arson, we can see similarities with Fineman's (1995) model of firesetting (see above), which proposes internal and external cognitive or sensory reinforcement. Within the action systems framework, four modes of functioning are proposed, labelled *expressive, integrative, adaptive* and *conservative* (see Table 2.1). In the first study to apply this model to criminal behaviour, Fritzon *et al* (2001) studied a sample of 230 individuals convicted of arson and 41 incidents of international

Table 2.1 Summary of action system modes of functioning

Source of action in relation to agent	Locus of effect in relation to agent	Mode	Behavioural examples
Internal	External	Expressive	Communicative, serial acts, with emotional trigger
Internal	Internal	Integrative	Self-harm: set fire to self or own home
External	External	Adaptive	Opportunistic burning of rubbish bins or cars, vandalism
External	Internal	Conservative	Outburst with trigger specific to target (often partner); use of accelerants

terrorist hostage-taking. The arson data for the study were drawn from the files of six UK police forces (rural and metropolitan). Subsequent studies have essentially replicated the same model using different samples, including an incarcerated population ($n = 65$; Almond *et al*, 2005) and a female population with mental disorder ($n = 50$; Miller & Fritzon, 2007). Below, findings from the arson studies are integrated with the generic descriptions of each of the four modes of action.

1 *Expressive mode.* The expressive model of functioning involves actions that have an internal source and external target. According to Shye (1985) this is the way in which the system 'exercises its power and influence on its surroundings [by trying to create] a reality which reflects in one way or another the system's own characteristics' (p. 102). In the context of criminal behaviour, this mode of functioning would be expected to reflect elaborate pre-offence fantasies and a fixation on particular forms of repetitive behaviours. This accords with Geller's (1992) emphasis on arson as a means of emotional acting out. Fritzon *et al* (2001) found that arsonists operating within this mode chose targets that provided the individual with vicarious attention, including hospitals and public buildings. The arsonist remained at the scene and was often a serial offender, presumably due to the positive reinforcement gained from the effects of the fire.

2 *Integrative mode.* The integrative mode describes adjustments that take place within the system itself. This is distinct from the expressive mode, in that the impact of the action is primarily internal, rather than necessarily having an observable external effect. In the presence of emotional disturbance, individuals operating in this mode might, for example, engage in life-threatening behaviours. Within arson this

internal distress results in firesetting that is directed at the arsonists themselves, often within their own home and involving a suicide note or gesture. These fires also involve multiple items and the arsonists tend to remain at the scene (Fritzon *et al*, 2001).

3   *Adaptive mode*. Functioning in this mode, the action system responds to external events in the environment by making adjustments to that environment. Crimes committed within this mode of action are expected to be opportunistic, with the selection of the actual target being less important than the desire to modify or gain from the act. In arson, the adaptive mode has been reflected in vandalism fires, or in attempts to cover up another crime, such as car theft or burglary. The variables that are associated with these fires are: setting fire to commercial premises, schools, cars and rubbish bins; breaking into the property; bringing material to the scene in order to set the fire; and multiple offenders (Fritzon *et al*, 2001).

4   *Conservative mode*. Shye describes this as 'events [that] constitute a fundamental aspect of [the system's] identity' and gives as examples the adoption of a constitution by an American state, or perpetuation of religious beliefs. Broadly, these involve events that originate externally but that are internally assimilated by the system. In the context of criminal behaviour, however, it may be more appropriate to adopt a slightly broader definition of acts that involve the conservative mode of functioning. For example, criminal acts perpetrated out of a desire for personal revenge may be seen as the individual responding to an external source of frustration that they wish to hurt or remove. This would be seen as conservative particularly where the retaliation was directed at someone with whom there was a close personal relationship, so that the act would be directed at redressing the individual's own state of emotional well-being. This form of firesetting could be inferred to carry the function of restoring power or control to the arsonist following what they consider to be a personal slight or affront, as shown by the variables 'outburst' (the fire was set while the arsonist was emotionally aroused and extensive property damage was carried out in addition to the fire), 'accelerant' (the arsonist used petrol or other flammable liquids), 'multiple seats' (fires were set in more than one location within the property) and 'witness' (the fire was set in the presence of another person, often the property owner or partner of the arsonist). In particular, the variable 'witness' indicates that by setting a fire in front of the protagonist, the arsonist obtains further emotional relief by making a direct impact on that person (Fritzon *et al*, 2001).

In summary, the action systems model provides hypotheses for distinguishing different forms of behaviours, thus fulfilling the criteria of *unifying power* and *fertility* for theory development (Newton-Smith, 2002).

The action systems model also provides structural hypotheses about the ways in which the four modes of action are expected to relate to each other empirically (*fertility*). The studies described above have used multidimensional scaling (MDS) to test the functional and structural hypotheses, and the resulting MDS plots have shown that, as predicted by the model, the variables associated with the expressive mode are located opposite the conservative variables, and the integrative opposite the adaptive. *External validity* and *empirical adequacy* have also been achieved by modelling different behaviours occurring across situations within the same individual (e.g., Miller & Fritzon, 2007; Neville *et al*, 2007; Fritzon & Miller, 2010). For example, Miller & Fritzon (2007) studied two forms of behaviour – self-harm and firesetting – exhibited by a group of 50 women with mental disorder incarcerated in a forensic psychiatric hospital. Behaviours were subjected to MDS. In the first set of findings, the hypotheses predicted by the action systems model were confirmed separately for both firesetting and self-harm. That is, four groups of variables associated with expressive, integrative, adaptive and conservative actions were found. For example, expressive forms of self-harm were characterised by the women exhibiting verbal and physical aggression at the same time as they engaged in self-harming actions, and these acts were often triggered by an emotionally disturbing event, such as an anniversary of an instance of abuse, or a birthday of a child with whom the patient did not have contact. Conservative forms of self-harm, on the other hand, were more often triggered by an argument with another person within the woman's living space, and involved self-harm in a private location, symbolising the internal locus of effect desired by conservative forms of action. The second set of findings illustrated correlations among the four modes of action system functioning *across* the two behavioural modalities. In other words, women who had set 'expressive' fires tended also to engage in 'expressive' forms of self-harm, whereas 'conservative' arsonists tended to be 'conservative' self-harmers, and so on.

Another way of testing the *external validity* of the action systems model is by reference to an already established and tested theory. As mentioned above, the current chapter seeks to do this in relation to Ward & Siegert's (2002) pathways model, which has been extensively referenced in relation to the research and treatment of sexual offenders. The next section outlines the pathways model and makes note of the similarities between it and the action systems model. Given that the action systems model is proposed to describe fundamental principles governing behaviour and that the model has already been found to apply to a variety of criminal behaviours (Fritzon & Brun, 2001; Fritzon & Garbutt, 2001; Fritzon *et al*, 2001), the existence of similar conceptual themes in the behaviour of sexual offenders would offer further validation for the proposed modes of action. This would be especially encouraging since the field of both conceptual and applied research in sexual offending is comparatively advanced.

Modes of functioning as pathways

Comparing the action systems model with Ward & Siegert's pathways to sexual offending

In their 'theory knitting' approach, Ward & Siegert (2002) develop a model of sexual offending that effectively combines a typology with a theory. Their model brought together a number of single theories of sexual offending into one comprehensive model. Ward & Beech (2006) extended this work into a developmental account of the process of sexual offending, combining levels of explanation from genetics, ecology, neuroscience and clinical features of sexual offending. While the action systems model outlined above does not describe all of these individual factors, it does explicitly account for the ecological and descriptive features of behaviour. On the other hand, the literature on the genetic and neuropsychological origins of firesetting behaviour is very sparse and thus there is currently no empirical basis upon which to integrate these factors within a generic explanatory model of firesetting.

A point of similarity between the action systems and pathways models is the proposal that there are four primary mechanisms by which offending occurs as a product of social learning, and environmental and biological factors. For example, Ward & Siegert argue that sexual offending is the result of (1) *intimacy deficits*, (2) *distorted sexual scripts*, (3) *emotional dysregulation*, and (4) *antisocial cognitions*. A fifth *multiple dysfunctional* mechanism also exists, although Ward & Siegert argue that in most cases one 'primary' factor will exert the most causal influence (see also Ward & Sorbello, 2003; Ward & Beech, 2006). Thus, when making comparisons, only the four pathways characterised by one primary deficit described by the pathways model will be examined.

In specific reference to sexual offending, the *intimacy deficits* pathway describes individuals whose offending occurs in the context of relationship difficulties, including rejection and isolation due to the absence of an adult intimate relationship. The *deviant sexual scripts* pathway describes situations in which sexual contact is the primary mechanism whereby individuals achieve interpersonal intimacy, and cognitive distortions facilitate inappropriate sexual contact, for example between adults and children, or other deviant sexual practices, including coercion of an adult sexual partner. The *dysregulation* pathway describes individuals who have difficulties in the self-regulation of emotions and behaviour. The *antisocial cognitions* pathway describes individuals who possess general pro-criminal attitudes and beliefs and their offending reflects these antisocial tendencies.

In a similar way to the action systems framework, the pathways model also fulfils many of the criteria for theory evaluation (Newton-Smith, 2002): it is supported by empirical research on the proximal and distal

37

risk factors for sexual offending, and has explanatory depth, unifying power and external consistency – in that it has formed the basis for the development of treatment programmes that target each area of risk and need, and these treatment programmes have themselves received strong empirical support, in the form of outcome research showing reductions in reoffending (Marshall *et al*, 1998; Beech *et al*, 1999). It is noted, however, in relation to empirical validation that, despite the popularity of the pathways model, only three studies have actually tested the model. One of these was a qualitative study of 13 child molesters (Connolly, 2004) in which ten were found, using grounded theory analysis, to fit one of the pathways. The second study, by Middleton *et al* (2006), applied the model to a sample of 72 internet child sexual offenders, with the result that not quite half the sample (46%) fitted one of the pathways, primarily due to a high proportion of the sample not showing high scores on any of the psychological tests affiliated with the pathways. Finally, Gannon *et al* (2011) employed cluster analysis on a set of ten psychometric tests completed by 97 contact child sexual offenders, and found only limited support for the pathways model, in that no clusters emerged that resembled the patterns that would be expected to support the 'emotional regulation' and deviant scripts' pathways.

Despite the possible limitations of the pathways model in relation to encapsulating all of the variations that exist among samples of sexual offenders, the following section shows that some similarities exist conceptually between the four pathways and the four-factor action systems framework. In applying this model to arson, it is hoped that many of the elements of the typological and theoretical research can be brought together, with the aim particularly of forming hypotheses about how existing approaches to the treatment of arson can be seen as theoretically robust. The following section outlines the similarities that exist between the description of the sexual pathways model and the action systems modes of functioning, and also draws on additional literature on the motives and characteristics of arsonists. The section explicitly examines the evidence for links between the four pathways of the Ward & Siegert (2002) model and the action systems model put forward by Fritzon and others (e.g., Fritzon *et al*, 2001), as well as other theoretical models, and thus offers evidence for the relative robustness of the action systems model as applied to arson.

The four modes described

(1) Intimacy deficits/conservative

According to the pathways model of sexual offending, offenders fitting this pathway experience significant difficulties in the area of developing and maintaining appropriate adult intimate relationships. Thus, inappropriate sexual partners, such as children, are selected as less threatening or more easily coerced into sexual contact than adult women.

In relation to arson, the conservative mode describes actions arising from conflict with a significant person in the arsonist's social network, often an intimate partner. These arsonists therefore have perhaps less severe difficulties in the area of intimacy deficits than their sexual offender counterparts, inasmuch as they are at least capable of initiating relationships, if not sustaining them. According to Canter & Fritzon (1998) the intimacy difficulties experienced by these arsonists are more often in relation to the maintenance, rather than the development, of relationships. Thus, these individuals have been able to initiate relationships but fires are set in the context of conflict in or the dissolution of the relationships. In the general literature, arsonists are often described as under-assertive (e.g., Harris & Rice, 1996) and lacking in social skills, and this may be particularly relevant for this group. In this way arson is seen as a goal-oriented, problem-solving strategy (e.g., revenge); it often occurs after alcohol consumption, which is in itself another example of a problematic coping mechanism. Swaffer (1993) also described a group of young firesetters with poor social skills who often used fire as a means of expressing anger and carrying out an act of revenge against a person whom they felt unable to confront.

(2) Deviant interest/expressive

Within the pathways model of sexual offending there is an identified subgroup of sexual offenders whose offending is driven by deviant sexual fantasies and preoccupations and for whom sexual behaviour may be used as a coping strategy. Similarly, some arsonists have a long-standing interest in fire and may use fire as a surrogate for emotional and possibly sexual expression. According to the action systems framework, the expressive arsonist often sets multiple fires and reports early experiences of fire, such as making false alarm calls or observing fire-related behaviour in family members or friends. This subtype of arsonist selects targets (e.g., public buildings and hospitals) to create a fire with particular properties (Canter & Fritzon, 1998). One bushfire arsonist whom the author treated described fires with particular physical properties resulting from burning different forms of vegetation, and had an almost encyclopaedic knowledge of the colours, smoke patterns and burning times associated with setting fire to various types of plant. Swaffer (1993) describes this 'pathological' group as fixated with fire and its properties, including the aftermath (arrival of fire services, gathering of crowds, etc.). Kocsis & Cooksey (2002) identified a possible direct overlap category of arsonists who set fires associated with sexual activity, suggesting a form of emotional relief similar to the expressive arson described by Fritzon et al (2001).

Fineman (1995) also describes a 'severely disturbed' subtype of arsonist for whom fire forms a major part of their fantasy life, and who obtain internal sensory reinforcement from firesetting. Fineman also observes that these arsonists are possibly the most resistant to treatment and are at high risk for future firesetting.

(3) Self-regulatory control problems/integrative

According to Ward & Siegert's (2002) pathways model of sexual offending this type of sexual offence is hypothesised to occur as a result of an insecure attachment style, whereby the individual has failed to develop appropriate regulatory mechanisms to deal with intense emotional arousal and uses sexual behaviour as a deviant coping mechanism. Sexual offenders operating in this pathway exhibit problems with mood management, low self-esteem, impaired problem-solving and reduced autonomy; they tend to distance themselves emotionally from other people.

Within the action systems model of arson, the integrative subtype appears to set fires under circumstances of heightened emotional sensitivity, resulting from a situational or personal trigger, such as a significant anniversary or date (Miller & Fritzon, 2007). These fires can be seen as acts of self-harm, as they are often targeted at the arsonists themselves, either within their own home or involving body parts or personal property of a significant nature, such as bedding or clothing. This subtype of arsonist is more commonly female and psychiatrically disturbed (Canter & Fritzon, 1998) and thus is rarely observed in prison samples (Kocsis & Cooksey, 2002; Gannon & Pina, 2010). Recent research indicates that, from an early age, girl arsonists are more likely to engage in firesetting in an effort to release internalised tension or to express emotional stress (Roe-Sepowitz & Hickle, 2011).

In line with other typologies that have identified a subgroup of arsonists called 'pathological', or 'psychiatric', both Canter & Fritzon (1998) and Lewis (1999) have found that the expressive and integrative forms of arson are those most likely to be set by people with mental disorder. On the other hand, Miller & Fritzon (2007) have found that all four subtypes of arson are set by individuals with mental disorder.

(4) Antisocial thinking patterns/adaptive

Within the pathways model of sex offending, there is a subgroup of individuals who exhibit generalised antisocial attitudes and behaviours. Similar to these offenders who are more likely to exhibit general recidivism rather than specifically sexual re-offending, many typologies of arson have described a so-called 'delinquent' or antisocial group of offenders (e.g., Swaffer, 1993; Kocsis & Cooksey, 2002). Within the action systems framework, this category is described as 'adaptive' in that the arsonists manipulate environmental opportunities that arise in the context of other illegal activities, such as car theft or breaking and entering properties. These individuals rarely present with fire-setting as their only behavioural problem, and thus intervention would focus not specifically upon the particular expression, but on the general underlying cognitions and attitudes supportive of offending/rule-breaking more broadly.

Empirical validity of the action systems model: behaviour maintenance/escalation

The action systems model provides a framework for understanding how individuals' behaviour results from internal and external cues, and there is evidence from recent studies that suggests that the modes of behaviour may represent characteristic ways of responding to these cues. For example, Jones (2004) has developed the term 'offence paralleling behaviour' to capture the consistencies that are observed between behaviours exhibited by offenders during incarceration or treatment and core functional aspects of their offending behaviours. Within the arson literature, Miller & Fritzon (2007) found such functional consistencies between the firesetting offence behaviours and the institutional self-harming behaviours of a group of 50 women detained in a forensic psychiatric hospital.

Within arson behaviour itself, consistency has also been noted among serial offenders. Fritzon (1998) found that 79% of 37 serial arsonists exhibited the same behavioural mode of action for each fire. Furthermore, the majority of serial arsonists set fires according to the expressive mode of action and many serial arsonists also displayed very specific behavioural consistency, such as setting fire to the same, or similar, target types. Other research has had similar findings (Dickens *et al*, 2009), with serial arsonists preferentially exhibiting certain crime behaviours more than one-off arsonists. These behaviours include certain targets, such as industrial or agricultural facilities, cars and rubbish, as well as involvement in the aftermath of the fire, such as self-extinguishing, staying to watch and assisting the fire brigade. These are all variables coded as 'expressive' within the action systems framework. Another relevant finding from the Fritzon (1998) research is that within nine of the cases where the serial offenders were not consistent, the latest offence in the series was classified as conservative. In many ways this is the most serious offence theme, containing the variables 'accelerants' and 'multiple items' (the fire was set using a variety of flammable objects that were often placed into a pile or spread around the property, which would also be coded as 'multiple seats'). This would suggest that, where there is a change in offence theme, it is in the direction of escalating seriousness. Furthermore, Fritzon found that there was a relationship between the number of offences in a series and the seriousness of those offences. One possible explanation for this is that as a series progresses, the psychological 'rewards' obtained from setting fires diminishes and that, rather like substance addiction, more of the stimulus is needed to provide the same benefits.

In terms of risk assessment, generally, then, the responses to specific environmental cues may be regarded as proximal risk factors, while the developmental circumstances that led to the adoption of a particular dominant operating style (one of the four action systems modes) would be considered distal risk factors. While the individual proximal risk factors may vary from one offence to another, the distal factors are considered relatively stable. In this way, the action systems framework offers a number of hypotheses for the development of a risk assessment instrument. See also Chapter 10 for a discussion of assessment and risk approaches for adult arsonists.

Treatment of firesetting

Clinical approaches to firesetting are less developed for adult arsonists than for juvenile arsonists (Gannon & Pina, 2010) and in part this reflects a lack of a suitable framework for understanding the risks and needs of arsonists (see Chapter 11). Again, the action systems model provides a possible basis for proposing different treatments for firesetters who operate according to each of the four modes of action.

The action systems framework suggests that offending behaviour has a number of very different psychological origins. Adaptive criminal events may be used by people who lack intellectual or psychological resources and who therefore rely on manipulating the environment to achieve their goals. On the other hand, integrative actions may be viewed primarily as a product of self-destructive tendencies, albeit that in some circumstances, as with firesetting, these events are also crimes. Persons who commit expressive acts may be serial offenders, who use crime as a characteristic way of communicating. Finally, conservative crimes are often caused by external agents and can be conceptualised as revengeful.

For clinical work with offenders, the principle of responsivity is important (Andrews & Bonta, 2003), as it provides a specific framework for understanding how offenders' therapeutic needs are likely to differ, and that topographical (offence) similarity does not imply functional similarity. Individuals operating within each of the four modes of the faceted action systems theory (FAST) are likely to respond to different modes of therapeutic interactions and even to require different theoretical orientations towards therapy. An alternative suggestion is that arsonists could benefit from an approach to group treatment that is similar to that adopted for sex offenders. The modular programmes outlined by Swaffer et al (2001) and Taylor et al (2002) in their treatment of arsonists take this approach and contain many of the elements suggested below.

Persons operating within an integrative mode of functioning are likely to have a tendency to direct the expression of emotions inwards and to dissociate and distance themselves from others. Perhaps they may perceive verbal communication as inadequate or difficult. Therapeutic work should therefore concentrate on the individual's difficulty in recognising, understanding and managing emotions. An approach that draws on ideas from dialectic behaviour therapy (e.g., Linehan, 1993) or acceptance commitment therapy (e.g., Eifert & Forsyth, 2005) would seem to meet the needs of this subgroup of arsonists. In particular, training in mindfulness and emotional regulation skills would seem to be of benefit for this subgroup.

Individuals who communicate expressively may have a similar constellation of clinical treatment requirements, in that there is a need to modify the valence of their emotional expression and to find alternative outlets. Treatment may also address the secondary gains of the behaviour, by changing environmental reinforcers. Group therapy may be helpful for maintaining a milieu where destructive behaviour is not valued but positive change is. Participation in therapeutic communities (Dolan, 1998) may be an effective treatment choice in such cases due to the emphasis on structured environmental contingencies and social rewards facilitated through the community.

For individuals with a tendency towards conservative acts, there may be a heightened interpersonal sensitivity and a cognitive bias towards perceiving others' actions as deliberately harmful or provocative. An objective of treatment would be to modify cognitive distortions, possibly through interpersonal or schema-focused therapy (e.g., Young et al, 2003), as well as incorporating elements from violent offender programmes, where the stages of anger/arousal are taught as well as cognitive reappraisal and restructuring techniques.

Finally, treatment oriented within the adaptive mode could concentrate on acknowledging the impact that external circumstances have and reducing the desirability of manipulating the environment and others. It has been found that adaptive crime is associated with juvenile offenders (e.g., Canter & Fritzon, 1998) and therefore early-intervention programmes, such as family and multisystemic therapies, are likely to be most effective here, coupled with environmental crime prevention strategies.

As noted by Gannon & Pina (2010), the majority of treatment offered to people who have set fires focuses on generic offending behaviour, which is surprising when specialised programmes exist for violent offenders and sexual offenders. The very sparse literature on the treatment of arsonists has generally focused on group treatment programmes, with evidence being drawn from research on other offending behaviour to show that this format can be effective. On the other hand, some of the subgroups of the action systems framework might respond better to individual treatment, especially those with clinical treatment needs as well as offence behaviour needs. As outlined above when discussing the integrative form of firesetting, perhaps a combined approach such as the format suggested by Linehan (e.g., 1993), which utilises group treatment for skills training and individual treatment for managing the problem behaviour, might be useful at least for certain types of individuals who set fires, especially those with a mental disorder which has contributed to the firesetting in some way.

One of the primary advantages of the action systems framework is the way in which it can facilitate an understanding of the underlying processes that give rise to behaviours. Therapy should aim to identify an individual's mode of functioning, and then specifically attempt to encourage the individual to deal with interpersonal situations in a more positive manner. The identification of the source and target of an individual's behaviour means that this encouragement can be specifically tailored to meet the interpersonal style of the individual, which would be expected to be more beneficial than the employment of generic therapeutic interventions.

Conclusions

The chapter has summarised a model for understanding the different behaviours of arsonists, and utilised research on other types of offender, notably sex offenders, to illustrate how common themes and patterns exist between these groups in terms of the psychological origins of their behaviour. There is a stark contrast in the breadth and depth of knowledge of these two types of offence and there is a need for a great deal of research and clinical focus on firesetting if we are fully to understand its origins and development, in order to inform practice.

The action systems model is essentially a typology, although it offers a more comprehensive and broader way of understanding human behaviour than a simple list of motives. Empirical research utilising the model has highlighted some potentially productive areas for further development, especially in the areas of risk assessment and clinical interventions with firesetters. This has included providing a framework for evaluating therapeutic progress, by understanding the functional consistencies in both the offending behaviour and institutional behaviour, such as self-harming (Miller & Fritzon, 2007), as well as behaviours occurring within a group treatment context that can be regarded as 'therapy interfering' behaviours versus 'cooperative' or 'therapy facilitative' behaviours (Neville *et al*, 2007). Thus, the action systems model represents a new way of conceptualising and possibly treating firesetting that is worthy of comprehensive exploration.

References

Almond, L., Duggan, L., Shine, J., *et al* (2005) Test of the arson action system model in an incarcerated population. *Psychology, Crime and Law*, **11**, 1–15.

Andrews, D. & Bonta, J. (2003) *The Psychology of Criminal Conduct* (3rd edn). Anderson.

Barker, A. (1994) *Arson: A Review of the Psychiatric Literature*. Oxford University Press.

Beech, A., Fisher, D. & Beckett, R. (1999) *STEP 3: An Evaluation of the Prison Sex Offender Treatment Programme*. Home Office. At http://rds.homeoffice.gov.uk/rds/pdfs/occ-step3.pdf (accessed 17 December 2010).

Canter, D. (1985) Introduction. In *Facet Theory Approaches to Social Research* (ed. D. Canter). Springer-Verlag.

Canter, D. & Fritzon, K. (1998) Differentiating arsonists: a model of firesetting actions and characteristics. *Legal and Criminological Psychology*, **3**, 73–96.

Connolly, M. (2004) Developmental trajectories and sexual offending: an analysis of the pathways model. *Qualitative Social Work*, **3**, 39–59.

Dickens, G., Sugarman, P., Edgar, S., *et al* (2009) Recidivism and dangerousness in arsonists: characteristics of repeat firesetters referred for psychiatric assessment. *Journal of Forensic Psychiatry and Psychology*, **20**, 621–639.

Dolan, B. (1998) Therapeutic community treatment for severe personality disorders. In *Psychopathy: Antisocial, Criminal, and Violent Behavior* (eds T. Millon, E. Simonsen, M. Birket-Smith & R. D. Davis), pp. 407–430. Guilford Press.

Doley, R. (2009) *A Snapshot of Serial Arson in Australia*. Lambert Academic Publishing.

Eifert, G. H. & Forsyth, J. P. (2005) *Acceptance and Commitment Therapy for Anxiety Disorders*. New Harbinger.

Fineman, K. R. (1995) A model for the qualitative analysis of child and adult fire deviant behaviour. *American Journal of Forensic Psychology*, **13**, 31–60.

Fish, J. S. (2004) The neglected element of human emotion in Talcott Parsons's 'The structure of social action'. *Journal of Classical Sociology*, **4**, 115–134.

Fritzon, K. (1998) *Differentiating Arsonists: An Action Systems Model of Malicious Firesetting*. Unpublished PhD thesis, University of Liverpool.

Fritzon, K. & Brun, A. (2005) Beyond Columbine: a faceted model of school-associated homicide. *Psychology, Crime and Law*, **11**, 53–71.

Fritzon, K. & Garbutt, R. (2001) A fatal interaction: the role of the victim and function of aggression in intrafamilial homicide. *Psychology, Crime and Law*, **7**, 309–331.

Fritzon, K. & Miller, S. (2010) Functional consistency in female forensic psychiatric patients: an actions systems theory approach. In *Offence Paralleling in Offender Populations* (eds L. Jones & M. Daffern), pp. 137–150. Wiley.

Fritzon, K., Canter, D. & Wilton, Z. (2001) The application of an action systems model to destructive behaviour: the examples of arson and terrorism. *Behavioral Sciences and the Law*, **19**, 657–690.

Gannon, T. A. & Barrowcliffe, E. (2011) Firesetting in the general population: the development and validation of the Fire Setting and Fire Proclivity Scales. *Legal and Criminological Psychology*. DOI: 10.1348/135532510X523203.

Gannon, T. A. & Pina, A. (2010) Firesetting: psychopathology, theory and treatment. *Aggression and Violent Behaviour*, **15**, 224–238.

Gannon, T. A., Terriere, R. & Leader, T. I. (2011) An evaluation of Ward and Siegert's pathways model: a cluster analysis approach. *Psychology, Crime and Law* (in press).

Geller, J. L. (1992) Communicative arson. *Journal of Hospital and Community Psychiatry*, **43**, 76–77.

Harris, G. T. & Rice, M. E. (1996) A typology of mentally disordered firesetters. *Journal of Interpersonal Violence*, **11**, 351–363.

Icove, D. J. & Estepp, M. H. (1987) Motive based offender profiles of arson and fire-related crimes. *FBI Law Enforcement Bulletin*, **56**, 17–23.

Inciardi, J. (1970) The adult firesetter. *Criminology*, **8**, 145–155.

Jackson, H. F. (1994) Assessment of firesetters. In *The Assessment of Criminal Behaviours in Secure Settings* (eds M. McMurran & J. Hodge), pp. 94–126. Jessica Kingsley.

Jackson, H. F., Glass, C. & Hope, S. (1987) A functional analysis of recidivistic arson. *British Journal of Clinical Psychology*, **26**, 175–185.

Jones, L. (2004) Offence paralleling behaviour (OPB) as a framework for assessment and intervention with offenders. In *Applying Psychology to Forensic Practice* (eds A. Needs & G. Towl), pp. 34–63. Blackwell.

Kerr, M. E. & Bowen, M. (1988) *Family Evaluation: An Approach Based on Bowen Theory*. Norton.

Kocsis, R. & Cooksey, R. W. (2002) Criminal psychological profiling of serial arson crimes. *International Journal of Offender Therapy and Comparative Criminology*, **46**, 631–656.

Kocsis, R., Irwin, H. J. & Hayes, A. F. (1998) Organised and disorganised behaviour syndromes in arsonists: a validation study of a psychological profiling concept. *Psychiatry, Psychology and Law*, **5**, 117–130.

Kolko, D. J. (2002) *Handbook on Firesetting in Children and Youth*. Academic Press.

Kolko, D. & Kazdin, A. (1990) Matchplay and firesetting in children: relationship to parent, marital, and family dysfunction. *Journal of Clinical Child Psychology*, **19**, 229–238.

Lewis, H. (1999) *Mentally Disordered Arsonists: Characteristics and Firesetting Behaviours*. Unpublished Masters thesis, University of Surrey.

Lewis, N. O. C. & Yarnell, H. (1951) *Pathological Firesetting (Pyromania)*. Nervous and Mental Disease Monographs no. 82. Coolidge Foundation.

Linehan, M. M. (1993) *Cognitive–Behavioral Treatment of Borderline Personality Disorder*. Guilford.

Lutes, C. (2001) *Al-Qaida in Action and Learning: A Systems Approach*. George Washington University. At http://www.au.af.mil/au/awc/awcgate/readings/al_qaida2.htm (accessed 17 December 2010).

Marshall, W., Fernandez, Y., Hudson, S., *et al* (1998) *Source Book of Treatment Programs for Sexual Offenders*. Plenum Press.

Megargee, E. (1977) A new classification system for criminal offenders. I: The need for a new classification system. *Criminal Justice and Behavior*, **4**, 107–114.

Middleton, D., Elliott, I. A., Mandeville-Norden, R., *et al* (2006) An investigation into the applicability of the Ward and Siegert pathways model of child sexual abuse with Internet offenders. *Psychology, Crime and Law*, **12**, 589–603.

Miller, S. & Fritzon, K. (2007) Functional consistency across two behavioural modalities: firesetting and self harm in female special hospital patients. *Criminal Behaviour and Mental Health*, **17**, 31–44.

Neville, L., Miller, S. & Fritzon, K. (2007) Understanding change in a prison therapeutic community: an action systems approach. *Journal of Forensic Psychiatry and Psychology*, **18**, 181–203.

Newton-Smith, W. (2002) *A Companion to the Philosophy of Science*. Blackwell.

Parsons, T. (1953) Some comments on the state of the general theory of action. *American Sociological Review*, **18**, 618–631.

Prins, H. (1994) *Fire-Raising: Its Motivation and Management*. Routledge.

Roe-Sepowitz, D. & Hickle, K. (2011) Comparing boy and girl arsonists: crisis, family, and crime-scene characteristics. *Legal and Criminological Psychology*, **16**, 277–288.

Santtila, P., Hakkanen, H. & Fritzon, K. (2003a) Inferring the characteristics of an arsonist from crime scene behaviour: a case study in offender profiling. *International Journal of Police Science and Management*, **5**, 1–15.

Santtila, P., Hakkanen, H., Alison, L., *et al* (2003b) Juvenile firesetters: crime scene actions and offender characteristics. *Legal and Criminological Psychology*, **8**, 1–20.

Shye, S. (1985) Nonmetric multivariate models for behavioural action systems. In *Facet Theory: Approaches to Social Research* (ed. D. Canter), pp. 97–148. Springer-Verlag.

Swaffer, T. (1993) A motivational analysis of adolescent fire setters. *Issues in Criminological and Legal Psychology*, **20**, 41–45.

Swaffer, T., Haggett, M. & Oxley, T. (2001) Mentally disordered firesetters: a structured intervention programme. *Clinical Psychology and Psychotherapy*, **8**, 468–475.

Taylor, J. L., Thorne, I., Roberston, A., *et al* (2002) Evaluation of a group intervention for convicted arsonists with mild and borderline intellectual disabilities. *Criminal Behaviour and Mental Health*, **12**, 282–293.

Vaughn, M. G., Fu, Q., DeLisi, M., *et al* (2010) Prevalence and correlates of fire-setting in the United States: results from the National Epidemiological Survey on Alcohol and Related Conditions. *Comprehensive Psychiatry*, **51**, 217–223.

von Bertalanffy, L. (1968) *General Systems Theory: Foundation, Development, Applications*. Braziller.

Ward, T. & Beech, A. (2006) An integrated theory of sexual offending. *Aggression and Violent Behavior*, **11**, 44–63.

Ward, T. & Siegert, R. J. (2002) Toward a comprehensive theory of child sexual abuse: a theory knitting perspective. *Psychology, Crime and Law*, **9**, 319–351.

Ward, T. & Sorbello, L. (2003) Explaining child sexual abuse: integration and elaboration. In *Sexual Deviance: Issues and Controversies in Sexual Deviance* (eds T. Ward, D. R. Laws & S. M. Hudson), pp. 1–18. Sage.

Ward, T., Polaschek, D., & Beech, A. (2006) *Theories of Sexual Offending*. Wiley.

Young, J. E., Klosko, M. E. & Weishaar, M. E. (2003) *Schema Therapy: A Practitioner's Guide*. Guilford.

CHAPTER 3

Differentiating firesetters: lessons from the literature on motivation and dangerousness

Geoff Dickens and Philip Sugarman

This chapter reviews in detail the long history of exploration of firesetters' motives and underlines the importance of revenge, vandalism and excitement. However, as fire is inherently somewhat unpredictable, research has only recently begun to identify the centrality of firesetting behaviour in the prediction of future firesetting risk. The courts rightly value the identification of recklessness and intention to endanger life, and look to mental health professionals for guidance. We conclude that the future direction of clinical assessment and research should centre on behaviour, intention and the prediction of risk.

It has long been established that the typical firesetter is young and male (e.g., Lewis & Yarnell, 1951), but in reality firesetters are a heterogeneous group who cut across categories of gender, age and intellectual ability. The characteristics of these groups (men and women, juveniles and adults, those with and without intellectual disability) are worth detailed, individual attention to identify different approaches to risk assessment and treatment. The advantage of such groupings is that they emerge from naturally occurring dichotomies and require little conceptual elucidation. Historically, however, research has not followed this approach. A favoured approach to firesetter differentiation, one that drove a considerable amount of enquiry from the 1970s to the 1990s, has been motivational typing. Motivation can be defined as: 'the driving force or forces responsible for the initiation, persistence, direction and vigour of goal directed behaviour' (Colman, 2009). More recently, motivational classification has been viewed as flawed (Prins, 1994; Gannon & Pina, 2010), primarily because clear *motives* (such as revenge) are often confused with *characteristics* (such as institutionalisation), but also because entirely different cases of firesetting, such as fires endangering and not endangering life, can be conflated under one heading, such as revenge (Soothill, 1990).

This chapter critiques the chequered history of motivational classification, before examining firesetting behaviour through a prism of forensic risk. We seek to examine what the literature on firesetting recidivism and destructiveness can tell us about identification of the most dangerous firesetters. Throughout, we use the term 'firesetting', but when talking about individual studies of people convicted for their intentional firesetting behaviour or when referring to legal issues, we use the term 'arson'. This distinction leads logically to a caveat: the literature on motivation, recidivism and dangerousness in firesetting has concerned convicted and clinical samples that may not be representative of all those who deliberately set fires and thus the generalisability of empirical research in this area is limited. Most research has been conducted with all-male or largely male samples and these results cannot be assumed to generalise to women.

Motivation

Given the problems with motivational classification outlined above, should motive concern the mental health practitioner? The answer is a pragmatic 'yes'. Psychiatric morbidity is common among those convicted of arson (Enayati *et al*, 2008; Anwar *et al*, 2011) and in order to assist in their determination of disposal the courts are generally inclined to call for psychiatric reports in all but the most straightforward cases (Prins, 2005; *R v. Calladine* [1975]). In the UK, case law (*R v. Hoof* [1980]) has established that there should be separate counts relating to: arson with intent to endanger life; arson reckless as to whether life was endangered; and simple arson. In effect, the court should attempt to distinguish between recklessley and intentionally destructive cases of arson, with the final decision being made by the jury. Further, this distinction will be reflected in sentencing, and cases of arson with intent to endanger life or aggravating features (including premeditation) are punishable by 8–10 years in prison (see Chapter 9). Practitioners, chiefly forensic psychiatrists, are required to make informed judgements about the presence or absence of mental disorder in referred firesetters and to comment about intentionality and motivation. Those who are required to advise the court thus need a clear grasp of the evidence base on the role of motivation in firesetting.

The historical context

Firesetting was viewed by 19th-century European scholars as strongly associated with young female domestic staff living and working in accommodation far from home and setting fires for reasons of 'nostalgia' (Barker, 1994). Later, firesetting was linked by Sigmund Freud to libidinal development and he proposed a strong role for sexual fetishism. He posited that the 'warmth radiated by fire evokes the same kind of glow as accompanies the state of sexual excitation, and the motion of the flame suggests the phallus in action' (Freud, 1932, p. 407). Freud proposed that men have a natural instinct to extinguish fire by the act of urination and that this act, involving both a real and a symbolic penis, represents suppressed homosexuality. Gold (1962), a US psychiatrist of the psychodynamic school, believed that setting fires was often a displaced sexual urge, the result of enforced sexual abstinence. Consequently, he argued, sexual excitement and masturbation would often accompany firesetting. These hypotheses have not been empirically supported and very few people have reported deriving sexual pleasure from firesetting (3% in the sample studied by Lewis & Yarnell, 1951; 2.5% in that studied by Rice & Harris, 1991). Phallometric testing has failed to differentiate between arsonists and non-arsonists when exposed to fire-related stimuli (Koson & Dvoskin, 1982; Quinsey *et al*, 1998), which further leads to rejection of the unconscious sexual motivation hypothesis. However, the failure of classification by sexual motivation did not discourage the search for a wider motivational typology.

Firesetter motivational typologies: some considerations

Classification of offender 'type', or typology, can result from conceptually driven inductive approaches or from deductive methods that examine measurable relationships between observed and reported firesetter charac-teristics and fire-scene variables. Firesetter typology is thus similar to other approaches to classification (Bailey, 1994). With notable exceptions (Harris & Rice, 1996; Canter & Fritzon, 1998), firesetter typologies have been inductive; and even though some have involved the examination of empirical data (Lewis & Yarnell, 1951; Inciardi, 1970; Icove & Estepp, 1987; Ravateheino, 1989), there is little evidence that the development of category headings for classificatory purposes has involved any more than *thinking about* the data, albeit from the informed perspective of clinical or investigative expertise. Nevertheless, the aim of both inductive and deductive approaches is to reduce complex information about a heterogeneous group with little in common beyond a superficial index behaviour into meaningful, homogeneous chunks. Put simply, typology is intended to make theory manageable (Helfgott, 2008). Classification can provide mental health practitioners, criminal justice officials and others with information to aid decision-, policy- and law-making, and to guide risk assessment and treatment interventions (Helfgott, 2008). Different typologies may be required to achieve different ends (Byrne & Roberts, 2007): those developed to assist police investigation and the detection of firesetters may not be informative about the assessment of recidivism risk or intervention strategy. Quantitative and qualitative differences between offender types may suggest differential aetiological factors, intervention strategies and management approaches and thus classificatory systems can inform more complex multifactor theories in due course (Gannon & Pina, 2010). In the absence of well-developed and empirically tested multifactor theories, firesetter classificatory systems have been a notable feature of the literature. Given their proliferation, a standard approach to evaluation is required and in the following section we comment on proposed firesetter typologies in respect of the following issues:

- *Clarity and objectivity*. There should be sufficiently detailed explication for each constituent category of the typology, including clear specifications of the criteria for category membership.
- As a corollary, assignment of category membership for individual firesetters should be *reliable* between raters.
- Category membership should be *mutually exclusive* and no individual should meet the criteria for membership of more than one category.
- A satisfactory typology will be *comprehensive*, allowing classification of all individuals within the categories, with no 'others' left over who remain unexplained.
- The best typology is the most *parsimonious*. It should have relatively few categories. All else being equal, the typology with the fewest categories is preferred.
- *Homogeneity* of behaviour of the target population. A satisfactory typology should attempt to describe or explain those who display a comparable set of behaviours.
- *Empirical congruence* demands that the typology is supported by available data (Gibbons, 1975; Helfgott, 2008).

Inductive firesetter typologies

Although Magee (1933) had already posited a dichotomous typology comprising *pathological* and *non-pathological* firesetters, the first classificatory system to present significant data on firesetting emerged from Lewis & Yarnell's (1951) classic work. The two Columbia University psychiatrists gathered details of cases of firesetting from records held by the US National Board of Fire Underwriters covering a 5-year period and for other representative cases dating back to 1919. Records included fire investigation details and, where conducted, psychiatric reports. The researchers were granted access to data from institutions and clinics where offenders were sent following conviction and they also personally interviewed 100 firesetters. Those who were believed to have set fires for profit (e.g., by defrauding insurance) were excluded. Details of 1145 adult male and 200 female firesetters resulted in a four-category classification: *unintentional firesetting* due to temporary confusion or lack of judgement; *delusional* in response to command voices or other delusional ideas; *erotic* due to sexual fetishism or pyromaniac traits; and *revenge* for real or perceived slights or because of jealousy. A fifth category, *children* who set fires for reasons of mischief or excitement, was included based on analysis of details of 200 additional cases of juvenile firesetting. Subgroups included 'vagrant' and 'institutionalised' firesetters, which constitute sociodemographic characteristics rather than motivators, and some psychotic firesetters were acknowledged by Lewis & Yarnell to be individuals 'who seemed to naturally belong with the revenge, pyromaniac, and so on groups' (p. 376) and thus the typology did not comprise *mutually exclusive* categories. The largest proportion of the adult male sample (60%) were described as 'pyromaniacs', fitting Lewis & Yarnell's *erotic* firesetter category. This finding has not been supported by subsequent research on the prevalence of pyromania (Koson & Dvoskin, 1982; Harmon *et al*, 1985; Prins *et al*, 1985; O'Sullivan & Kelleher, 1987; Rice & Harris, 1991; Leong, 1992; Ritchie & Huff, 1999) and thus the classification lacked *empirical congruence*. Finally, Gannon & Pina (2010) have noted that Lewis & Yarnell did not offer any explanation of the implications of their categorisations for risk assessment or intervention. Despite these limitations, most publications in the subsequent 60 years have cited this influential work.

Inciardi (1970), a sociologist with a background as a parole officer, examined detailed case reports of 138 convicted arsonists released from New York state prisons between 1961 and 1966, of whom 97% were male; their median age range was 21–29 years and their median IQ 80–89. From these cases he devised a six-category behavioural typology comprising:

- *revenge* (58%)
- *excitement* (e.g., from watching the fire itself or seeing the fire officers in action) (13%)
- *institutionalisation* (e.g., residents of psychiatric hospitals) (6%)
- *insurance claim* (e.g., to collect the insurance on property) (6%)
- *vandalism* (e.g., wilful destruction of property for fun) (5%)
- *crime concealment* (e.g., setting a fire to conceal evidence of a burglary) (3%).

The high frequency of *revenge* has been mirrored in other studies (Lewis & Yarnell, 1951; Koson & Dvoskin, 1982; O'Sullivan & Kelleher, 1987; Ravateheino, 1989; Rix, 1994). Inclusion of 'for profit' arsonists increased the *heterogeneity* of the sample in relation to Lewis & Yarnell's study, but restriction to convicted arsonists limited its generalisability to firesetters as a population. The definitions that Inciardi proposed for each category are clear and succinct (e.g., a *revenge* firesetter 'is a person who, because of a quarrel or a feeling of hatred or jealousy, seeks revenge upon the victim by means of fire', p. 148). Interestingly, individuals categorised as *revenge* firesetters were felt by Inciardi to represent the most dangerous subgroup but it was not clearly articulated why this was the case. This group were usually intoxicated at the time of their firesetting and often had serious alcohol problems. Inciardi's category of *institutionalised* firesetters constitutes a sociodemographic category and not a motive. Further, Inciardi stated that this subgroup largely comprised individuals with grievances against the institution in which they were held and, intuitively, this seems to best fit the revenge category and thus the typology has limitations related to *mutual exclusivity*. This typology appears to have been influential, however, and a number of subsequent firesetter classifications differed only in minor ways, or refined Inciardi's typology with the addition of one or two new categories.

Dennett (1980), an experienced fire investigator, described firesetters' motives under similar headings to Inciardi but with the addition of a heroism category (e.g., firesetters deliberately creating circumstances whereby they can display heroic qualities by saving people). Ravateheino (1989) categorised by motivation 180 people (86% male, mean age 27.7 years, age range 5–59 years) arrested for arson in Helsinki over a 15-year period and added discrete categories for pyromaniacs (defined as those without motive) and children. Like Inciardi (1970), the reported motivational categories in fact comprised a mixture of offender motives ('revenge, jealousy, hatred, envy, grudges') and characteristics ('alcoholics, mental patients, and temporarily disturbed'). The typology therefore fails to achieve mutual exclusivity as an individual could be both alcoholic and motivated from revenge.

Icove & Estepp (1987) examined qualitative records of interviews conducted with 737 juveniles and 279 adults arrested for arson. The proportion of offenders fitting in each motive category were: *vandalism* (49%); *excitement* (25%); *revenge* (14%); *profit* (1%); *crime concealment* (2%); and *other motives* (8%). The preponderance of vandalism- and excitement-motivated firesetting in the sample probably reflected the high proportion of juveniles studied. A subsequent investigation of adult firesetters involving Icove (Sapp *et al*, 1996), a senior instructor with the US Federal Bureau of Investigation (FBI), supports this: the researchers interviewed 83 adult serial arsonists (94% male, median age 27 years) and reported that the most common motivation was *revenge* (27%), then *excitement* (23%), *profit* (12%) and *vandalism* (10%). The inclusion of a group comprising 'other motives' indicates that Icove & Estepp's typology failed to be *comprehensive*. The obvious strength of the work is its large sample size and a data-set that describes a wide range of sociodemographic and offence-related variables.

A six-category typology detailed in the FBI *Crime Classification Manual* (Douglas *et al*, 1997) is largely based on Icove & Estepp's (1987) system, with an additional category for *extremist-motivated arson* (e.g., deliberate burning of a research laboratory by animal rights activists). This classification is well explicated and therefore appears more *clear and objective* than some competing typologies. However, like most typologies, the underlying assumption is that the motivation for firesetting can be assigned to discrete categories and is not inherently multifactorial. Finally, the classification was developed for offender profiling and to aid in the investigation and detection of firesetters, and it is unclear whether the typology has implications for risk assessment or intervention.

In a novel study, Swaffer & Hollin (1995) conducted semi-structured interviews with 17 adolescents in a UK youth treatment service to investigate why they set fires; the approach taken was to ask in detail about the *antecedents* to the firesetting, the firesetting itself and its *consequences*. All but one participant reported setting a fire for just one of five emergent themes and there was little overlap between reported reasons: *revenge, crime concealment, self-injury, peer pressure* and *fascination with fire*. One small group *denied* involvement in firesetting. While this was a small study of adolescents and cannot be generalised to all firesetters, it is surprising that this type of research has not been conducted with adults in order to gain a more detailed picture of motivation using a transparent and structured self-report method.

Subsequent typologies have differed more fundamentally from Inciardi's (1970) basic template and are exemplified by multiple additional categories. While these typologies are more *comprehensive,* this is achieved at the cost of reduced *parsimony* and concurrent failure to solve issues related to *mutual exclusivity.* Based on his earlier work with imprisoned arsonists (Prins *et al*, 1985), Prins (1994) proposed a ten-category typology which added to Inciardi's (1970) template the following motive types: *arson committed for political purposes* (e.g., terrorism); *self-immolation as a political gesture; arson committed as an attention-seeking act;* and *arson for mixed motives;* and refined other categories. The last category is an interesting distinction and acknowledged what is intrinsically implied by the common lack of mutual exclusivity in many typological systems: the motives for any single act of firesetting may be multiple and almost certainly beyond the explanatory power of a simple unitary classification system. Prins (1994) transfomed Inciardi's *institutionalised firesetter* group into the item *arson due to mental disorder,* adding several subcategories to it, and refined Inciardi's *revenge* category to include subtypes for person-directed acts and those directed at society more widely. Prins (1994) acknowledged the weaknesses of his typology, specifically that *mutual exclusivity* is compromised by categories comprising a mixture of both motives and characteristics.

Cooke & Ide's (1985) classification further delineated between two types of 'torch': those who set fires to defraud insurance; and those who are hired by another to commit the crime. They also distinguished between those fires set by employees and those set by business rivals.

Rix (1994) examined existing classification systems (Inciardi, 1970; Prins *et al*, 1985) in order to ascribe motivation in his study of 153 people (84% male; mean age for men 25 years, women 31 years) referred for psychiatric examination following arrest for arson and found them wanting. He added multiple new categories, all accounting for fewer than 5% of the total: *rehousing* (individual sets fire to a domestic property in the hope of being resituated); *attempted suicide; antidepressant* (i.e., fires set in an attempt to lighten the firesetter's mood); and *heroism* (fires set so that the perpetrator could rescue people or raise the alarm and thus attract praise). The most common motives reported by Rix were *revenge* (31%); *excitement* (11%); *vandalism* (6%); and a *cry for help* (7%). By Rix's admission, it was not always clear how best to categorise arsonists and, once again, the typology, though *comprehensive,* failed to define *mutually exclusive* categories.

In the most extreme example of category inflation, Ritchie & Huff (1999) examined the case files of 283 arsonists (83% male; median age range 18–29 years) from FBI, prison and psychiatric hospital records and assigned motives to six main categories and 33 discrete subcategories. The most common motives were *revenge* (37%), *crime concealment* (17%), *vandalism* (16%), *profit* (6%) and *other* (18%), the last including murder, attempted suicide, juvenile firesetters and incompetent adults.

Finally, two studies (Geller & Bertsch, 1985; Geller *et al*, 1992) examined firesetting behaviour among psychiatric in-patients in two US hospitals and assigned individuals to seven groups, namely those who: *set a fire; threatened to set a fire; were careless with smoking; set off a false fire alarm; threw lighted matches or cigarettes; falsely called in a fire report;* or *set a fire to self or others*. While clearly not a motivational typology, these two studies illustrate the problem of too much heterogeneity in the target study group because it is not at all clear that members of categories share many underlying psychological characteristics.

Other classification systems have attempted to simplify the problem of category proliferation by conducting deeper conceptual analyses of the underlying commonalities of different motives in order to produce *parsimonious* typologies with, typically, two to four categories. Scott (1974) proposed that firesetting was either *motivated* (for profit, political or suicidal purposes) or *motiveless* (usually by children, or those with a mental disturbance, and who those set fires for sensual satisfaction). This is intuitively appealing, but a lack of *clarity* and *objectivity* is suggested by Scott's categorisation of those who set fire for revenge under *motiveless* firesetting (Willis, 2004). Kidd (1997) proposed a three-category system: *motivated arson* (for purposes of insurance fraud, intimidation or crime concealment), apparently *motiveless arson* (including in the context of pyromania, psychosis, mental illness or intellectual disability, vandalism or alcohol or drug use), and *juvenile fire involvement*. Gannon & Pina (2010) have highlighted the semantic contradiction arising from the classification of firesetting by some groups as motiveless. Vreeland & Levin (1990) described three categories: *for-profit* firesetters, *solitary* firesetters and *group* firesetters. These groups are clearly not mutually exclusive and therefore the categorisation is of questionable value. Muckley (1997) suggested also three categories: *curiosity* (mainly comprising children and adolescents), *deliberate* (comprising revenge firesetters and those for whom firesetting is part of a wider criminal repertoire) and the *career arsonist* (those for whom arson becomes an obsession). Faulk (1994) suggested two groupings based on whether the firesetter's motivation was *instrumental* (to achieve an end including profit, crime concealment, revenge, heroism, a cry for help, to enhance self-esteem or to relieve boredom) or *intrinsic* (fire being the object of interest itself, as in cases of pyromania or sexual fetishism). This was nuanced by Barker's (1994) application of Edmunds' (1978) typology of aggressive behaviour to firesetting, which categorised motives under four headings: *acquisitive* (setting fires for financial gain), *vindictive* (setting fires with the intention of causing harm to a person or people), *instrumental* (to achieve some other non-financial end, such as boredom release) and *cathartic* (fires set as an expression of emotion but at a random target).

In brief, a period between 1970 and 2000 saw a proliferation of inductively generated motivational classificatory systems for firesetters and arsonists.

These typologies frequently implicated motives including *revenge* (Lewis & Yarnell, 1951; Inciardi, 1970; Ravateheino, 1989), *vandalism* (Icove & Estepp, 1987; Ritchie & Huff, 1999) and *excitement* (Inciardi, 1970; Icove & Estepp, 1987; Rix, 1994). Unfortunately, these systems largely assumed that the reasons or motives that people have for setting fires are unidimensional, although Prins (1994) hinted at a *mixed motive* category, which, in reality, may better describe a far larger proportion of firesetters.

Commonly, typologies mix motives and characteristics among their category headings and it is often unclear how a motive has been assigned, although this usually seems to amount to firesetter self-report and professional opinion. There is very little evidence that category assignment can be made reliably. Some classificatory systems have been exhaustively detailed (Rix, 1994; Ritchie & Huff, 1999) and describe small numbers of cases very well but have little explanatory power. Authors of classificatory systems rarely spell out the implications that category membership holds for risk assessment and treatment. Finally, while a number of the studies detailed above have compared differently motivated groups across a range of sociodemographic, psychopathological, offending and other characteristics (Inciardi, 1970; Icove & Estepp, 1987; Pettiway, 1987; Ravateheino, 1989; Dickens *et al*, 2009), given the problematical nature of motivation-based classificatory systems it seems pointless to examine these findings in great detail beyond the inference that *revenge* appears to be associated with adult firesetters, and firesetting for reasons of *vandalism* and *excitement* with juveniles (Icove & Estepp, 1987; Sapp *et al*, 1996).

Deductive firesetter typologies

Deductive typologies comprise categories derived from observable and measurable relationships between variables that relate to firesetters' characteristics, behaviour, intention or motivation. Canter & Fritzon (1998) did not include motivation as a variable in their analysis and thus avoided many of the pitfalls described above. They analysed details of 175 arson cases where the offender was known and had been dealt with by the courts. A total of 42 offence variables (relating to target of fire, evidence of planning or intent, firesetting behaviour, fire outcome, timing etc.) and 23 offender variables (sociodemographic, psychopathological, offending) were developed which could be rated as present/absent from crime-scene or witness reports. Five variables occurred in more than 60% of cases (*offence within one mile of offender's home; offender did not raise alarm; the fire was set as opposed to a missile thrown; offender knew the owner of fired property; offence occurred on a weekday*) and are argued to indicate 'a significance and involvement of the arsonist and a determination to ensure the fire had some real destructive effect' (Canter & Fritzon, 1998, p. 80). Smallest-space analysis (SSA) was conducted to plot a matrix of observed relationships between variables. Commonly occurring items occupy the centre of the plot and less frequently occurring variables the outer portions.

The resulting pattern indicated congruence with an underlying two-axis model of firesetting: first, firesetting is targeted at objects *or* at people; and second, it has some instrumental end (e.g., the firesetting is associated with theft) *or* is of itself an expressive act (e.g., associated with a suicide attempt). Offence and offender variables associated with instrumental acts are least related to those associated with expressive acts; those who set person-targeted fires had fewer variables in common with those who set object-targeted fires. Based on this, Canter & Fritzon classified firesetters under one of four headings:

- *Instrumental person.* These often arise from a dispute between the firesetter and a partner or employer and frequently involve prior threats. They are associated with a discernible trigger and the use of accelerants. They appear to serve a specific purpose, usually revenge.
- *Expressive person.* Here, fires are set in an attempt to restore emotional equilibrium or alleviate distress. The firesetting may be coupled with a need for attention and deliberate endangerment of life.
- *Instrumental object.* This category is associated with opportunistic firesetting and achieving criminal ends.
- *Expressive object.* This category includes serial offences and those targeting particular public buildings.

These themes have been replicated in a study of incarcerated offenders (Almond *et al*, 2005), and while the categories do not suggest particular treatment strategies, they do support a common-sense position that *person-directed acts*, both expressive and instrumental, indicate particular dangerousness.

Rice & Harris (1995) examined 243 male firesetters with mental disorders (mean age 28.7 years; mean IQ 93) admitted over an 11-year period to a maximum-security psychiatric institution (for firesetting). Cluster analysis of the presence or absence of the following 11 firesetting-related variables was conducted: childhood aggression, school adjustment problems, separation from parents, time in correctional facilities, criminal history, adult aggression, IQ, employment history, childhood firesetting, total number of fires set and motive for firesetting recorded as one of four categorical variables (anger and revenge; acute psychosis/delusions; excitement and release of tension; attention seeking). Data were extracted from very complete records, including information from police, family, other institutions and patient self-report and interrater reliability was tested on a subsample. Subsequent criminal arrests, reconvictions and returns to institution were also recorded for the 208 firesetters who had been discharged. The average follow-up period during which reconviction could occur was 89 months. Analysis suggested four subtypes:

- *Psychotics* (33%). This group was typified by the fewest previous incidents of firesetting and their lack of use of accelerants in their firesetting.

- *Unassertives* (28%). This group had little history of aggression and little criminal history but were the least assertive and the most likely to be judged to set fires for reason of anger or revenge.
- *Multi-firesetters* (23%). This group had the most disturbed childhood histories, were young, had more versatile criminal careers and were most likely to commit another offence.
- Criminals (16%). This group also had disturbed backgrounds, a history of parental abuse, were the most likely to have a diagnosis of personality disorder, were the most assertive and were most likely to commit new offences following release.

Validity was strengthened by statistically significant differences between these groups on 25 of 30 additional variables relating to previous childhood and adult fires, as well as the index fire. In total, 66% of firesetters displayed any recidivism following discharge, 16% failed by lighting a fire, 31% by committing a violent offence and 57% by committing a non-violent criminal offence. *Multi-firesetters* and *criminals* had the highest recidivism for firesetting, or violent or any other offending. This is interesting because it suggests particular dangerousness among those with profiles similar to these two groups. Intervention strategies to increase assertiveness are indicated for those with similar profiles to *unassertives* and *multi-firesetters* but not for *criminals*.

In summary, a few studies have suggested that different types of firesetter can be reliably distinguished using data-driven methods. These studies draw on broader data-sets recording firesetters' characteristics, behaviour and imputed motive or intentionality than inductive motivational typologies. They also tend to focus on repeat offending as a crucial behavioural variable.

Recidivism and dangerousness in firesetting

We now move on from typology to examine firesetting through a prism of forensic risk. This section is not intended as a detailed guide to firesetter risk assessment, which is covered in depth in Chapter 10, but as an exploration of the firesetting literature in the context of the constituent elements of risk. 'Risk' is understood in multiple ways; in the field of mental health it is generally taken to refer to potential adverse events involving violence and aggression or self-harm. More precisely, elements of risk include estimation of the likelihood of dangerous behaviour based both on actuarial data and clinical experience (or subjective fear) and the potential destructiveness or consequences of the behaviour (Gunn, 1982, 1993; Pagani & Pinard, 2000; Kettles, 2004). One way of understanding forensic risk, therefore, is as a product of the likelihood of repeated dangerous behaviour or *recidivism* and the potential severity or *destructiveness* of that behaviour in terms of death, injury or psychological distress (Doyle, 1999; Kettles, 2004).

Firesetting recidivism

Reported recidivism rates across almost 30 studies (see Brett, 2004; Lindberg *et al*, 2005; Dickens *et al*, 2009) range from 4% (Soothill & Pope, 1973) to 60% (Rice & Harris, 1991), the disparity reflecting varying definitions, samples and methods. Studies associated with high recidivism use a definition of 'any history of repeated firesetting' (28% for males, 13% for females, Lewis & Yarnell, 1951; 38%, Koson & Dvoskin, 1982; 49%, Geller & Bertsch, 1985; 35%, O'Sullivan & Kelleher, 1987; 60%, Rice & Harris, 1991; 43%, Geller *et al*, 1992; 49%, Dickens *et al*, 2009). Quite simply, many people in clinical and offending samples who have set one fire are known to have set multiple fires. Even so, the true rate may be underestimated because these studies are dependent upon the quality of case notes. Unfortunately, these studies are not informative about repeated firesetting following a therapeutic or punitive intervention. Studies that report lower rates use the definition 'history of reconviction for arson' (10%, Hurley & Monahan, 1969; 18%, Sapsford *et al*, 1978; 11%, Harmon *et al*, 1985; 30%, Stewart, 1993 (females only); 20% for males, 4% for females, Rix, 1994; 16%, Repo & Virkkunen, 1997; 25%, Ritchie & Huff, 1999; 22%, Lindberg *et al*, 2005) or, in the small number of prospective studies, 'reconviction for arson during follow-up' (e.g., 4.4% of 67 arsonists convicted in England and Wales in 1951 reconvicted of arson by 1970, Soothill & Pope, 1973; 7.8% of 1352 individuals convicted in 1963–65 reconvicted of arson by 2001, Soothill *et al*, 2004).

Studies of firesetting recidivism have looked at samples of general psychiatric in-patients (Geller & Bertsch, 1985; O'Sullivan & Kelleher, 1987; Geller *et al*, 1992), secure psychiatric in-patients (Tennent *et al*, 1971; Rice & Chaplin, 1979; Koson & Dvoskin, 1982; Rice & Harris, 1991), people referred for pre-trial psychiatric assessment (Bourget & Bradford, 1989; Rix, 1994; Dickens *et al*, 2009) and prisoners (Soothill & Pope, 1973; Sapsford *et al*, 1978; Stewart, 1993; Soothill *et al*, 2004). Follow-up periods vary from 1 to 37 years (Rice & Chaplin, 1979; Soothill *et al*, 2004). There is considerable doubt whether those who are convicted of arson are representative of firesetters defined more broadly; rather, they comprise a skewed sample of a minority – those firesetters who fail to evade detection, prosecution and conviction despite the fact that only a very small proportion of deliberately set fires lead to a conviction.

To illustrate, a recent study (Hopkins, 2009) demonstrated that fire and rescue services (FRS) in England and Wales recorded 77700 deliberate primary fires (i.e., reportable fires or any fires involving casualties, and rescues or fires attended by five or more appliances) and 256000 deliberate secondary fires (i.e., reportable fires that were not in primary fire locations, not chimney fires, did not involve casualties and were attended by four or fewer appliances) in 2004–05. Contrastingly, the police recorded 48038 fires in total, or just over 14% of deliberate fires recorded by FRS, as arson during the same period. This discrepancy is thought to be the result of

59

different recording practices, whereby FRS merely have to suspect a fire was deliberately ignited, while police have to prove that a person behaved intentionally, recklessly or intended to damage property (Sugg, 2003). There are further opportunities for attrition at every subsequent stage of the criminal justice process. Hopkins examined a random sample of 1399 cases identified by police as arson, weighted to reflect the prevalence of cases of arson endangering life (12%) and arson not endangering life (88%). A suspect was identified by the police in 22.3%, charged in 8.4% and convicted in 3.2% of cases. A higher rate of detection was achieved in cases of arson endangering life (30.8%) than in cases of simple arson (5.5%), suggesting that in the most serious cases the greatest effort will be made to clear up the crime. It is also clear that detection and conviction rates for arson are very low relative to those for other serious offences. The conviction rate for arson of 5.5% in England and Wales compares with rates of 12% for criminal damage, 31% for sexual offences and 42% for offences of violence against the person (Home Office, 2007).

Given the inherently problematic nature of the recidivism literature there is limited utility to an in-depth examination of reported differences between recidivists and non-recidivists and the following represents a summary. In both Soothill & Pope's (1973) and Soothill et al's (2004) prospective studies, while reconviction was rare, it did occur for a small minority a considerable time after the original conviction. For example, of 1352 people convicted of arson in England and Wales between 1963 and 1965, 106 (7.8%) had been reconvicted by 2001; 54 of these 106 (50.9%) had been reconvicted by 1969, a further 34 (32.1%) by the end of 1979 and 18 more from 1980 onwards. The number of 'years at risk' between convictions (i.e., years out of prison or secure hospital) was unavailable but this finding does demonstrate that, for some, firesetting is persistent across the lifespan. Dickens et al (2009) examined 167 adult arsonists referred for forensic psychiatric assessment in one English region over a 24-year period (77% male; mean age 29 years, range 18–77 years). In total, there was evidence in the case notes that 81 (49%) individuals had set fires before the index offence. These multiple firesetters differed on a range of sociodemographic factors, childhood and family background, psychiatric morbidity and firesetting behaviour, which reflected findings from previous studies. Repeat firesetters were on average 5 years younger than once-only firesetters; they were more likely to be single and to have greater documented childhood history, including school problems and a family history of violence; they were more likely to have a diagnosis of personality disorder or psychosis; they were 6 years younger (mean age 21 years) at first conviction for any crime and were more likely to have previous convictions for property crime but not for violent crime.

Recidivism has been reported to be associated with family-reported childhood fire interest (Rice & Harris, 1991), maternal alcoholism (DeJong et al, 1992), parental absence in childhood (Virkkunen et al, 1996), intoxication at firesetting (Repo et al, 1997; Lindberg et al, 2005) and alcohol dependence (Koson & Dvoskin, 1982; Repo et al, 1997).

In Germany, where all defendants are tried in court and subsequently classified as 'fully responsible' for their actions, or as having diminished responsibility for the offence (the power to distinguish between right and wrong being assessed as gravely compromised at the time of the act), or being not responsible (had lost the power to distinguish between right and wrong at the time of the act) for psychiatric reasons, it has been possible to compare recidivism between clinical and non-clinical samples. Barnett *et al* (1997) examined reconviction rates of a random sample of 470 arsonists convicted in West Germany in 1983–85 and reconvicted by 1994 (mean follow-up 10 years). While 4% of the fully responsible group had been reconvicted of arson, 10% of the rest had been reconvicted (i.e., a trend towards higher recidivism in the psychiatric firesetter groups).

Importantly, firesetters commonly exhibit a range of antisocial offending behaviours (Blanco *et al*, 2010; Vaughn *et al*, 2010), so the risk of non-firesetting recidivism should be considered. Most convicted firesetters are not known to be violent, although a significant minority are. Soothill *et al* (2004) noted that 20% of those convicted of arson in England and Wales in 2000–01 had previous convictions for violent offences. A significant proportion of firesetters in clinical samples are also reported to have some history of violence (e.g., 54% by Rice & Harris, 1991). Some recidivist arsonists also reoffend violently. Soothill *et al* (2004) found that 68% of those convicted of arson in England and Wales in 1980–81 had a subsequent conviction by 2000–01; rates by crime type included 12.2% a violent crime, 4.9% a sexual offence, 17.9% burglary, 36.4% theft, 6.9% fraud or forgery and 21.6% criminal damage.

Soothill *et al* (2008) examined subsequent convictions among those arrested for arson and a range of other serious crimes (blackmail, kidnapping, threats to kill) in England and Wales between 1979 and 2001. Reconviction for any of these target crimes, or for homicide, among those first convicted of arson (9.6%) was higher than for those first convicted of blackmail (7.6%), kidnapping (5.5%) or threats to kill (7.0%). Mean follow-up periods were slightly longer for arsonists (12.9 years) and blackmailers (12.4 years) than for kidnappers (8.2 years) and those who made threats to life (5.6 years), which may explain the higher recidivism in these groups. More interestingly, although arsonists had the highest recidivism of any group, they also appeared to be the most specialised offenders: the vast majority of reconvictions among arsonists were also for arson (87%); blackmailers' subsequent convictions included blackmail less frequently (64%) and kidnappers (70%) and those who made threats to kill (69%) were also less frequently reconvicted of the same crime.

In a second study of their West German cohort, Barnett *et al* (1999) found that fewer of those convicted arsonists who had been found to be 'not responsible' for their actions (48%) than those who had been found to be fully responsible (75%) had been reconvicted of crimes other than arson. The psychiatric sample were more likely to be 'pure firesetters' than the non-psychiatric sample, who were more likely to be 'mixed firesetters'. Taken together these findings suggest that a core group of recidivist firesetters are 'pure firesetters' and that this group are more likely to have mental disorder.

In summary, the literature on recidivism is beset by difficulties of definition, low detection rates and non-comparable samples. However, we can reasonably confidently assert that the key psychopathological features associated with firesetting in general are associated with recidivist fire-setting: chiefly, psychosis, personality disorder, alcohol and substance misuse. A proportion of arsonists will recidivate violently, while some seem to be 'pure firesetters'.

Dangerousness and destructiveness

It is commonly believed that fire is so unpredictable that any attempt to differentiate between firesetters on the basis of the outcome, or severity, of their behaviour is pointless. Brett (2004) states that arson does not lend itself to empirical research because of the discontinuity between the apparent intentions of the arsonist and the outcome of the crime. Barker reports the received truth among firefighters that 'a large fire is one that started as a small fire and was not brought under control' and 'the final *quantum* of damage may thus bear little relevance to the initial intention, and a carelessly dropped match may wreak as much havoc as a fire deliberately started with gallons of petrol' (Barker, 1994, p. 5). Certainly, the first half of this proposition is reasonable; the London King's Cross Underground fire in November 1987, in which 31 people died, was the result of someone dropping a lighted match on a wooden escalator (Donald & Canter, 1990). However, while we agree that there *may* be equal destructiveness because fire is unpredictable, we do not accept that the most devastating outcome is equally likely across all cases of firesetting. The firesetter who is armed with gallons of petrol and, crucially, destructive person-oriented intent should logically be regarded as dangerous. The concept of risk is designed to help us cope with unpredictable situations in which we can nevertheless find some pointers of likelihood.

The destruction caused by fire may be, as at King's Cross, counted in the human costs of injuries and burns sustained or deaths caused (Cassuto & Tarnow, 2003) but quantifiable costs can also be attached to the increased load on emergency hospital services and damage caused to property in financial (Jacobson, 1985; Doley, 2003) or structural terms (Adler *et al*, 1994; Slavkin, 2004). Potential endangerment of life (Jacobson, 1985) and increased public fear (Gunn, 1982) will be among the less easily quantifiable costs of firesetting. The total sum of destructiveness may effectively be unknowable and it is thus unsurprising that studies that have aimed to differentiate between firesetters in terms of fire destructiveness have had limited success. In an extension of their deductive typology of 243 firesetters in maximum-security psychiatric hospital, Harris & Rice (1996) found that 20 (8%) index fires had led to high levels of injuries and property damage.

There were few differences across a range of childhood and adult variables between those involved in the most and least destructive fires except for youth and the presence of an extensive firesetting history. Dickens *et al* (2009) also rated fires as causing more or less extensive damage among their sample of 167 adults referred for forensic psychiatric examination and found that very few firesetter characteristics could differentiate between the two groups. However, evidence that there is some quantifiable difference in dangerousness between firesetters can be inferred from Soothill *et al's* (2004) study of reconviction rates among 5584 people convicted for arson in England and Wales in 1980–81. A similar proportion (10.0%) of those convicted of arson endangering life (AEL) were reconvicted for arson over the next 20 years as those for those convicted of arson but with no evidence of endangering life (ANEL) (10.8%). However, 41.3% of those originally convicted of AEL were reconvicted of AEL, while just 14.8% of those originally convicted of ANEL were reconvicted of AEL. Although Soothill *et al* (2004) note that there is considerable overlap between the two types of arson, and a significant minority of those convicted of ANEL go on to commit AEL, these findings do suggest that a number of arsonists are simply very dangerous and repeatedly set fires that endanger life.

While informed, professional opinion does not equate to actual risk, it is notable that, in a survey of 54 forensic mental health professionals, largely psychiatrists, the *apparent intention to endanger* life was viewed as the variable (of 11 alternatives, including *repeat firesetting* and *diagnosis of pyromania*) indicating the greatest dangerousness in a firesetter (Sugarman & Dickens, 2009).

Discussion and conclusions

Despite the difficulties encountered in identification of the most dangerous firesetters from a psychiatric or psychological perspective, since 1980 (with *R v. Hoof*) the legal system has required distinction between those guilty of simple arson and those guilty of the aggravated offence of intentionally or recklessly endangering life (see Chapter 9). This legal distinction is a sensible one and, as noted above, while outcome may not map precisely onto the original intention of the firesetter, researchers should further examine the distinguishing features of arsonists categorised in this dichotomous way. Psychiatrists are routinely required by the courts to inform them about the constituent elements of the legal formulation: intent and recklessness. However, as this chapter has demonstrated, the literature offers only a little useful information and it has focused on motivation rather than intentionality and recklessness. For practitioners who are looking for a practical solution, Gannon & Pina (2010) recommend use of the HCR-20 manual (Webster *et al*, 1997) for risk prediction as a structured clinical guide to predicting future violent behaviour in the form of firesetting. The manual

(p. 25) views arson as a 'less clear' case of violence and advises that risk assessors should consider the obvious likelihood of the fire causing extensive harm when taking a decision to rate firesetting as a violent behaviour.

More satisfying classificatory systems have emerged from the examination of observable relationships between fire-related variables. Canter & Fritzon (1998) usefully removed motivation from the equation and, by concentrating on crime-scene characteristics and evidence of specific behaviours, put intentionality centre stage through the inclusion of variables indicating planning (e.g., whether materials were brought to the scene, such as petrol or matches; attempting to avoid detection by wearing gloves to avoid leaving fingerprints) or deliberate life endangerment (fires in residential properties with no attempt to alert the occupants). However, this classification system represented an attempt to uncover underlying psychological types rather than to inform assessments of dangerousness or risk and intervention strategies. With regard to risk, the evidence base on recidivism is equivocal because of limitations in terms of detection rates and varying samples and definitions. Clearly, if firesetting is repeated then the risk that any one of those fires will cause extensive damage is increased, but repeated firesetting of itself may not best identify the most dangerous firesetters. The fact alone that someone has set a destructive fire may be relatively uninformative about future dangerousness, but indicators that the firesetter intends to be destructive, particularly of life, should be treated with the utmost gravity.

In summary, the literature on firesetting concentrates on classification by motive, often rather subjectively. Meanwhile, the orthodoxy is that the consequences of fire are totally unpredictable. However, research on classification by behaviour lends weight to legal concepts of recklessness, intention and the endangerment of property and of life. Clinical practice and research should build on the behavioural analysis of firesetting, and begin to elucidate intention as a cognitive concept in clinical practice. In this way it will be possible to improve both the prediction of future risk from firesetting and the resultant clinical and legal decision-making.

References

Adler, R., Nunn, R., Northam, E., *et al* (1994) Secondary prevention of childhood firesetting. *Journal of the American Academy of Child and Adolescent Psychiatry*, **33**, 1194–1202.

Almond, L., Duggan, L., Shine, J., *et al* (2005) Test of the arson action systems model in an incarcerated population. *Journal of Psychology, Crime and Law*, **11**, 1–15.

Anwar, S., Långström, N., Grann, M., *et al* (2011) Is arson the crime most strongly associated with psychosis? A national case–control study of arson risk in schizophrenia and other psychoses. *Schizophrenia Bulletin*, **37**, 580–586.

Bailey, K. D. (1994) *Typologies and Taxonomies. An Introduction to Classification Techniques.* Sage.

Barker, A. F. (1994) *Arson: A Review of the Psychiatric Literature.* Oxford University Press.

Barnett, W., Richter, P., Sigmund, D., *et al* (1997) Recidivism and concomitant criminality in pathological firesetters. *Journal of Forensic Science*, **42**, 879–883.

Barnett, W., Richter, P. & Tenneberg, B. (1999) Repeated arson: data from criminal records. *Forensic Science International*, **101**, 49–54.

Blanco, C., Alegria, A. A., Petry, N. M., *et al* (2010) Prevalence and correlates of fire-setting in the United States: results from the National Epidemiologic Survey on Alcohol and Related Conditions (NESARC). *Journal of Clinical Psychiatry*, **71**, 1218–1225.

Bourget, D. & Bradford, J. M. (1989) Female arsonists: a clinical study. *Bulletin of the American Academy of Psychiatry and the Law*, **17**, 293–300.

Brett, A. (2004) 'Kindling theory' in arson: how dangerous are firesetters? *Australian and New Zealand Journal of Psychiatry*, **38**, 419–425.

Byrne, J. M. & Roberts, A. R. (2007) New directions in offender typology design, development and implementation: can we balance risk, treatment and control? *Aggression and Violent Behavior*, **12**, 483–492.

Canter, D. & Fritzon, K. (1998) Differentiating arsonists: a model of firesetting actions and characteristics. *Legal and Criminological Psychology*, **3**, 73–96.

Cassuto, J. & Tarnow, P. (2003) The discotheque fire in Gothenburg 1998. A tragedy among teenagers. *Burns*, **29**, 405–416.

Colman, A. (2009) *A Dictionary of Psychology* (3rd edn). Oxford University Press.

Cooke, R. A. & Ide, R. H. (1985) *Principles of Fire Investigation* (chapter 16, pp. 248–260). *Institute of Fire Engineers*.

Dennett, M. F. (1980) *Fire Investigation*. Pergamon Press.

DeJong, J., Virkkunen, M. & Linnoila, M. (1992) Factors associated with recidivism in a criminal population. *Journal of Nervous and Mental Disease*, **180**, 543–550.

Dickens, G., Sugarman, P., Edgar, S., *et al* (2009) Recidivism and dangerousness in arsonists. *Journal of Forensic Psychiatry and Psychology*, **20**, 621–639.

Doley, R. (2003) Making sense of arson through classification. *Psychiatry, Psychology and the Law*, **10**, 346–352.

Donald, I. & Canter, D. (1990) Behavioural aspects of the King's Cross disaster. In *Fires and Human Behaviour* (2nd edn) (ed. D. Canter), pp. 15–30. David Fulton Publishers.

Douglas, J., Burgess, A. W., Burgess, A. G., *et al* (1997) *Crime Classification Manual: A Standard System for Investigating and Classifying Violent Crimes* (revised edn). Jossey Bass.

Doyle, M. (1999) Organisational response to crisis and risk: issues and implications for mental health nurses. In *Managing Crisis and Risk in Mental Health Nursing* (ed. T. Ryan), pp. 42–56. Stanley Thomas.

Edmunds, G. (1978) Judgements of different types of aggressive behaviour. *British Journal of Social and Clinical Psychology*, **17**, 121–125.

Enayati, J., Grann, M., Lubbs, S., *et al* (2008) Psychiatric morbidity in arsonists referred for forensic psychiatric assessment in Sweden. *Journal of Forensic Psychiatry and Psychology*, **19**, 139–147.

Faulk, M. (1994) *Basic Forensic Psychiatry* (2nd edn). Blackwell Science.

Freud, S. (1932) The acquisition of power over fire. *International Journal of Psychoanalysis*, **13**, 405–410.

Gannon, T. A. & Pina, A. (2010) Firesetting: psychopathology, theory and treatment. *Aggression and Violent Behavior*, **15**, 224–238.

Geller, J. & Bertsch, G. (1985) Fire-setting behaviour in the histories of a state hospital population. *American Journal of Psychiatry*, **142**, 464–468.

Geller, J. L., Fisher, W. H. & Bertsch, G. (1992) Who repeats? A follow-up study of state hospital patients' firesetting behaviour. *Psychiatric Quarterly*, **63**, 143–157.

Gibbons, D. C. (1975) Offender typologies – two decades later. *British Journal of Criminology*, **15**, 140–156.

Gold, L. H. (1962) Psychiatric profile of the firesetter. *Journal of Forensic Sciences*, **7**, 404–417.

Gunn, J. (1982) An English psychiatrist looks at dangerousness. *Bulletin of the American Academy of Psychiatry & the Law*, **10**, 143–153.

Gunn, J. (1993) Dangerousness. In *Forensic Psychiatry: Clinical, Legal and Ethical Issues* (eds J. Gunn & P. Taylor), pp. 624–645. Butterworth Heinemann.

Harmon, R. B., Rosner, R. & Wiederlight, M. (1985) Women and arson: a demographic study. *Journal of Forensic Sciences*, **30**, 467–477.

Harris, G. T. & Rice, M. E. (1996) A typology of mentally disordered firesetters. *Journal of Interpersonal Violence*, **11**, 351–363.

Helfgott, J. B. (2008) *Criminal Behaviour: Theories, Typologies and Criminal Justice*. Sage.

Home Office (2007) *Home Office Statistical Bulletin: Crimes Detected In England & Wales 2006/07*. At http://rds.homeoffice.gov.uk/rds/pdfs07/hosb1507.pdf (accessed 17 December 2010).

Hopkins, M. (2009) Why are arson detection rates so low? A study of the factors that promote and inhibit the detection of arson. *Policing*, **3**, 78–88.

Hurley, W. & Monahan, T. M. (1969) Arson: the criminal and the crime. *British Journal of Criminology*, **9**, 4–21.

Icove, D. J. & Estepp, M. H. (1987) Motive-based offender profiles of arson and fire-related crimes. *FBI Law Enforcement Bulletin*, **56**, 17–23.

Inciardi, J. (1970) The adult firesetter. *Criminology*, **8**, 145–155.

Jacobson, R. (1985) The subclassification of child firesetters. *Journal of Child Psychology and Psychiatry*, **26**, 769–775.

Kettles, A. (2004) A concept analysis of forensic risk. *Journal of Psychiatric and Mental Health Nursing*, **11**, 484–493.

Kidd, S. (1997) Arson – the problem that won't go away. *Fire Prevention*, **298**, 27–34.

Koson, D. F. & Dvoskin, J. (1982) Arson: a diagnostic study. *Bulletin of the American Academy of Psychiatry and the Law*, **10**, 39–49.

Leong, G. B. (1992) A psychiatric study of persons charged with arson. *Journal of Forensic Science*, **37**, 1319–1326.

Lewis, N. O. C. & Yarnell, H. (1951) *Pathological Firesetting (Pyromania)*. Nervous and Mental Disease Monographs no. 82. Coolidge Foundation.

Lindberg, N., Holi, M. M., Tani, P., *et al* (2005) Looking for pyromania: characteristics of a consecutive sample of Finnish male criminals with histories of recidivist firesetting between 1973 and 1993. *BMC Psychiatry*, **47**, 1–5.

Magee, J. (1933) Pathological arson. *Scientific Monthly*, **37**, 358–361.

Muckley, A. (1997) Burning up the town. *Fire Prevention*, **298**, 33–34.

O'Sullivan, G. H. & Kelleher, M. J. (1987) A study of firesetters in the south-west of Ireland. *British Journal of Psychiatry*, **151**, 818–823.

Pagani, L. & Pinard, G-F. (2000) Clinical assessment of dangerousness: an overview of the literature. In *Clinical Assessment of Dangerousness: Empirical Contributions* (eds G-F. Pinard & L. Pagani), pp. 1–22. Cambridge University Press.

Pettiway, L. E. (1987) Arson for revenge: the role of environmental situation, age, sex and race. *Journal of Quantitative Criminology*, **3**, 169–184.

Prins, H. (1994) *Fire-Raising: Its Motivation and Management*. Routledge.

Prins, H. (2005) The motivation of arsonists – reflections on research and practice. *British Journal of Forensic Practice*, **1**, 6–11.

Prins, H., Tennent, G. & Trick, K. (1985) Motives for arson (fire-raising). *Medicine, Science and the Law*, **25**, 275–278.

Quinsey, V. L. E., Harris, G. T., Rice, M. E., *et al* (1998) *Violent Offenders: Appraising and Managing Risk* (1st edn). American Psychological Association.

Ravateheino, J. (1989) Finnish study of 180 arsonists arrested in Helsinki. *Fire Prevention*, **233**, 30–34.

Repo, E. & Virkkunen, M. (1997) Criminal recidivism and family histories of schizophrenic and non-schizophrenic firesetters. Co-morbid alcohol dependence in schizophrenic firesetters. *Journal of the American Academy of Psychiatry and the Law*, **25**, 207–215.

Repo, E., Virkkunen, M., Rawlings, R., *et al* (1997) Criminal and psychiatric histories of Finnish arsonists. *Acta Psychiatrica Scandinavica*, **95**, 318–323.

Rice, M. E. & Chaplin, T. (1979) Social skills training for hospitalized male arsonists. *Journal of Behavior Therapy and Experimental Psychiatry*, **10**, 105–108.

Rice, M. E. & Harris, G. T. (1991) Firesetters admitted to a maximum security psychiatric institution. *Journal of Interpersonal Violence*, **6**, 461–475.

Rice, M. E. & Harris, G. T. (1995) Violent recidivism: assessing predictive validity. *Journal of Consulting and Clinical Psychology*, **63**, 364–375.

Ritchie, E. C. & Huff, T. G. (1999) Psychiatric aspects of arsonists. *Journal of Forensic Science*, **44**, 733–740.

Rix, K. J. B. (1994) A psychiatric study of adult arsonists. *Medicine, Science and the Law*, **34**, 21–34.

Sapp, A. D., Huff, T. G., Gary, G. P., *et al* (1996) *Essential Findings from a Study of Serial Arsonists*. Federal Bureau of Investigation.

Sapsford, R. J., Banks, C. & Smith, D. D. (1978) Arsonists in prison. *Medicine, Science and the Law*, **18**, 247–254.

Scott, D. (1974) *The Psychology of Fire*. Charles Scribner's Sons.

Slavkin, M. L. (2004) Characteristics of juvenile firesetting across childhood and adolescence. *Forensic Examiner*, **13**, 6–18.

Soothill, K. (1990) Arson. In *Principles and Practice of Forensic Psychiatry* (eds R. Bluglass & P. Bowden), pp. 779–786. Churchill Livingstone.

Soothill, K. L. & Pope, P. J. (1973) Arson: a twenty-year cohort study. *Medicine, Science and the Law*, **13**, 127–138.

Soothill, K., Ackerley, E. & Francis, B. (2004) The criminal careers of arsonists. *Medicine, Science and the Law*, **44**, 27–40.

Soothill, K., Francis, B. & Liu, J. (2008) Does serious offending lead to homicide? *British Journal of Criminology*, **48**, 522–537.

Stewart, L. A. (1993) Profile of female firesetters: implications for treatment. *British Journal of Psychiatry*, **163**, 248–256.

Sugarman, P. & Dickens, G. (2009) Dangerousness in firesetters: a survey of psychiatrists' views. *Psychiatric Bulletin*, **33**, 99–101.

Sugg, D. (2003) *Arson: From Reporting to Conviction*. Arson Control Forum Research Bulletin no. 1. Office of the Deputy Prime Minister.

Swaffer, T. & Hollin, C. R. (1995) Adolescent firesetting: why do they say they do it? *Journal of Adolescence*, **18**, 619–623.

Tennent, T. G., McQuaid, A., Loughnane, T., *et al* (1971) Female arsonists. *British Journal of Psychiatry*, **119**, 497–502.

Vaughn, M. G., Qiang, F., DeLisi, M., *et al* (2010) Prevalence and correlates of fire-setting in the United States: results from the National Epidemiological Survey on Alcohol and Related Conditions. *Comprehensive Psychiatry*, **51**, 217–223.

Virkkunen, M., Eggert, M., Rawlings, R., *et al* (1996) A prospective follow-up of alcoholic violent offenders and firesetters. *Archives of General Psychiatry*, **53**, 523–529.

Vreeland, R. G. & Levin, B. M. (1990) Psychological aspects of firesetting. In *Fires and Human Behaviour* (2nd edn) (ed. D. Canter), pp. 31–46. David Fulton Publishers.

Webster, C. D., Douglas, K. S., Eaves, D., *et al* (1997) *HCR-20: Assessing Risk for Violence* (version 2). Simon Fraser University.

Willis, M. (2004) *Bushfire Arson: A Review of the Literature*. Research and Public Policy Series no. 61. Australian Institute of Criminology.

Legal cases

R v. Calladine [1975] *Psychiatric reports should be obtained before sentencing.* The Times Law Reports, 3 December 1975 English Court of Appeal Decision.

R v. Hoof [1980] 2 Cr. App. R. (S.) 299. *There should be separate counts alleging arson with intent to endanger life and arson reckless as to whether life was endangered.*

CHAPTER 4

The potential relevance of brain dysfunction in arson

Mairead Dolan and Troy E. McEwan

There is a very limited literature linking firesetting with abnormalities in brain function. In this chapter we review the literature on the relevance of brain dysfunction and neuropathology in firesetting. We conducted Medline and PsycINFO searches on the neurobiology and neuropathology of firesetting. In summary, firesetting is largely associated with childhood conduct problems, antisocial personality pathology and alcohol misuse rather than with major mental illness. Although there are anecdotal reports of an association between organic brain syndromes and firesetting, most literature focuses on epilepsy and autistic-spectrum disorders and intellectual impairment. There are few studies investigating the neurobiology of arson, but available work points to evidence of reduced serotonergic function and a hypoglycaemic tendency in arsonists which appears to be associated with type 2 alcoholism. The neuropsychology of arson has not been extensively investigated, but one study suggests that arsonists may have greater impairments in executive function than do violent and sex offenders. We conclude that further work is needed to explore the neurobiology of firesetting and the potential roles of genes, environment and brain structure and function in the aetiology and maintenance of this behaviour.

Arson is a crime with significant impacts in terms of financial loss, serious injury and death (Geller, 1992, 2008; Barker, 1994; Gaynor, 1996). 'Arson' is a forensic/legal classification (Gaynor & Hatcher, 1987) referring to deliberate firesetting and using the key criteria of wilful and malicious motive and intent (Gaynor & Hatcher, 1987; Ritchie & Huff, 1999). The true extent of the problem is unknown, as it is often difficult to determine whether or not a fire has been deliberately set and only a small proportion of arson offences come to prosecution. Nonetheless, the incidence of arson appears to have increased in the USA and in most European countries in recent years (Prins, 1994; Räsänen et al, 1995; Soothill et al, 2004). In England and Wales there were 39 318 cases in 2007–08 (Home Office, 2008). 'Firesetting' is used to describe a broader range of fire-lighting behaviour, which may not involve the conscious intent to commit a crime (Barnett et *al*, 1999; Ritchie & Huff, 1999). 'Firesetting' is often used in the clinical literature to denote 'fire-lighting' in the absence of a diagnosis of pyromania. 'Pyromania' refers to a pathological form of firesetting. In DSM-IV-TR (see Chapter 12, Box 12.1, p. 228) it is defined as:

multiple episodes of deliberate and purposeful firesetting ... [with] tension or affective arousal before setting a fire ... fascination with, interest in, curiosity about, or attraction to fire and its situational contexts (e.g., paraphernalia, uses, consequences) ... pleasure, gratification, or a release of tension when setting the fire, witnessing its effect, or participating in its aftermath. (American Psychiatric Association, 2000; see also Barnett *et al*, 1999)

DSM-IV-TR excludes firesetting engaged in for monetary gain, political expression, expression of anger or to mask criminal activity. It also excludes firesetting that is better accounted for by conduct disorder, a manic episode or an antisocial personality disorder or any form of judgement impairment, including intoxication, dementia or mental retardation.

Despite the differences between the concepts of arson, firesetting and pyromania, they are not always distinguished in the literature. The true incidence of pyromania in the general population remains unknown. Of the six impulse control disorders listed in DSM-IV-TR, only trichotillomania and pathological gambling appear to be common in the general population (4% and 3%, respectively) (American Psychiatric Association, 2000). Pyromania, like intermittent explosive disorder and pathological gambling, is diagnosed more frequently in men than in women (American Psychiatric Association, 2000). The clinical and experimental evidence for pyromania as a disorder is not strongly supported (Kolko, 2002), as it is actually extremely rare (Geller, 2008). Given the high level of comorbidity between repetitive firesetting and conduct disorder in juvenile firesetters (Kolko & Kazdin, 1986) its application to children is thought to be questionable (Kolko, 1985). A 2005 report on a sample of 90 Finnish adult male criminals with recidivist firesetting between 1973 and 1993 indicated that 56 met exclusion criteria for pyromania (psychosis, mental retardation, organic brain syndromes and antisocial personality disorder) and only 12 of the remaining 34 fulfilled DSM-IV-TR inclusion criteria (Lindberg *et al*, 2005). However, 9 of these 12 were intoxicated with alcohol at the time of the index offence. If substance misuse is taken as a further exclusion criterion, there were only three individuals in this sample who could be diagnosed with pyromania, and all three worked as volunteer firefighters, so their fascination with fire may be qualitatively different from that of pyromanic arsonists (see Chapter 11). This work and that of Grant & Kim (2007) suggest that pyromania is extremely rare if comorbidity is an exclusion criterion.

Internationally, studies suggest that firesetting as a wider concept appears to be mainly committed by males, with a male:female ratio of between 6:1 and 9:1 (Lewis & Yarnell, 1951; Bourget & Bradford, 1989; Stewart, 1993; Dickens *et al*, 2007). The majority are White (Bennett & Hess, 1984; Harris & Rice, 1984; Rix, 1994; Ritchie & Huff, 1999), from low socioeconomic groups with poor education (Wolford, 1972; Rice & Harris, 1991; Räsänen *et al*, 1995; Ritchie & Huff, 1999; Doley, 2003) and are younger than non-firesetting criminals (Rice & Harris, 1991). Studies looking at offending patterns suggest that firesetters may have more in common with property offenders than violent offenders (Vreeland & Levin, 1980; Hill *et al*, 1982) in that they have low levels of interpersonal violence (McKerracher & Dacre, 1966; Hill *et al*, 1982; Bennett & Hess, 1984; Jackson *et al*, 1987; Jackson, 1994; Räsänen *et al*, 1995; Rice & Harris, 1996; Soothill *et al*, 2004). Studies looking at recidivist juvenile firesetters suggest they have high rates of conduct disorder and attention-deficit hyperactivity disorder (McCardle *et al*, 2009). Recidivism in adult firesetters appears to be associated with younger age at first onset of firesetting, low IQ, school failure, enuresis and personality disorder (Rice & Harris, 1991; Repo *et al*, 1997; Dickens *et al*, 2009), but some studies focusing on psychiatrists' perceptions of dangerousness have highlighted the importance of physical characteristics of the firesetting, such as multiple set points and the use of accelerants in addition to the intent to endanger life (Sugarman & Dickens, 2009). From a psychiatric perspective, the literature generally suggests that conduct disorder and antisocial personality disorder are the most prevalent diagnoses in firesetters (Bradford, 1982; Kolko, 1985; Geller, 1987; Barnett & Spitzer, 1994; Repo & Virkkunen, 1997*a,b*; Sakheim & Osborn, 1999; Martin *et al*, 2004; Mackay *et al*, 2006) and that these disorders increase the risk of recidivistic behaviour (Martin *et al*, 2004; Lindberg *et al*, 2005). While comorbid Axis I pathology has been reported in some studies (McKerracher & Dacre, 1966; Geller, 1987; Virkkunen *et al*, 1987; Ritchie & Huff, 1999), there are also anecdotal reports of organic brain lesions and neuropathology in firesetters (Prins, 1994; Heidrich *et al*, 1996; Shirahama *et al*, 2010).

Firesetting from a neurobiological and neuropathological perspective

Firesetting behaviour, including arson, is thought to be the result of the interaction of a complex but poorly understood set of factors that includes individual temperament, parental psychopathology and possibly neurochemical predispositions (Blumberg, 1981; Soltys, 1992; Barnett & Spitzer, 1994; Ritchie & Huff, 1999; American Psychiatric Association, 2000). Although there are many typologies of arson, Geller (1992) proposed that arsonists could be divided into four major categories:

- arson unassociated with psychobiological disorders
- arson associated with mental disorders
- arson associated with medical or neurological disorder
- juvenile firesetters.

Others have suggested that although organic disorders may occur in firesetters, they may not be directly associated with fire-raising (Prins *et al*, 1985). In some of these cases motivations may be based on revenge or sexually motivated firesetting.

While there are a number of psychoanalytic, psychological and social learning theories about firesetting (Gannon & Pina, 2010), this chapter focuses first on the potential role of alcohol intoxication in firesetting and then on the evidence that there may be a link between brain pathology or dysfunction and firesetting.

Alcohol and firesetting

Laubichler & Kühberger (1995) looked at the role played by alcohol in pyromania and arson. They examined a series of 103 arsonists (95 men, 8 women). Seventy were under the influence of alcohol at the time of the arson and 54 were alcohol dependent. Alcohol intoxication at the material time was seen in adults but not adolescent offenders and was not found to be associated with psychosis or major mental illness, but was associated with married rather than single status. They noted that fires set at night were particularly associated with alcohol problems and that there was a significant correlation between the frequency and level of alcohol consumption and the number of previous convictions for arson. They also noted that the association between alcohol misuse and firesetting was most striking in those with underlying personality pathology. Subsequent work by this group (Räsänen *et al*, 1994; Laubichler *et al*, 1996) confirmed the association between alcohol and firesetting but further suggested that frustration and aggression were motives and alcohol intoxication was a disinhibitory factor. Other studies point to the significance of hereditary issues in the association between alcohol and arson, as firesetters often have a paternal history of alcoholism (Repo *et al*, 1997; Virkkunen *et al*, 1996).

Few studies have systematically assessed personality pathology in samples of alcoholic firesetters. However, the descriptive characteristics of the samples in the majority of studies suggest that the alcoholic firesetters appear to fit into type 2 alcoholism, which is characterised by high heritability, early onset, frequent social complications, high levels of impulsiveness and sensation-seeking behaviour, and low platelet monoamine oxidase (MAO) activity (Von Knorring *et al*, 1991). Given that type 2 alcoholism tends to be associated with antisocial personality pathology and criminality (Blumberg, 1981; Von Knorring *et al*, 1991; Laubichler & Kühberger, 1995; Virkkunen *et al*, 1996) it is possible that many of the key neurobiological correlates of antisocial personality pathology and criminality will be relevant in our understanding of the neuropathology of type 2 alcoholic firesetters.

Neurochemical theories

Studies of Scandinavian samples of forensic patients have explored the notion that there is a central monoamine (particularly serotonin) deficit in alcoholic impulsive (type 2) violent offenders and firesetters. In one of the earliest reports (Virkkunen et al, 1987) researchers examined cerebrospinal fluid (CSF) monoamine levels in 20 arsonists, 20 habitually violent offenders and 10 healthy in-patient volunteers. The raw data and data adjusted for confounding factors such as age, height, gender and season of lumbar puncture showed significantly lower concentrations of 3-methoxy-4-hydroxyphenylglycol (MHPG) and 5-hydroxyindoleacetic acid (5-HIAA) in the arsonists than in the other groups. Although CSF concentrations of MHPG or 5-HIAA did not correlate with the severity of repeated firesetting behaviour, low blood glucose nadir in an oral glucose tolerance test did. The findings suggested that firesetting is associated with low levels of monoamines and a hypoglycaemic tendency. The monoamine abnormalities were replicated in a number of other studies by this group (Roy et al, 1986; Virkkunen et al, 1989a,b) but a key finding to emerge was that recidivism at 3 years was particularly associated with low 5-HIAA level at baseline assessment (Virkkunen et al, 1989a). The glucose abnormalities reported by Virkkunen (1984) were also noted in other studies from this group (Roy et al, 1986; Virkkunen et al, 1989a), suggesting a potentially robust association between firesetting and hypoglycaemia.

A later study by the same group (Virkkunen et al, 1994) specifically examined psycho-physiological and biochemical correlates of aggressive and impulsive behaviours in alcoholic firesetters and violent offenders. Participants underwent lumbar punctures and oral glucose and aspartame challenges and their diurnal activity rhythms were recorded with physical monitors. Discriminant function analyses revealed that impulsive offenders (who included arsonists) with antisocial personality disorder had low mean CSF 5-HIAA and corticotropin levels, but high mean CSF testosterone levels. Impulsive offenders with intermittent explosive disorder had a low mean CSF 5-HIAA concentration and low blood glucose nadir after glucose challenge and a desynchronised diurnal activity rhythm. Overall, the findings suggested that low CSF 5-HIAA was consistently associated with impulsivity, regardless of the diagnostic group, and high testosterone was associated with aggression and interpersonal violence.

The findings also suggest that alcoholic firesetters, who are considered to be suffering from an impulse control disorder, have impairments in serotonergic function and abnormalities in glucose metabolism, which may account for their recidivistic behaviour. There is now a fairly extensive literature supporting the notion that serotonergic deficits are associated with psychometrically measured impulsivity and impulsive aggressive behaviour across a number of studies of antisocial samples (Coccaro, 1989; Dolan et al, 2001; Seo et al, 2008). The specificity of this association for firesetters may be questionable, as few studies have systematically measured impulsive or aggressive traits in samples of firesetters or violent offenders. The association between central serotonin deficits in impulsive males who started fires noted by Virkkunen et al (1987) is well established; however, the findings from the above Scandinavian studies need to be interpreted with caution, as they were conducted in samples with alcohol misuse issues, which may have confounded the findings, as alcohol misuse in itself is associated with impairments in serotonergic function.

Genetics

From a general perspective, offending behaviour and criminality are thought to be heritable and much of this heritability is linked with antisocial personality traits (Ferguson, 2010). While no genetic studies have specifically looked at arson or firesetting there is evidence that conduct disorder and antisocial personality disorder are highly prevalent in firesetters (Repo & Virkkunen, 1997a; Sakheim & Osborn, 1999; Kolko, 2002; Lindberg et al, 2005; Martin et al, 2004; Mackay et al, 2006). There is also evidence from behavioural genetic studies to support the notion that a significant amount of the variance in antisocial personality and behaviour (including firesetting) is due to genetic contributions. Ferguson (2010) in a meta-analytic review of behavioural genetic aetiological studies of antisocial behaviour found that 56% of the variance can be explained through genetic influences, with 11% due to shared non-genetic influences and 31% due to unique non-genetic influences. This would suggest that there may be an important genetic contribution to repetitive firesetting where it is present in conjunction with a range of other antisocial behaviours.

There are reports of an association between chromosomal abnormalities, particularly Klinefelter's (XYY) syndrome, and firesetting (Neilsen, 1970; Kaler et al, 1989; Eytan et al, 2002) but all three of these are based on case series rather than large cohorts, so there is no clear evidence that this syndrome is specifically linked with firesetting.

Brunner et al (1993) identified a large Dutch kindred with an X-linked non-dysmorphic mild intellectual disability and a range of impulsive offending behaviours, including arson. The family had a genetic defect in Xp11–21 and a maximum multipoint lod score of 3.69 was obtained with a CA repeat polymorphism in the structural gene for monoamine oxidase A (MAOA). This led to renewed interest in the role of monoamines in disorders characterised within the impulse control disorders, including pyromania and repeat firesetting.

Several, but not all, studies have shown that a functional polymorphism on the monoamine oxidase A gene (MAOA-LPR) interacts with childhood adversity to predict adolescent and adult antisocial behaviour, which may include firesetting in the context of conduct disorder (Foley et al, 2004; Reif et al, 2007; Weder et al, 2008; Prom-Wormley et al, 2009). The Avon Longitudinal Study of Parents and Children, UK (Enoch et al, 2010) examined whether MAOA-LPR interacted with early life stressors (from before birth to 3 years) to influence behaviour in prepubertal children. The impact on behavioural disinhibition of family adversity from pre-birth to age 3 years, and of stressful life events from 6 months to 7 years, was determined in 7500 girls and boys. Measures of behavioural disinhibition included hyperactivity and conduct disturbances at ages 4 and 7 years. In both sexes, exposure to family adversity and stressful life events in the first 3 years of life predicted behavioural disinhibition at age 4, persisting until age 7. In girls, MAOA-LPR interacted with stressful life events experienced from 6 months to 3.5 years to influence hyperactivity at ages 4 and 7. In boys, the interaction of MAOA-LPR with stressful life events between 1.5 and 2.5 years predicted hyperactivity at age 7 years. The low-activity MAOA-LPR variant was associated with increased hyperactivity in girls and boys exposed to high stress. In contrast, there was no MAOA-LPR interaction with family adversity. This suggests that exposure to common stressors from pre-birth to 3 years predicted behavioural disinhibition and interactions between MAOA-LPR and stressful life events specifically predicted hyperactivity. Although there have been no genetic studies looking at firesetting behaviours specifically, it is possible that interactions between MAOA-LPR and stressful events may be important in accounting for the relatively high rates of conduct problems and hyperactivity associated with firesetting (Kolko, 2002; McCardle et al, 2009).

In recent years there has been significant interest in the roles of other specific genes in the development and maintenance of antisocial behaviour. While there are reports that catechol-O-methyltransferase (COMT) polymorphisms may be associated with impulsive violence in those diagnosed with antisocial personality disorder (ASPD) (Vevera et al, 2009), there have been no studies looking at COMT as a modifying gene that plays a role in determining inter-individual variability in the proclivity for impulsive firesetting behaviour, despite its association with ASPD. Given reports that firesetting may be associated with reduced 5-HT function there may also be value in exploring polymorphisms in the serotonin transporter gene (5HTTLPR). Some support for an association between 5HTTLPR, marijuana use and property offending was reported in the National Longitudinal Study of Adolescent Health (Vaske et al, 2009).

Arson and intellectual disability

The first large study to look at psychopathology and arson found that approximately 50% of male and 66% of female arsonists had low IQ (Lewis & Yarnell, 1951). Early work suggested that intellectual disability may be over-represented in juvenile female firesetters (Inciardi, 1970). Low IQ has been reported to be associated with firesetting in a number of studies (Geller, 1987; Jackson, 1994; Lowenstein, 2003; Räsänen et al, 1994; Rice & Harris, 1996). The actual prevalence of arson among offenders with intellectual disability is thought to be higher than it is in the general population (Walker & McCabe, 1973; Bradford & Dimock, 1986; Räsänen et al, 1994). In samples of firesetters the rate of intellectual disability has been reported to be 1.36% (Devapriam et al, 2007), 3% (Puri et al, 1995),

11% (Räsänen *et al*, 1994; Rix, 1994) and 15% (Leong & Silva, 1999). Taylor *et al* (2002) and Lindsay & Taylor (2005), however, have questioned these rates on the basis of variability in the assessment of intellectual disability.

Intellectual disability may be associated with a range of underlying neuropsychiatric disorders, including heritable conditions that warrant further investigation. The latter notion was highlighted in a recent report (Shirahama *et al*, 2010) on a 23-year-old woman with a history of intellectual disability and recidivist firesetting who was found to be the third generation in her family to suffer from Fahr disease, which a characterised by intracranial calcification of the basal ganglia (globus pallidus).

Arson and neuropsychological function

There is now an extensive literature highlighting evidence of deficits in executive function and memory in offender samples with conduct problems and antisocial personality pathology (Moffitt & Henry, 1991; Dolan, 1994; Morgan & Lilienfeld, 2000). There are, however, no studies specifically looking at the neuropsychological profiles of arsonists, despite case reports of executive deficits in firesetters generally (Calev, 1995).

Dolan *et al* (2002*a*) examined the neuropsychological test performance of 27 violent offenders, 20 sex offenders and 13 arson offenders who were detained in high-security hospitals and matched on age, intelligence and DSM-IV cluster B personality disorder profile. All patients completed a variety of self-report measures of cognitive, affective and behavioural dispositions relevant to offender populations. Trait impulsivity was further assessed and composite impulsivity scores were derived. Assessments of emotional state were administered prior to neuropsychological testing. The researchers found few differences in the personality profile of the offender groups, although sex offenders scored higher on trait anxiety, depression and tension measures than arson offenders and violent offenders. The offender groups did not significantly differ in their performance on neuropsychological tests, except that arsonists had poorer set-shifting ability, through perseverative error. This impairment may adversely influence arsonists' ability to learn from experience and increase their risk of recidivistic behaviour.

More generally, offenders with DSM-IV cluster B personality pathology tend to have greater impairments in executive function than healthy controls (Dolan & Park, 2002; Dolan *et al*, 2002*b*). Although the studies had relatively small sample sizes, the findings did not support the notion that arson as an offence is specifically associated with high scores on self-report measures of trait impulsivity. Despite the classification of pyromania as an impulse control disorder in DSM-IV, further work is needed to examine the relevance of trait impulsivity to recidivistic firesetting.

Arson and epilepsy

A number of case reports and series have suggested there is an association between epilepsy and arson (Byrne & Walsh, 1989; Carpenter & King, 1989; Brook & Dolan, 1996; Pontius, 1999) but few studies have specifically looked at the association between ictal activity and firesetting. Milrod & Urion (1992) reported on three boys with firesetting, photoparoxysmal responses to intermittent photic stimulation and temporal lobe electro-encephalographic abnormalities. Their firesetting resolved and behaviour improved after the administration of anticonvulsants. More recently, Reuber & Mackay (2008) specifically explored the relationship between epilepsy and criminal behaviour, including arson. They looked at all criminal cases where the finding was 'not guilty by reason of insanity (NGRI) because of epilepsy' in England and Wales between 1975 and 2001. Thirteen cases were identified, accounting for 7.3% of all verdicts of NGRI. Charges included murder, attempted murder, assault, arson, abduction/kidnapping and burglary. Of the defendants, 92.3% were male, 76.9% had neuropsychological impairments and 84.6% had psychiatric comorbidity. Over two-thirds of offences probably occurred during the post-ictal period. This case series suggested that arson as an offence was not specifically associated with epilepsy and that it was rare for epileptic seizures to cause criminal acts or omissions. The relatively low standard of proof required meant that some of the cases were not actually related to seizures. Of particular interest, there were no definite examples of ictal criminal behaviour that could be classified as automatisms. In cases of arson where the defendant has epilepsy, pre-trial assessments need to be thorough as a defence of automatism may be raised.

Arson and autism-spectrum disorders

The prevalence of autism-spectrum disorders (ASD) in the general population is thought to be around 0.60% (Constantino & Todd, 2003; Chakrabarti & Fombone, 2005) but rates are believed to be higher in forensic samples. Scragg & Shah (1994) screened all male patients in Broadmoor high-security hospital and found a prevalence of 1.5%, which increased to 2.3% with the inclusion of equivocal cases. More recently, Hare *et al* (2004) screened 1305 patients in all three high-security English hospitals and found the prevalence of ASD to be 2.4%, with an additional 2.4% for equivocal cases. An examination of the criminal histories indicated that while homicide rates were similar to the hospital base rates, arson was over-represented (16% v. 9%).

It has been argued that criminal activity in ASD, including arson, may be explained by 'theory of mind' (ToM) deficits, with associated abnormalities in amygdala–prefrontal circuitry, and by the abnormal, repetitive narrow interests often associated with ASD (Haskins & Silva, 2006). Several case reports highlight the association between arson and ASD, particularly Asperger syndrome (Everall & Leconteur, 1990; Murrie *et al*, 2002; Barry-Walsh & Mullen, 2004), and many of the people in these reports exhibited either a repetitive narrow fixation on fire or a deficit in ToM that impaired their ability to understand the impact on the victims of their firesetting. There is now an extensive literature on the neuropsychiatry of ASD which suggests significant alterations in brain function associated with social cognition (Baron-Cohen, 1995; Critchley *et al*, 2000; Grady & Keightley, 2002; Baron-Cohen & Belmonte, 2005).

Brain imaging studies support the notion that brain areas involved in social cognition, including the amygdala, prefrontal cortex and fusiform gyrus, are affected in ASD (Critchley *et al*, 2000; Baron-Cohen & Belmonte, 2005) and these abnormalities may account for firesetting. Further research is needed on the relevance of ToM deficits and low empathy in ASD offenders in the assessment of culpability and future risk. To date, most studies of ToM have focused on ASD children and there have been no studies looking at ToM deficits in adult arson offenders. Given the growing evidence that ASD are associated with impairments in brain function in areas involved in social cognition, forensic assessments for court may ultimately include comprehensive neuropsychiatric assessments, which will contribute to the debate on the association between ASD psychopathology and criminal intent (Haskins & Silva, 2006).

Psychopharmacological treatment

The literature of treatment of firesetting behaviour generally focuses on psycho-educational approaches or cognitive–behavioural therapy (Palmer *et al*, 2005). There are, however, anecdotal reports of firesetters who have responded to olanzapine (Parks *et al*, 2005). Given suggestions that pyromania is an impulse control disorder and that it is frequently associated with antisocial personality pathology, it is possible that serotonergic agents may have relevance for the treatment of recidivistic firesetting (Gabbard, 1995). Patients who have comorbid addictive disorders may also benefit from opiate antagonists. Studying the relationships between repeated firesetting and other psychiatric conditions (affective disorders, addictive disorders and personality disorder) will help provide a better conceptualisation of these disorders and lead to the development of pharmacological treatments that are targeted to the symptom profile of the patients.

Conclusions

To date, there has been very little study of the neurobiology of firesetting behaviour. Research on the characteristics and background of offenders who

77

have committed arson suggests that there are high rates of comorbidity with antisocial personality disorder, conduct disorder and alcohol misuse. These disorders are in turn associated with subtle impairments in serotonergic and executive function. Future studies should examine how arson offenders can be distinguished from other offenders with these impairments. The role of genes, neurotransmitters and brain structure and function in recidivistic firesetters has yet to be systematically examined. With advances in imaging technology it may be possible to study the effects of psychological and pharmacological treatments on firesetters (Grant, 2006; Grant & Kim, 2007).

Acknowledgements

The authors are members of the Australian Bushfire Arson Prevention Initiative, which receives support from Monash University and the Royal Automobile Club of Victoria (RACV).

References

American Psychiatric Association (2000) *Diagnostic and Statistical Manual of Mental Disorders* (4th edn, text revision) (DSM-IV-TR). APA.

Barker, A. F. (1994) *Arson: A Review of the Psychiatric Literature*. Oxford University Press.

Barnett, W. & Spitzer, M. (1994) Pathological firesetting 1951–1991: a review. *Medicine, Science and the Law*, **34**, 4–20.

Barnett, W., Richter, P. & Renneberg, B. (1999) Repeated arson: data from criminal records. *Forensic Science International*, **101**, 49–54.

Baron-Cohen, S. (1995) *Mindblindness: An Essay on Autism and Theory of Mind*. MIT Press.

Baron-Cohen, S. & Belmonte, M. K. (2005) Autism: a window onto the development of the social and the analytic brain. *Annual Review of Neuroscience*, **28**, 109–126.

Barry-Walsh, J. B. & Mullen, P. E. (2004) Forensic aspects of Asperger's syndrome. *Journal of Forensic Psychiatry and Psychology*, **15**, 96–107.

Bennett, W. M. & Hess, K. M. (1984) *The Arsonist: A Closer Look*. Charles C. Thomas.

Blumberg, N. H. (1981) Arson update: a review of the literature on firesetting. *Bulletin of the American Academy of Psychiatry and the Law*, **9**, 255–265.

Bourget, D. & Bradford, J. M. (1989) Female arsonists: a clinical study. *Bulletin of the American Academy of Psychiatry and the Law*, **17**, 293–300.

Bradford, J. M. W. (1982) Arson: a clinical study. *Canadian Journal of Psychiatry*, **27**, 188–193.

Bradford, J. & Dimock, J. (1986) A comparative study of adolescents and adults who wilfully set fires. *Psychiatric Journal of the University of Ottawa*, **11**, 228–234.

Brook, R. & Dolan, M. (1996) Arson and epilepsy. *Medicine, Science and the Law*, **36**, 268–271.

Brunner, H. G., Nelen, M. R., van Zandoort, P., *et al* (1993) X-linked borderline mental retardation with prominent behavioural disturbance: phenotype, genetic localization, and evidence for disturbed monoamine metabolism. *American Journal of Human Genetics*, **52**, 1032–1039.

Byrne, A. & Walsh, J. B. (1989) The epileptic arsonist. *British Journal of Psychiatry*, **155**, 268.

Calev, A. (1995) Pyromania and executive frontal dysfunction. *Behavioural Neurology*, **8**, 163–167.

Carpenter, P. K. & King, A. L. (1989) Epilepsy and arson. *British Journal of Psychiatry*, **154**, 554–556.

Chakrabarti, S. & Fombone, F. (2005) Prevalence of development disorders in pre-school children: confirmation of high prevalence. *American Journal of Psychiatry*, **162**, 1113–1141.

Coccaro, E. F. (1989) Central serotonin and impulsive aggression. *British Journal of Psychiatry*, **155**, 52–62.

Constantino, J. N. & Todd, R. D. (2003) Autistic traits in the general population: a twin study. *Archives of General Psychiatry*, **60**, 524–530.

Critchley, H. D., Daly, E. M., Bullmore, E. T., *et al* (2000) The functional neuroanatomy of social behaviour: changes in cerebral blood flow when people with autistic disorder process facial expressions. *Brain*, **123**, 2203–2212.

Devapriam, J., Bala Raju, L., Singh, N., *et al* (2007) Arson: characteristics and predisposing factors in offenders with intellectual disabilities. *British Journal of Forensic Practice*, **9**, 23–27.

Dickens, G., Sugarman, P., Ahmad, F., *et al* (2007) Gender differences amongst arsonists at psychiatric assessment. *Medicine, Science and the Law*, **47**, 233–238.

Dickens, G., Sugarman, P., Edgar, S., *et al* (2009) Recidivism and dangerousness in arsonists. *Journal of Forensic Psychiatry and Psychology*, **20**, 621–639.

Dolan, M. (1994) Psychopathy – a neurobiological perspective. *British Journal of Psychiatry*, **165**, 151–159.

Dolan, M. & Park, I. (2002) The neuropsychology of antisocial personality disorder. *Psychological Medicine*, **32**, 417–427.

Dolan, M., Anderson, I. M. & Deakin, J. F. W. (2001) Relationship between 5-HT function and impulsivity and aggression in male offenders with personality disorders. *British Journal of Psychiatry*, **178**, 352–359.

Dolan, M., Deakin, W. J. F., Roberts, N., *et al* (2002*a*) Serotonergic and cognitive impairment in impulsive aggressive personality disordered offenders: are there implications for treatment? *Psychological Medicine*, **32**, 105–117.

Dolan, M., Millington, J. & Park, I. (2002*b*) Personality and neuropsychological function in violent, sexual and arson offenders. *Medicine, Science and the Law*, **42**, 34–43.

Doley, R. (2003) Pyromania: fact or fiction? *British Journal of Criminology*, **43**, 797–807.

Enoch, M. A., Steer, C. D., Newman, T. K., *et al* (2010) Early life stress, MAOA, and gene–environment interactions predict behavioural disinhibition in children. *Genes, Brain, and Behaviour*, **9**, 65–74.

Everall, I. P. & Leconteur, A. (1990) Firesetting in an adolescent boy with Asperger's syndrome. *British Journal of Psychiatry*, **157**, 284–288.

Eytan, A., Paoloni-Guacobino, A., Thorens, G., *et al* (2002) Firesetting behaviour associated with Klinefelter syndrome. *International Journal of Psychiatry in Medicine*, **32**, 395–399.

Ferguson, C. J. (2010) Genetic contributions to antisocial personality and behaviour: a meta-analytic review from an evolutionary perspective. *Journal of Social Psychology*, **150**, 160–180.

Foley, D. L., Eaves, L. J., Wormley, B., *et al* (2004) Childhood adversity, monoamine oxidase A genotype and risk for conduct disorder. *Archives of General Psychiatry*, **61**, 738–744.

Gabbard, G. O. (1995) *Treatments of Psychiatric Disorders*. American Psychiatric Press.

Gannon, T. A. & Pina, A. (2010) Firesetting: psychopathology, theory and treatment. *Aggression and Violent Behaviour*, **15**, 224–238.

Gaynor, J. (1996) Firesetting. In *Child and Adolescent Psychiatry: A Comprehensive Textbook* (ed. L. Melvin), pp. 601–611. Williams & Wilkins.

Gaynor, J. & Hatcher, C. (1987) *The Psychology of Child Firesetting: Detection and Intervention*. Brunner/Mazel.

Geller, J. L. (1987) Firesetting in the adult psychiatric population. *Hospital and Community Psychiatry*, **38**, 501–506.

Geller, J. L. (1992) Arson in review: from profit to pathology. *Psychiatric Clinics of North America*, **15**, 623–645.

Geller, J. L. (2008) Firesetting: a burning issue. In *Serial Murder and the Psychology of Violent Crime* (ed. R. N. Koscis), pp. 141–178. Humana Press.

Grady, C. L. & Keightley, M. L. (2002) Studies of altered social cognition in neuropsychiatric disorders using functional neuroimaging. *Canadian Journal of Psychiatry*, **47**, 327–336.

Grant, J. E. (2006) SPECT imaging and treatment of pyromania. *Journal of Clinical Psychiatry*, **67**, 998.

Grant, J. E. & Kim, S. W. (2007) Clinical characteristics and psychiatric co-morbidity of pyromania. *Journal of Clinical Psychiatry*, **68**, 1717–1722.

Hare, D. J., Gould, J., Mills, R., *et al* (2004) *A Preliminary Study of Individuals with Autistic Spectrum Disorders in Three Special Hospitals in England*. National Autistic Society. At http://www.autism.org.uk/~/media/F6C03DB687454477AF51EC0285B11209.ashx (accessed 17 December 2010).

Harris, G. T. & Rice, M. E. (1984) Mentally disordered firesetters: psychodynamic versus empirical approaches. *International Journal of Law and Psychiatry*, **7**, 19–34.

Haskins, B. G. & Silva, J. A. (2006) Asperger's disorder and criminal behaviour: forensic-psychiatric considerations. *Journal of the American Academy of Psychiatry and the Law*, **34**, 374–384.

Heidrich, A., Schmidtke, A., Lesch, K. P., *et al* (1996) Cerebellar arachnoid cyst in a firesetter: the weight of organic lesions in arson. *Journal of Psychiatry and Neuroscience*, **21**, 202–206.

Hill, R. W., Langevin, R., Paitich, D., *et al* (1982) Is arson an aggressive act or a property offence? A controlled study of psychiatric referrals. *Canadian Journal of Psychiatry*, **27**, 648–654.

Home Office (2008) *Findings from the British Crime Survey and Police Recorded Crime*. Home Office. At http://www.homeoffice.gov.uk/rds/pdfs08/hosb0708.pdf (accessed 20 December 2010).

Inciardi, J. A. (1970) The adult firesetter – a typology. *Criminology*, **8**, 145–155.

Jackson, H. F. (1994) Assessment of firesetters. In *The Assessment of Criminal Behaviours in Secure Settings* (eds M. McMurran & J. Hedge), pp. 94–126. Jessica Kingsley.

Jackson, H. F., Glass, C. & Hope, S. (1987) A functional analysis of recidivistic arson. *British Journal of Clinical Psychology*, **26**, 175–185.

Kaler, S. G., White, B. J. & Kruesi, M. J. P. (1989) Firesetting and Klinefelter syndrome. *Pediatrics*, **84**, 749–750.

Kolko, D. J. (1985) Juvenile firesetting: a review and methodological critique. *Clinical Psychology Review*, **5**, 345–376.

Kolko, D. J. (ed.) (2002) *Handbook on Firesetting in Children and Youth*. Academic Press.

Kolko, D. J. & Kazdin, A. E. (1986) A conceptualization of firesetting in children and adolescents. *Journal of Abnormal Child Psychology*, **14**, 49–61.

Laubichler, W. & Kühberger, A. (1995) The role of alcohol in 'pyromania' and arson. *Blutalkohol*, **32**, 208–217.

Laubichler, W. A., Kühberger, P. & Sedlmeier, P. (1996) 'Pyromania' and arson. A psychiatric and criminologic data analysis. *Nervenarzt*, **67**, 774–780.

Leong, G. B. & Silva, J. A. (1999) Revisiting arson from an out-patient forensic perspective. *Journal of Forensic Science*, **44**, 558–563.

Lewis, N. O. C. & Yarnell, H. (1951) *Pathological Firesetting (Pyromania)*. Nervous and Mental Disease Monographs no. 82. Coolidge Foundation.

Lindberg, N., Holi, M. M., Tani, P., *et al* (2005) Looking for pyromania: characteristics of a consecutive sample of Finnish male criminals with histories of recidivist firesetting between 1973 and 1993. *BMC Psychiatry*, **47**, 1–5.

Lindsay, W. R. & Taylor, J. L. (2005) A selective review of research on offenders with developmental disabilities: assessment and treatment. *Clinical Psychology and Psychotherapy*, **12**, 201–214.

Lowenstein, L. F. (2003) Recent research into arson (1992–2000). Incidence, causes and associated features, predictions, comparative studies and prevention and treatment. *Psychiatry, Psychology and Law*, **10**, 192–198.

Mackay, S., Henderson, J., Del Bove, G., *et al* (2006) Fire interest and antisociality as risk factors in the severity and persistence of juvenile firesetting. *Journal of the American Academy of Child and Adolescent Psychiatry*, **45**, 1077–1084.

Martin, G., Bergen, H. A., Richardson, A. S., *et al* (2004) Correlates of firesetting in a community sample of young adolescents. *Australian and New Zealand Journal of Psychiatry*, **38**, 148–154.

McCardle, S., Lambie, I., Barker-Collo, S., *et al* (2009) *Adolescent Firesetting. A New Zealand Case-Controlled Study of Risk Factors for Adolescent Firesetting*. New Zealand Fire Service Commission Research Report no. 46. At http://www.fire.org.nz/Research/Published-Reports/Documents/85ef271de5e12e5d7e143d153ea1fc39.pdf (accessed 17 December 2010).

McKerracher, D. W. & Dacre, J. I. (1966) A study of arsonists in a special security hospital. *British Journal of Psychiatry*, **112**, 1151–1154.

Milrod, L. M. & Urion, D. K. (1992) Juvenile firesetting and the photoparoxysmal response. *Annals of Neurology*, **32**, 222–223.

Moffitt, T. E. & Henry, B. H. (1991) Neuropsychological studies of juvenile delinquency and juvenile violence. In *Neuropsychology of Aggression* (ed. J. S. Milner), pp. 131–146. Klewer.

Morgan, A. B. & Lilienfeld, S. O. (2000) A meta-analytic review of the relation between antisocial behaviour and neuropsychological measures of executive functioning. *Clinical Psychology Review*, **20**, 113–136.

Murrie, D. C., Warren, J. L., Kristiansson, M., *et al* (2002) Asperger's syndrome in forensic settings. *International Journal of Forensic Mental Health*, **1**, 59–70.

Neilsen, J. (1970) Criminality among patients with Klinefelter's syndrome and the XYY syndrome. *British Journal of Psychiatry*, **118**, 365–369.

Palmer, E. J., Caulfield, L. S. & Hollin, C. R. (2005) *Evaluation of Interventions with Arsonists and Young Firesetters*. Office of the Deputy Prime Minister.

Parks, R. W., Green, R., Girgis, S., *et al* (2005) Response of pyromania to biological treatment in a homeless person. *Neuropsychiatric Disease and Treatment*, **1**, 277–280.

Pontius, A. A. (1999) Motiveless firesetting: implicating partial limbic seizure kindling by revived memories of fires in 'limbic psychotic trigger reaction'. *Perceptual and Motor Skills*, **88**, 970–982.

Prins, H. (1994) *Fire Raising: Its Motivation and Management*. Routledge.

Prins, H., Tennent, G. & Trick, K. (1985) Motives for arson (fire raising). *Medicine, Science and the Law*, **25**, 275–278.

Prom-Wormley, E. C., Eaves, L. J., Foley, D. L., *et al* (2009) Monoamine oxidase and childhood adversity as risk factors for conduct disorder in females. *Psychological Medicine*, **39**, 579–590.

Puri, B. K., Baxter, R. & Cordess, C. C. (1995) Characteristics of fire-setters. A study and proposed multi-axial psychiatric classification. *British Journal of Psychiatry*, **166**, 393–396.

Räsänen, P., Hirvenoja, R., Hakko, H., *et al* (1994) Cognitive functioning ability of arsonists. *Journal of Forensic Psychiatry*, **5**, 615–620.

Räsänen, P., Hakko, H. & Väisänen, E. (1995) Arson trend increasing: a real challenge to psychiatry. *Journal of Forensic Science*, **40**, 976–979.

Reif, A., Rösler, M., Freitag, C. M., *et al* (2007) Nature and nurture predispose to violent behaviour: serotonergic genes and adverse childhood environment. *Neuropsychopharmacology*, **32**, 2375–2383.

Repo, E. & Virkkunen, M. (1997a) Criminal recidivism and family histories of schizophrenic and non-schizophrenic firesetters: co-morbid alcohol dependence in schizophrenic firesetters. *Journal of the American Academy of Psychiatry and the Law*, **25**, 207–215.

Repo, E. & Virkkunen, M. (1997b) Outcomes in a sample of Finnish firesetters. *Journal of Forensic Psychiatry*, **8**, 127–137.

Repo, E., Virkkunen, M., Rawlings, R., *et al* (1997) Criminal and psychiatric histories of Finnish arsonists. *Acta Psychiatrica Scandinavia*, **95**, 318–323.

Reuber, M. & Mackay, R. D. (2008) Epileptic automatisms in the criminal courts: 13 cases tried in England and Wales between 1975 and 2001. *Epilepsia*, **49**, 138–145.

Rice, M. E. & Harris, G. T. (1991) Firesetters admitted to a maximum security psychiatric institution: offenders and offences. *Journal of Interpersonal Violence*, **6**, 461–471.

Rice, M. E. & Harris, G. T. (1996) Predicting the recidivism of mentally disordered firesetters. *Journal of Interpersonal Violence*, **11**, 364–375.

Ritchie, E. L. & Huff, T. G. (1999) Psychiatric aspects of arsonists. *Journal of Forensic Science*, **44**, 733–740.

Rix, K. J. B. (1994) A psychiatric study of adult arsonists. *Medicine, Science and the Law*, **34**, 21–34.

Roy, A., Virkkunen, M., Guthrie, S., *et al* (1986) Indices of serotonin and glucose metabolism in violent offenders, arsonists and alcoholics. In *Psychology of Suicidal Behaviour* (eds J. J. Mann & M. Stanley), pp. 202–220. New York Academy of Sciences.

Sakheim, G. A. & Osborn, E. (1999) Severe versus non-severe firesetters revisited. *Child Welfare*, **78**, 411–434.

Scragg, P. & Shah, A. (1994) Prevalence of Asperger's syndrome in a secure hospital. *British Journal of Psychiatry*, **165**, 679–682.

Seo, D., Patrick, C. & Kennealy, P. J. (2008) Role of serotonin and dopamine system interactions in the neurobiology of impulsive aggression and its comorbidity with other clinical disorders. *Aggression and Violent Behaviour*, **13**, 383–395.

Shirahama, M., Akiyoshi, J., Ishitobi, Y., *et al* (2010) A young woman with visual hallucinations, delusions of persecution and a history of performing arson with possible three-generation Fahr disease. *Acta Psychiatrica Scandinavica*, **121**, 75–77.

Soltys, S. M. (1992) Pyromania and firesetting behaviours. *Psychiatric Annals*, **22**, 79–83.

Soothill, K., Ackerley, E. & Francis, B. (2004) The criminal careers of arsonists. *Medicine, Science and the Law*, **44**, 27–40.

Stewart, L. A. (1993) Profile of female firesetters: implications for treatment. *British Journal of Psychiatry*, **163**, 248–256.

Sugarman, P. & Dickens, G. (2009) Dangerousness in arsonists: a survey of psychiatrists' views. *Psychiatric Bulletin*, **33**, 99–101.

Taylor, J. L., Thorne, I., Robertson, A., *et al* (2002) Evaluation of a group intervention for convicted arsonists with mild and borderline intellectual disabilities. *Criminal Behaviour and Mental Health*, **12**, 282–293.

Vaske, J., Newsome, J., Makarios, M., *et al* (2009) Interaction of 5HTTLPR and marijuana use on property offending. *Biodemography and Social Biology*, **55**, 93–102.

Vevera, J., Stopkova, R., Bes, M., *et al* (2009) COMT polymorphisms in impulsively violent offenders with antisocial personality disorder. *Neuroendocrinology Letters*, **30**, 753–756.

Virkkunen, M. (1984) Reactive hypoglycaemic tendency among arsonists. *Acta Psychiatrica Scandinavica*, **46**, 600–603.

Virkkunen, M., Nuutila, A., Goodwin, F. K., *et al* (1987) Cerebrospinal fluid monoamine metabolite levels in male arsonists. *Archives of General Psychiatry*, **44**, 241–247.

Virkkunen, M., DeJong, J., Bartko, J., *et al* (1989a) Relationship of psychobiological variables to recidivism in violent offenders and impulsive fire setters. A follow-up study. *Archives of General Psychiatry*, **46**, 600–603.

Virkkunen, M., DeJong, J., Bartko, J., *et al* (1989b) Psychobiological concomitants of history of suicide attempts amongst violent offenders and impulsive fire setters. *Archives of General Psychiatry*, **46**, 604–606.

Virkkunen, M., Kallio, E., Rawlings, R., *et al* (1994) Personality profiles and state aggressiveness in Finnish violent offenders, impulsive firesetters and healthy volunteers. *Archives of General Psychiatry*, **51**, 28–33.

Virkkunen, M., Eggert, M., Rawlings, R., *et al* (1996) A prospective follow-up study of alcoholic violent offenders and fire setters. *Archives of General Psychiatry*, **53**, 523–529.

Von Knorring, A. L., Hallman, J., von Knorring, L., *et al* (1991) Platelet monoamine oxidase activity in type 1 and type 2 alcoholism. *Alcohol*, **26**, 409–416.

Vreeland, R. & Levin, B. M. (1980) Psychological aspects of firesetting. In *Fires and Human Behaviour* (ed. D. Canter), pp. 31–46. Wiley.

Walker, N. & McCabe, S. (1973) *Crime and Insanity in England, Vol. 2*. Edinburgh University Press.

Weder, N., Yang, B. Z., Douglas-Palumberi, H., *et al* (2008) MAOA genotype, maltreatment, and aggressive behaviour: the changing impact of genotype at varying levels of trauma. *Biological Psychiatry*, **65**, 417–424.

Wolford, B. (1972) Some attitudinal, psychological and sociological characteristics of incarcerated arsonists. *Fire and Arson Investigator*, **22**, 1–30.

CHAPTER 5

The developmental aspects of firesetting

Sherri MacKay, Erin M. Ruttle and Ashley K. Ward

Thousands of injuries, hundreds of fatalities and millions of dollars in property loss are among the annual costs of youth firesetting in North America and the UK (Hall, 2005; Arson Prevention Bureau, 2006). Given the scope of the negative outcomes associated with juvenile firesetting, it is surprising that there is so little empirical study of this behaviour. One central reason for the lack of research may be that fire involvement by children and adolescents is relatively common. Almost half of all boys will engage in some unsanctioned fire-starting (Kafry, 1978; Grolnick *et al*, 1990), which may have led to the perception that juvenile fire involvement is a normal behaviour of little clinical relevance (Pollack-Nelson *et al*, 2006). Indeed, the average caregiver does not report their child's fire involvement (Kafry, 1978) or view it as requiring expert consultation (Webb *et al*, 1990). As only about 5% of 300 randomly polled mental health workers received any training about juvenile firesetting (Sparber, 2005), many mental health professionals also may believe that juvenile firesetting is benign.

Juvenile firesetting is a heterogeneous behaviour that occurs during all developmental periods (i.e., pre-school, childhood, adolescence) and many children and adolescents stop their fire involvement without intervention. However, there is a small subgroup whose firesetting will persist, to the peril of both themselves and their communities. Fire involvement or even just fire interest during childhood is an important predictor of both adolescent arson (Hanson *et al*, 1994) and adult arson (Rice & Harris, 1991). One central task for researchers and clinicians working with youth firesetters has been to differentiate juveniles at low risk for further fire involvement from those at high risk, in order to develop and implement programmes that fit the needs of the individual. Much of the scant empirical literature on juvenile firesetting has examined the characteristics of juvenile firesetters, how they differ from non-firesetters and more recently the differences within the firesetting group. The empirical advances have been slow and the knowledge base remains small. Although specific risk factors have been identified, a comprehensive multifactorial biopsychosocial profile has yet to emerge.

Despite heterogeneity in youth firesetters, most specialists working with this population agree that any juvenile with firesetting behaviour requires some form of intervention, brief or otherwise, because of the injury risk associated with this behaviour. Juvenile fire involvement can result in significant burn injury, and children and youths are more likely to die in fires they start themselves than any other cause.

The aim of this chapter is to provide readers with an understanding of child and adolescent firesetting through: an overview of the research literature on the terms used and the prevalence rates associated with youth firesetting; the theoretical underpinnings of the behaviour; the psychosocial, fire-specific and mental health factors that co-occur in this population; recidivism; and a review of current assessment and treatment approaches.

Definitions and prevalence rates

Definitions

Operational definitions and descriptions of fire-related behaviour by youths are often unclear or missing in the research literature. This can lead to confusion about the nature of the behaviour in question, its severity and clinical significance, as well as a lack of consistency between studies (MacKay et al, 2011). 'Fire involvement' is an umbrella term that includes all unsanctioned or dangerous behaviours involving fire that have been threatened, planned or carried out, regardless of intent or motivation (MacKay et al, 2004). Some examples of unsanctioned fire involvement by youths are match play, lighter play, fire play, firesetting, arson and bomb-making. Generally, youth 'firesetting' is defined as an event where property or a person was targeted in a fire that was ignited by a youth without the supervision or permission of an authority figure (Strachan, 1981; Showers & Pickrell, 1987).

Fire involvement may be motivated by boredom, curiosity, impulsivity, attention-seeking, maliciousness, emotion dysregulation, pathological interest in fire, or some combination of these. In theory, a description of the motivation for the fire involvement can help clarify the severity of the behaviour and the diagnoses that may be relevant. DSM-IV-TR (American Psychiatric Association, 2000) includes firesetting as one of 15 criteria for the diagnosis of conduct disorder but further specifies that the firesetting is committed 'with the intention of causing serious damage' (p. 99), implicitly ruling out more benign motives such as curiosity or boredom. Although very little is actually known about children's and adolescents' motivations for firesetting, there is strong evidence that supports the co-occurrence of firesetting and antisocial behaviour.

One of the most common psychiatric diagnoses provided in this population is conduct disorder (Kolko & Kazdin, 1991). DSM-IV (American

Psychiatric Association, 1994) field trials demonstrated that firesetting had high predictive utility for the diagnosis of conduct disorder (Lahey *et al*, 1994). As well, firesetting has been linked to poor outcomes in prospective studies of boys with aggressive conduct disorder (Kelso & Stewart, 1986). Of importance, however, is that only a minority of youths with conduct disorder engage in repetitive firesetting (Jacobson, 1985) and conduct disorder *per se* is not a strong predictor of firesetting recidivism in juvenile arsonists (Repo & Virkkunen, 1997). Variables other than behaviour disorder are necessary to understand the onset and persistence of firesetting.

Firesetting also is the main criterion for diagnosing pyromania, defined in DSM-IV-TR as 'deliberate and purposeful fire setting on more than one occasion that is attributed to an individual's fascination with, interest in, curiosity about, or attraction to fire and the arousal or pleasure associated with firesetting' (American Psychiatric Association, 2000, p. 671). Similar criteria are described for the diagnosis of pathological firesetting in ICD-10 (World Health Organization, 2007). DSM-IV-TR suggests that this form of firesetting is quite rare in children (p. 670). This low rate may, in part, be explained by the exclusion criterion 'that the firesetting is not done to express anger or vengeance and that the firesetting is not better accounted for by Conduct Disorder' (p. 671). Unfortunately, the utility of pyromania as both a construct and a diagnosis for children and adolescents is limited, as there is very little research evaluating pyromania in younger age groups and no empirical data on the comorbidity of pyromania and serious conduct problems in youths who set fires. Fire-specific interest has certainly emerged as an important construct in understanding the onset and persistence of juvenile firesetting. Importantly, neither of the aforementioned DSM-IV-TR diagnostic criteria for firesetting includes the most prevalent forms of fire involvement by youth, such as match play or firesetting that is committed without intent to cause serious damage or injury (Martin *et al*, 2004; MacKay *et al*, 2011).

Prevalence rates

Since the results of studies of child and adolescent firesetting are largely influenced by several methodological factors (e.g., population from which the study sample is drawn, operational definition of firesetting and type of informant recruited to provide data), prevalence estimates of firesetting in children and adolescents vary substantially. Self-report rates of firesetting are particularly important to consider because caregivers may under-report this often covert behaviour (Kolko, 1985; Loeber *et al*, 1993). For example, only 28% of community parents of fire-involved children are aware of their child's interest (Del Bove *et al*, 2008).

Firesetting appears to be common among the general population of children and adolescents. Self-report studies that employ inclusive definitions of firesetting (e.g., unsanctioned or unsupervised use of ignition materials to burn targets) indicate that, during the elementary school years, approximately 10–57% of children will have set a fire without a supervising adult present (Kafry, 1978; Cole *et al*, 1986; Martin *et al*, 2004). By high school, 88% of boys and 81% of girls have played with fire (Jones & Jackson, 1999) and approximately 27% of adolescents will have set a fire on at least one occasion during the preceding 12 months (MacKay *et al*, 2009). In contrast, low rates of firesetting are reported when caregivers are the informants (Achenbach & Edelbrock, 1981; Del Bove *et al*, 2008) and when firesetting is strictly defined as with intent to cause serious damage to objects or persons, the latter with rates of, for example, 0.1% and 0.4% (Lahey *et al*, 1994; Gelhorn *et al*, 2009).

Sex and age are moderators of firesetting. Males tend to engage in firesetting more frequently than females; among children and adolescents the male:female ratio of fire involvement is between 6:1 (Perrin-Wallqvist & Norlander, 2003) and 9:1 (Fineman, 1980). The prevalence rates of fire involvement appear to decline during the course of development; reportedly, more younger children are involved with fire than are adolescents (Chen *et al*, 2003; Dadds & Fraser, 2006; MacKay *et al*, 2009). Although firesetting is rarely (4%) the primary presenting problem in child and adolescent clinical settings (Stewart & Culver, 1982), the prevalence rate of firesetting in clinical samples varies widely, from 2% (Jacobson, 1985) to 52% (Kolko & Kazdin, 1988), depending on the setting (out-patient or in-patient), the sex and age of the child and the definition employed.

Of all offences, arson has the greatest rate of youth participation. Youths aged 12–17 account for 42–47% of all police contact and arrests for arson in Canada (Canadian Centre for Justice Statistics, 2004; Office of the Ontario Fire Marshal, 2009), approximately 50% of all fire-related charges in the USA (Snyder, 2008) and 40% of those cautioned or arrested for arson in the UK (Arson Prevention Bureau, 2006). Of note is that a large proportion of serious fires are committed by pre-adolescent youths; more than one-third of US arson arrests in 1997 were of children aged 12 or less (Snyder, 1999).

Theoretical perspectives

Several models of the aetiology and maintenance of firesetting behaviour in children and adolescents have been put forth by theorists and researchers. The psychodynamic framework of firesetting dominated conceptualisations during the first half of the 20th century. Early psychodynamic interpretations of firesetting, as described by Freud (1932), proposed a link between firesetting, enuresis and sexual desire. While some support is provided in the literature (Kaufman *et al*, 1961), several studies have failed to replicate a relationship between firesetting and enuresis in juveniles (Bradford, 1982; Heath *et al*, 1983; Jacobson, 1985). Further, in samples that include youths, extremely low rates of sexual arousal associated with firesetting have been reported (Lewis & Yarnell, 1951). Tests for differences in sexual response patterns to fire-related stimuli between firesetters and non-firesetters have not been conducted in juveniles.

In the past few decades, perspectives on youth firesetting have shifted from psychodynamic models to models that apply behavioural, cognitive–behavioural and social learning principles. The development, maintenance, and persistence of youth firesetting have been reconceptualised to incorporate: individual characteristics; family, parenting and social circumstances; and environmental factors. Fineman's dynamic behaviour theory of firesetting (Fineman, 1980, 1995) views it as the result of the interaction of risk factors from three domains: personality and individual factors (e.g., demographic, physical and psychological factors); family and social factors (e.g., family variables such as parental supervision, peer variables); and immediate environmental conditions (i.e., events, thoughts and feelings that occur immediately before, during and after the firesetting). Risk for firesetting is thought to accrue as a result of predisposing and reinforcing historical factors, as well as the dynamic factors in the immediate environment. This model identifies two main groups of firesetting individuals: non-pathological and pathological firesetters. Non-pathological firesetters set fires out of curiosity or by accident; pathological firesetters are motivated to set fires with malicious or criminal intent and often display other antisocial behaviours or concurrent psychopathology. Within both broad groups are subtypes of firesetters. For example, pathological firesetters include delinquent, cognitively impaired and seriously disturbed subtypes. Fineman's theory is recognised as one of the first to carefully specify the broad range of variables that lead to firesetting (Gaynor, 1996) but his specific typology of firesetters has yet to be tested.

Patterson's (1982) social learning approach provides a developmental account that places firesetting at an advanced level on the trajectory of child and adolescent antisocial behaviour. This framework proposes that a child develops antisocial behaviour through learning and experience in two general stages. The first stage begins at home, with ineffective parenting, characterised by parental distance, a lack of involvement in the child's life and limited monitoring and supervision of the child. Caregivers who experience social disadvantage and who have substance misuse or dependence or a high level of stress are at risk for ineffective parenting practices (Patterson *et al*, 1992). Dysfunctional parenting practices – which include the absence of clear rules and expectations for children and inappropriate strategies for monitoring and responding to child compliance or disobedience – set the stage for learning antisocial behaviours in the home. The child's antisocial behaviour progresses through disobedience, fighting, tantrums, lying and stealing, with firesetting occurring later in this developmental chain. Numerous struggles over discipline as well as confrontations between the caregiver and child lead to a cycle of coercive exchanges. A coercive exchange models aggressive behaviour and often ends with the emotionally dysregulated parent giving way to the child, negatively reinforcing the child's aggressive behaviour as well as the ineffective parenting. In adolescence, ongoing lax parental monitoring of the youth, caregiver–child conflict, association with deviant peers and school problems all increase the likelihood of further progression of antisocial behaviour and criminality (Patterson & Dishion, 1985). This model has been widely tested and has empirical support from several studies (e.g., Patterson & Dishion, 1985; Ramsey et al, 1990). Although evidence supporting the hypothesis that firesetting represents an advanced level of antisocial behaviour has been found (Forehand et al, 1991; Stickle & Blechman, 2002), the richness of Patterson's developmental model has yet to be investigated in firesetting samples and very little is known about the natural history or developmental course of firesetting.

An alternative social learning perspective on juvenile firesetting is that firesetting youths have poor social skills and are ineffective at gaining social reinforcement and solving interpersonal disputes. They are thought to use firesetting as an alternative to pro-social problem-solving and as a mechanism for gaining immediate reinforcement and revenge (Vreeland & Levin, 1980) without the need for interpersonal confrontation (Jackson et al, 1987).

Kolko & Kazdin (1986) developed an ecological risk model for juvenile firesetting and began to operationalise fire-specific constructs in their research. They describe three groups of risk factors for firesetting: learning experiences and cues (e.g., early modelling of fire behaviours, early interest in fire and direct experience with fire); the child's cognitive, behavioural and motivational profile (e.g., limited fire safety skills, deficits in social skills, impulsivity, presence of covert antisocial behaviours); and parental and family influences and stressors (e.g., limited parental supervision and monitoring, inconsistent or harsh discipline strategies, parental emotional distance, stressful life events). In younger children, exposure to ignition materials, heightened curiosity, excitement about fire and impulsivity may lead to increased experimentation and play with matches and lighters. Furthermore, heightened emotional arousal, coupled with a limited understanding of the cause and effect and potential consequences of fire play, can impede the learning and use of basic fire safety skills. In older children and adolescents, difficulties with attention, impulsivity and anger management are factors hypothesised to contribute to firesetting (Kolko & Kazdin, 1991).

Characteristics of youth firesetters

Psychosocial factors

Many research studies of youth firesetting have focused on identifying the factors that co-occur with firesetting. Gaining an understanding of these factors has been particularly important for mental health professionals who work with these youths. For example, this information provides practitioners with possible explanations for the onset and maintenance of fire-related behaviour as well as targets for fire-specific and general mental health intervention. The psychosocial factors linked to youth firesetting largely overlap with the factors linked to general maladaptive outcomes, such as antisocial behaviour and delinquency (e.g., Hawkins *et al*, 1998; Lipsey & Derzon, 1998; Farrington & Welsh, 2007; Leschied *et al*, 2008). Further, the characteristics of juvenile firesetters appear to be similar to those of adult firesetters (Gannon & Pina, 2010).

Several individual factors have been identified to precede or co-occur with child and adolescent firesetting. The most common characteristic noted is prior or concurrent antisocial behaviour (Kolko *et al*, 2001; MacKay *et al*, 2006). A number of studies have reported associations between firesetting and cruelty to animals (Moore *et al*, 1996; Sakheim & Osborn, 1999; Slavkin, 2001; Dadds & Fraser, 2006), sexual misbehaviour (Jacobson, 1985), lack of empathy (Sakheim & Osborn, 1999), conduct problems and disorder (Kolko & Kazdin, 1988, 1989*a*; Forehand *et al*, 1991; Kolko *et al*, 2001; Martin *et al*, 2004; McCarty & McMahon, 2005; MacKay *et al*, 2006) and delinquency (Forehand *et al*, 1991; Stickle & Blechman, 2002; Becker *et al*, 2004). Firesetting youths also are more likely than their non-firesetting peers to have a history of aggression (Sakheim & Osborn, 1999) or to display current aggression (Jacobson, 1985; Forehand *et al*, 1991; Stickle & Blechman, 2002; Chen *et al*, 2003; McCarty & McMahon, 2005). Even when matched for the presence of conduct disorder, firesetting youths have more extreme levels of antisocial behaviour (Forehand *et al*, 1991; Stickle & Blechman, 2002).

Additionally, a significant proportion of these youths exhibit hyperactive (McCarty & McMahon, 2005; Dadds & Fraser, 2006) and impulsive traits (Kolko & Kazdin, 1991; McCarty & McMahon, 2005) as well as greater levels of emotion dysregulation and anger (Kolko & Kazdin, 1991). Higher anger levels differentiate high-risk from low-risk firesetters (Sakheim & Osborn, 1999). Firesetting youths reportedly experience more social problems and peer rejection than non-firesetting youths (Chen *et al*, 2003; Sakheim & Osborn, 1999) and more impairment in their primary attachments (Nurcombe, 1964; Sakheim *et al*, 1985).

Generally, family and parenting factors are not well researched in the youth firesetting population. Some family variables have been linked to firesetting, such as single-parent households (Pollinger *et al*, 2005; Root *et al*, 2008) and households without a biological mother or father (Ritvo *et al*, 1983). Reportedly, firesetting youths experience more frequent caregiver disruption (Strachan, 1981). Several studies have found that harsh, dysfunctional and physically abusive parenting practices are observed more frequently in firesetting children and adolescents than in non-firesetting youths (Ritvo *et al*, 1983; Bradford & Dimock, 1986; Bailey *et al*, 2001; Becker *et al*, 2004; McCarty & McMahon, 2005; Dadds & Fraser, 2006).

Maltreated firesetters commit more fire-related acts, demonstrate greater versatility in their firesetting and are more likely to remain involved with firesetting than non-maltreated firesetters (Root *et al*, 2008). Also, firesetting youths report less parental warmth (McCarty & McMahon, 2005). Severe maternal rejection has been linked to high-risk firesetting (Sakheim & Osborn, 1999). Cross-sectional and longitudinal evidence has shown that parental mental health problems, such as depression (Kolko & Kazdin, 1986; McCarty & McMahon, 2005) and substance use (Showers & Pickrell, 1987; Becker *et al*, 2004), occur frequently in caregivers of children involved with fire.

Fire-specific factors

Fire-specific factors, including age of onset of fire involvement, curiosity about fire and severity of firesetting, play an important role in understanding and describing the characteristics of youth fire involvement. For example, fire-specific variables have been found to contribute to the maintenance of firesetting behaviour (MacKay *et al*, 2006) and differentiate high-rate firesetters from low-rate firesetters and desisters (Martin *et al*, 2004). Demographic factors, such as sex and age, moderate certain fire-specific variables. A higher proportion of children who endorse fire play and firesetting are male (Kolko & Kazdin, 1989*b*; Grolnick *et al*, 1990) and males are more likely to have greater involvement and interest in fire than females (Block *et al*, 1976; Kolko *et al*, 2001; Chen *et al*, 2003; Martin *et al*, 2004; Dadds & Fraser, 2006). Female youths express a greater level of fear of fire than males (Block *et al*, 1976) and are more likely to initiate their fire involvement at an older age (McCarty & McMahon, 2005). Research has consistently found that, compared with older children, younger children express greater interest in fire (Block *et al*, 1976; Chen *et al*, 2003; Dadds & Fraser, 2006) and more frequently engage in match play, fire play and firesetting than their older counterparts (Dadds & Fraser, 2006; MacKay *et al*, 2009).

Exposure to inappropriate models of fire-related behaviour, curiosity about fire, greater knowledge of items that burn (Kolko & Kazdin, 1989*a,b*, 1991), current fire involvement (Kolko & Kazdin, 1989*a,b*; MacKay *et al*, 2009) and a history of fire involvement differentiate firesetting youths from their non-firesetting peers (Hanson *et al*, 1994). Firesetting recidivism is linked to a greater degree of firesetting severity, firesetting interest and antisocial behaviour (MacKay *et al*, 2006; Repo & Virkkunen, 1997). Attentional bias for fire-related stimuli has been shown to relate to greater firesetting frequency (Gallagher-Duffy *et al*, 2009). Additionally, firesetting recidivists are more likely to experience a neutral or positive feeling about their previous firesetting and to acknowledge the potential for future fire involvement than youths who commit a single act of firesetting (Kolko & Kazdin, 1994).

Longitudinal research has provided evidence that early-starting, recidivist firesetters differ from their late-starting and non-firesetting peers on a number of variables, such as knowledge about fire and community complaints about the youth's firesetting (Kolko & Kazdin, 1992). High-risk firesetters differ from low-risk firesetters in that they have a greater history of fire play and higher levels of excitement about fire (Sakheim & Osborn, 1999).

Mental health problems

Relative to non-firesetting adolescents, firesetting youths evince more out-of-home placements (Bailey *et al*, 2001), including psychiatric out-patient (Moore *et al*, 1996) and residential care (Ritvo *et al*, 1983), more contact with psychologists and mental health services (Räsänen *et al*, 1995; Moore *et al* 1996; Bailey *et al*, 2001) and more contact with social services (Bailey *et al*, 2001). As well, firesetting adolescents more frequently report greater psychological distress (MacKay *et al*, 2009), self-injurious behaviour (Moore *et al*, 1996), suicidal thoughts and behaviour (Räsänen *et al*, 1995; Martin *et al*, 2004; MacKay *et al*, 2009) and alcohol and substance use problems (Räsänen *et al*, 1995; Bailey *et al*, 2001; Martin *et al*, 2004; MacKay *et al*, 2009) than their non-firesetting counterparts. Their alcohol and substance use also may be more serious in nature (Martin *et al*, 2004).

Symptoms of psychopathology, including attention-deficit hyperactivity disorder (ADHD), oppositional defiant disorder, conduct disorder, anxiety and depression, occur in greater rates in firesetting youths (Jackson *et al*, 1987; Becker *et al*, 2004; Dadds & Fraser, 2006). Conduct disorder appears to be the most common mental health diagnosis found in children and adolescents who set fires (Kolko & Kazdin, 1989*a*, 1991; Forehand *et al*, 1991; Becker *et al*, 2004; McCarty & McMahon, 2005; Dadds & Fraser, 2006; MacKay *et al*, 2006). Personality disorders, such as antisocial personality disorder and borderline personality disorder, and substance use disorders have been noted in samples of youth firesetters with court contact (Repo & Virkkunen, 1997). Maltreated firesetting youths show greater internalising and externalising psychopathology than non-maltreated firesetters (Root *et al*, 2008) and youth firesetters in residential care are more likely to have more severe externalising and internalising symptoms relative to firesetting out-patients (Pollinger *et al*, 2005). It is noteworthy that serious parental psychopathology has been reported in this population, including substance use (Becker *et al*, 2004) and maternal depression (Jacobson, 1985; Linnoila *et al*, 1989; McCarty & McMahon, 2005). Compared with individuals with minor histories of firesetting, children and adolescents with severe firesetting behaviour are characterised by lower IQ, sexual conflicts, lack of empathy, history of physical aggression, poor social judgement, anger towards a paternal caregiver and maternal rejection (Sakheim & Osborn, 1999).

Continuity of firesetting

Very few studies on the rates and correlates of firesetting continuity or recidivism have been completed. Del Bove *et al* (2008) noted a 15% firesetting recidivism rate in the 2–6 years following an initial assessment in a community sample of Italian youths, and firesetting recidivism was related to greater externalising and internalising psychopathology. MacKay *et al* (2006) reported a 26% recidivism rate in their sample of clinic-referred firesetters who received a brief intervention; a greater degree of antisocial behaviour and firesetting severity and interest at assessment predicted recidivism at follow-up. Adler *et al* (1994) reported a 40% recidivism rate in their treated sample of child and adolescent firesetters. Kolko *et al* (2001) noted a 50% rate of recidivism in their clinic sample at 2-year follow-up. The authors found that the children's initial level of covert behaviour and involvement in firesetting predicted recidivism. In a subsequent study, Kolko *et al* (2006) examined the specificity, moderators and predictors of firesetting recidivism. Fire history, fire interest/attraction and externalising behaviours were all found to predict firesetting recidivism. McCarty & McMahon (2005) found in their longitudinal study of a community sample that, compared with non-firesetters, persistent firesetters experienced a greater frequency of less appropriate and harsh discipline, physical abuse and lower parental warmth. Those who desisted from firesetting had greater academic achievement. In their sample of convicted youths and adults, Repo & Virkkunen (1997) found that 15.6% of offenders committed a new act of arson over a 6-year follow-up.

Assessment techniques

In North America, the evaluation of child and adolescent firesetters is most often undertaken by fire service professionals. One of the most well known fire service organisations, the United States Fire Administration (USFA) of the Federal Emergency Management Agency (FEMA), developed and revised the *Juvenile Firesetter Intervention Handbook* on the assessment of firesetting youths (Federal Emergency Management Agency, 1979, 1983, 2002). The FEMA programme is based on risk assessment and utilises structured interviews and questionnaires to classify youths as being at 'low', 'definite' or 'extreme' risk for further firesetting. The level of firesetting risk is used to determine the nature of recommended interventions. Specifically, youths classified as low risk are provided with fire safety education, while youths rated as definite or extreme risk are referred to mental health or other social service agencies for assistance. Determining a youth's level of risk for further firesetting is perhaps the most consistent feature of the fire service professional's work with juvenile firesetters.

The current version of the FEMA manual offers two formats for assessing firesetting risk: a comprehensive format (Comprehensive Fire Risk Evaluation) and an abbreviated format (Juvenile Firesetter Risk Survey). Both formats involve structured interviews with the youth and with a parent or caregiver. The interviews include questions about fire-specific variables (e.g., fire history and characteristics of the presenting fire) as well as questions about general psychosocial variables (e.g., behavioural, family, peer, school and trauma issues), which are combined in risk equations. Of note is that these instruments require fire service personnel to make clinical ratings of the juvenile's appearance, intelligence, mental status and psychopathology. Although the FEMA instruments have been widely used for over 30 years, there are, to date, no peer-reviewed studies on their reliability or concurrent or predictive validity (DiMillo, 1996). However, there are currently no alternative peer-reviewed instruments that have been fully validated and disseminated to assess firesetting severity or to predict firesetting recidivism.

In addition to the FEMA assessment instruments, a number of fire-specific measures are available for empirical studies of juvenile firesetters. Several instruments to assess firesetting were developed by Kolko & Kazdin through their research with children aged 6–12 years. The 14-item Firesetting History Screen (Kolko & Kazdin, 1988) evaluates the frequency of match play and firesetting in the past year and lifetime. The Firesetting Risk Interview (Kolko & Kazdin, 1989a,b) is an 86-item caregiver-completed questionnaire with eight fire-specific subscales (including Curiosity, Early experience, Fire competence, Fire knowledge and Exposure) and seven general factors (e.g., Supervision/discipline, Frequency of harsh punishment). Additionally, the Fire Incident Analysis (Kolko & Kazdin, 1991, 1994) provides a quantitative assessment of a specific fire incident. This tool asks 50 questions from four broad domains about the fire incident itself, behavioural and emotional correlates in the 2 weeks preceding the incident, motivations for the fire, and consequences of the fire.

MacKay and colleagues also have developed a battery of fire-specific assessment tools (MacKay et al, 2004; Henderson et al, 2006). The Fire Involvement Interview (FII; MacKay et al, 2006; Root et al, 2008) is a semi-structured interview that can be used to obtain detailed information about a youth's past and current fire involvement (e.g., specific information about frequency, versatility and age of onset). The Fire Interest Questionnaire (FIQ; MacKay et al, 2006, 2009) measures fire interest and fire-related behaviours and is completed independently by the youth and his or her caregiver. MacKay and colleagues also developed a fire-specific Stroop task to provide an experimental measure of fire interest (Gallagher-Duffy et al, 2009). Indices of fire-specific behaviours (e.g., age of onset, frequency, versatility, interest) derived from these instruments have been found to predict firesetting recidivism in youths. Additionally, MacKay & Henderson (2009) designed the Fire Involvement Risk Evaluator for Youth (FIRE-Y). This tool identifies and operationalises the fire-specific risk factors to be evaluated. Additionally, it provides a structured format for mental health professionals to organise this information to assist their clinical judgements about an individual's firesetting risk as well as the targets for intervention. Preliminary evidence from their clinical research programme indicates that the probability of firesetting recidivism is related to the cumulative number of fire-specific risk factors present.

Recently, Robert Stadolnik developed the Firesetting Risk Assessment Tool for Youth (FRAT-Y; Stadolnik, 2010). The FRAT-Y may be used with children aged 5–17 and, similar to the MacKay & Henderson (2009) tool, is completed by a mental health clinician at the end of an assessment to organise information collected during the assessment and to make a rating of estimated risk (low, moderate or high). The tool also allows clinicians to assign primary and secondary firesetting motivations and guides them in identifying appropriate intervention and treatment recommendations for the child and family.

Information about a youth's fire-related history, interest and firesetting incidents is important for understanding firesetting behaviour and aids in the estimation of risk for further firesetting behaviour. Although several instruments are available to evaluate fire-specific factors, research on their diagnostic and prognostic reliability and validity is still limited. Therefore, it is important that existing fire-specific instruments be used in conjunction with standardised measures of youth and family psychosocial functioning to ensure a comprehensive and valid summary of the youth's mental health. Ideally, a comprehensive assessment of a firesetting child or youth will incorporate an evaluation of general psychosocial risk factors in addition to fire-specific factors. From a clinical perspective, case formulation and planning involve understanding the broad psychosocial context as well as the history and specifics of the firesetting itself.

Interventions for youth firesetting

In response to the negative consequences of firesetting, many communities in North America and the UK have developed and implemented interventions for children and adolescents who set fires. The most common intervention is fire safety education (FSE), which is provided by fire service professionals (Bumpass *et al*, 1985; Kolko, 1988; Adler *et al*, 1994; Johnstone *et al*, 2004; Palmer *et al*, 2007). Some communities offer multi-modal, firesetting-specific treatment programmes that include a psychological intervention. These treatments typically involve two components: a psychological intervention, typically behavioural therapy or cognitive–behavioural therapy (CBT), that targets actual firesetting behaviour and problem areas of child and family mental health functioning; and an educational intervention in the form of FSE (Bumpass *et al*, 1985; Adler *et al*, 1994; Kolko, 2001). Case studies using multi-component psychological treatments were the stepping stones to the mental health treatments delivered today (McGrath *et al*, 1979; Koles & Jenson, 1985; Cox-Jones *et al*, 1990). These case studies included satiation, contingency management, social skills training, relaxation and FSE to eliminate firesetting behaviour. Aside from satiation, recent treatments tend to incorporate many of these same techniques as well as CBT-based methods to promote new cognitive and behavioural skills to address the deficits exhibited by juvenile firesetters and their caregivers (MacKay *et al*, 2004; Kolko *et al*, 2006). Firesetting treatments are often administered by mental health professionals but also sometimes by fire service professionals (e.g., Adler *et al*, 1994). It remains to be determined what type and level of professional training is required to successfully implement firesetting interventions of a psychological nature, as no research is available on this topic.

A need for collaborative, multi-modal treatments

In their national survey of fire intervention programmes in England and Wales, Palmer *et al* (2007) noted that, although there is a lack of established treatments for firesetters, practice appeared to be at its best when firesetting interventions were collaborative and made use of information-sharing protocols between agencies, such as partnerships between fire and rescue services and youth offending services. It has also been argued that multidisciplinary interventions that are collaborative across community agencies are likely to have the greatest impact in serving children and families with complex needs, prompting calls for a multi-agency approach that includes the fire service as well as mental health and child welfare agencies (Kolko, 2002; Lambie *et al*, 2002; McCarty & McMahon, 2005; Putnam & Kirkpatrick, 2005; Henderson *et al*, 2006; Sharp *et al*, 2006).

A survey of juvenile firesetting interventions in North America found that while most programmes consist of a firesetting risk assessment (88%) and at least one session of FSE, almost half of the programmes also provided access to mental health components such as brief counselling with the child or caregivers (Kolko *et al*, 2008). Of these, 30% provided access to short-term counselling and 24% provided extended therapy. Some programmes provided group counselling, specialised restitution, residential treatment, special graphing techniques (see 'Review of treatment studies' below), satiation or mentoring.

After identifying a broad array of risk factors for persistent youth firesetting, including characteristics from the child, family and parenting domains, McCarty & McMahon (2005) highlighted the need for multi-component interventions to adequately address the needs associated with these broad risk factors. The authors noted that FSE interventions will often need to be supplemented with general mental health interventions, such as CBT, to address child externalising problems, and parent training, to address parental factors such as disciplinary strategies. There is evidence to suggest that a combination of parent management training and CBT interventions for children and adolescents with disruptive behaviours is more effective than the application of either component delivered alone (Kazdin *et al*, 1992).

Review of treatment studies

Although treatment outcome studies have been completed for children and adolescents with externalising behaviour problems such as disruptive behaviour and conduct disorder (Estrada & Pinsof, 1995; Feinfeld & Baker, 2004; Kazdin & Wassell, 2000), empirical investigations of interventions for juvenile firesetters are rare. Notably, there are no peer-reviewed studies that specifically examine treatment outcomes for adolescent firesetters. Therefore, the efficacy of fire service, mental health or collaborative/ combined approaches for this age group remains unknown. The available evidence on treatment effectiveness has come from studies of children under the age of 13 (Bumpass *et al*, 1985; Kolko *et al*, 2006) or from studies using combined child and adolescent samples (Bumpass *et al*, 1983; Adler *et al*, 1994). The first treatment studies that appeared in the literature that went beyond single case reports (Adler *et al*, 1994; Bumpass *et al*, 1985) reinforced the primary role of the fire service in dealing with juvenile firesetters by showing decreased firesetting as the result of fire service interventions.

One early study reported on a new firesetting prevention programme used by the Dallas Fire Department (Bumpass *et al*, 1985). The programme was both administered and run by fire service professionals. Its main component was a psychological technique called 'graphing', which was intended to help firesetting youths recognise the association between events that trigger firesetting and feelings that lead to firesetting behaviour. The study found that, after the first year of the programme, only 2% of participants had set subsequent fires, marking a substantial reduction from the 32% recidivism rate found for 198 youth firesetters treated over the 3 years before the new programme was implemented. While the programme appears to have been effective in preventing the recurrence of firesetting, the study did not use a controlled design and it lacked long-term follow-up. Nevertheless, the work by Bumpass *et al* (1983, 1985) was important because it provided some of the first empirical data showing that fire department interventions could significantly reduce firesetting recidivism in youths. Additionally, it provided initial support for the therapeutic use of systematic interviewing and analysis of the events and feelings involved in a firesetting sequence.

An Australian study subsequently examined a multi-modal intervention programme for firesetting children and adolescents (Adler *et al*, 1994). The brief control condition consisted of fire safety information given to caregivers in the form of a pamphlet. The experimental condition consisted of two or three sessions of home intervention comprising FSE, a behaviour-modification component taught to parents and the Bumpass graphing procedure, all administered by a trained fire service professional. This study found a significant decrease in the frequency and severity of firesetting in both groups over the 12 months after the intervention was completed. The mean rate of firesetting for the entire sample fell from 7.1 fires in the year before referral to 1.5 fires in the 12 months after participants had joined the programme. However, there were no significant differences found between the control condition and the experimental condition. That is, participation in the fire service 'psychological' intervention provided no additional improvement. Despite significant design limitations (e.g., no tracking of treatment fidelity in the experimental condition), the study is important as it was the first controlled study to report that brief intervention by fire service professionals can have an impact on firesetting, even for youths with serious recurrent firesetting. However, it is worth emphasising that the rate of firesetting during follow-up was 40% (40/99), underscoring the recurrent nature of juvenile firesetting despite intervention, brief or otherwise.

A third firesetting intervention study was conducted with hospitalised young children in the USA (Kolko *et al*, 1991). A brief CBT group-based intervention focusing on fire safety and prevention skills training comprising instruction and practice in fire safety concepts and preventive activities was found to be more effective than individual fire assessment and awareness discussions with a nurse in reducing fire involvement and increasing fire safety knowledge post-training and at 6-month follow-up, according to parental reports (Kolko *et al*, 1991).

Kolko (2001) subsequently completed the first and only randomised clinical trial to date comparing FSE and CBT interventions with a control intervention. The study sample included children up to the age of 13 years who were referred to a clinic for their firesetting. Referred firesetters and their parents were randomly assigned to either an FSE condition, comprising eight sessions of instruction in fire safety and prevention skills by trained fire service personnel, or a CBT condition consisting of eight sessions of trained mental health professionals providing youths with exposure to the graphing technique and instruction in problem-solving skills and parents with instruction on the motives of firesetting, the promotion of pro-social activities and behaviour management principles. These conditions were then compared with a brief intervention designed to parallel 'routine service', consisting of a two-contact home visit by a firefighter. Improvements were found in all three intervention groups post-intervention and at 1-year follow-up; however, while FSE and CBT were both more efficacious than the home visit at reducing the frequency of reported fires post-intervention, CBT was only marginally better. Of note, the FSE in this study provided more intensive, structured and monitored training of fire safety skills than is typically provided by the fire service in its FSE interventions. This could explain why the FSE and CBT conditions showed similar results. Nevertheless, follow-up data from this study indicated that the recidivism rate for juvenile firesetting is substantial (15–24%), even after multi-session intervention. Additionally, and in contrast to the findings of Adler *et al* (1994), while the brief fire service intervention was followed by some reduction (50%) in firesetting recidivism, the skills-focused and manualised multi-session FSE and CBT treatments produced significantly better outcomes.

In a follow-up to the Kolko (2001) study, Kolko *et al* (2006) examined moderators, specificity and predictors of firesetting recidivism. They found that FSE exerted specific effects on knowledge about fire and fire safety skills, whereas CBT tended to show specific effects only on problem-solving skills. Exposure to fire models/materials, the child's general fire knowledge and family functioning were suggested as moderators of the effects of FSE and CBT in an exploratory analysis. Fire history, fire interest/attraction and externalising behaviours were found to be predictors of firesetting recidivism. Follow-up analyses provided preliminary evidence that fire-specific as well as general mental health factors are important mediators and moderators of treatment outcome. Additional study of these factors and their remediation may lead to improvements in intervention programmes for juvenile firesetting.

Case examples

Three brief case vignettes, in the form of fictional case notes, are provided to help illustrate the heterogeneity of cases that present with youth firesetting and the different intervention approaches that may be used.

Example 1

The evaluation of fire-specific factors reveals the presence of one or two episodes of fire involvement that are of relatively recent onset and there is no indication of malicious intent to damage property or injure persons. The fire involvement appears to have occurred without much forethought or planning and when ignition materials were easily accessible to the child. A brief general mental screen indicates the absence of other problem behaviours and risk factors for childhood psychopathology, such as parental psychopathology or maltreatment. The parent appears to be concerned about the fire involvement and motivated to do what is necessary to ensure that further fire episodes do not occur. The child appears to be remorseful and states that he will not set another fire. Typically, this type of case will respond well to a brief educational intervention provided by trained fire service professionals. The fire safety education should focus on the active learning of fire safety rules and procedures by child and caregiver and a home safety check should ensure that the home is fire safe in case another fire should occur and act as a strong message to the child and family that fire safety is important.

Example 2

The evaluation of fire-specific factors reveals more than two fire incidents that involved different ignition materials, targets and locations. Planning or intent to cause damage or harm is evident. Heightened fire interest and fire involvement have been sustained over a period of time. Ignition materials are freely available in the home as family members and the youth smoke. The child and caregiver feel that intervention is not necessary and do not appear to appreciate the danger the firesetting behaviour presents. The general mental health screen suggests the presence of other problem behaviours (some antisocial behaviours) in the child and risk factors for childhood psychopathology (poor parental monitoring). Typically, this type of case will respond best to a collaborative fire service intervention combined with a brief mental health intervention. The mental health intervention will focus first on motivating the youth and caregiver to work on preventing further fire involvement. The caregiver and youth will benefit from psychoeducation about the precipitants, concomitants and reinforcers of youth firesetting. Negative outcomes like burn injury and involvement in the juvenile justice system may need to be highlighted. Functional analysis of the fire history will be used to identify and provide personalised feedback about the precipitants and reinforcing consequences of the fire involvement as well as to identify treatment targets and strategies for reducing the probability of further occurrences. Caregiver strategies will focus on clear rules about fire involvement, monitoring of fire-related behaviours as well as rewarding fire-safe behaviours and setting out the negative consequences for inappropriate fire-related behaviours. Child strategies will focus on impulse control and problem-solving, with past fire incidents as the context in which to embed and practise skills.

Example 3

The youth presents with dangerous fire involvement (a single serious fire start but multiple and long-standing firesetting, with extreme fire fascination) and poor motivation to change, as well as a lack of remorse and understanding of the dangerousness of the firesetting behaviour. There are indications of serious individual psychopathology (e.g., aggression, substance misuse, psychopathy, emotion dysregulation, obsessional preoccupation with fire) and caregiver psychopathology (e.g., substance misuse, maltreatment). The family requires immediate intervention to manage the risk of burn injury to self or others. Procedures for ensuring a safe home in which access to ignition materials and opportunities for further firesetting are eliminated are paramount. The youth and caregiver require specialised treatment to address the concurrent mental health and substance misuse issues as well as fire-specific treatment. Accountability for further fire involvement will be an important component.

Summary and future directions

Despite the significant and devastating costs of firesetting by children and youths, the subject has received relatively little empirical investigation. Although studies suggest a link between firesetting in childhood and adolescence and adult firesetting, an understanding of the life span trajectories of firesetting has yet to be established. Prospective longitudinal studies following child firesetters into adulthood would provide insight into the development and continuity of firesetting. Further research on the role of general mental health factors and fire-specific factors in the onset and maintenance of firesetting is of both theoretical and practical importance, as are studies to evaluate the efficacy of various methods and tools for evaluating firesetting risk and intervention approaches for firesetting youths. The high recidivism rates cited in existing empirical studies raise questions about the relative efficacy of popular firesetting intervention and treatment programmes and highlight the need for more outcome data.

The specific effects of different treatment components on treatment outcomes also remain unclear. Although reductions in firesetting recidivism and severity have been reported subsequent to brief as well as more intensive fire service and mental health interventions, more research evaluating the strengths and weaknesses of these interventions is clearly warranted. Efficacious intervention may better relate to the quality and extent of training and the use and monitoring of empirically based interventions rather than the professional discipline delivering the intervention. Given the multiple vulnerabilities of firesetting youths and their caregivers, empirically supported risk assessment protocols and intervention programmes are sorely needed.

References

Achenbach, T. M. & Edelbrock, C. S. (1981) Behavior problems and competencies reported by parents of normal and disturbed children aged four through sixteen. *Monographs of the Society for Research*, **46**, 1–82.

Adler, R. G., Nunn, R. J., Northham, E. A., *et al* (1994) Secondary prevention of childhood firesetting. *Journal of the American Academy of Child and Adolescent Psychiatry*, **33**, 1194–1202.

American Psychiatric Association (1994) *Diagnostic and Statistical Manual of Mental Disorders* (4th edn) (DSM-IV). APA.

American Psychiatric Association (2000) *Diagnostic and Statistical Manual of Mental Disorders* (4th edn, text revision) (DSM-IV-TR). APA.

Arson Prevention Bureau (2006) *Arson Control Forum Annual Report*. At http://www.communities.gov.uk/documents/fire/pdf/154145.pdf (accessed 20th December 2010).

Bailey, S., Smith, C. & Dolan, M. (2001) The social background and nature of 'children' who perpetrate violent crimes: a UK perspective. *Journal of Community Psychology*, **29**, 305–317.

Becker, K. D., Stuewig, J., Herrera, V., *et al* (2004) A study of firesetting and animal cruelty in children: family influences and adolescent outcomes. *Journal of the American Academy of Child and Adolescent Psychiatry*, **43**, 905–912.

Block, J. H., Block, J. & Folkman, W. S. (1976) *Fire and Children: Learning Survival Skills*. US Department of Agriculture.

Bradford, J. M. W. (1982) Arson: a clinical study. *Canadian Journal of Psychiatry*, **27**, 188–193.

Bradford, J. & Dimock, J. (1986) A comparative study of adolescents and adults who wilfully set fires. *Psychiatric Journal of the University of Ottawa*, **11**, 228–234.

Bumpass, E. R., Fagelman, F. D. & Brix, R. J. (1983) Intervention with children who set fires. *American Journal of Psychotherapy*, **37**, 328–345.

Bumpass, E. R., Brix, R. & Preston, D. A. (1985) A community-based program for juvenile firesetters. *Hospital Community Psychiatry*, **36**, 529–533.

Canadian Centre for Justice Statistics (2004) *Canadian Crime Statistics 2003*. Canadian Centre for Justice Statistics.

Chen, Y. H., Arria, A. M. & Anthony, J. C. (2003) Firesetting in adolescence and being aggressive, shy, and rejected by peers: new epidemiologic evidence from a national sample survey. *Journal of the American Academy of Psychiatry and the Law*, **31**, 44–52.

Cole, R. E., Grolnick, W. S., Laurenitis, L. R., *et al* (1986) *Children and Fire: Rochester Fire-Related Youth Project Progress Report*. University of Rochester.

Cox-Jones, C., Lubetsky, M. J., Fultz, S. A., *et al* (1990) Inpatient psychiatric treatment of a young recidivist firesetter. *Journal of American Academy of Child and Adolescent Psychiatry*, **29**, 936–941.

Dadds, M. R. & Fraser, J. A. (2006) Fire interest, fire setting and psychopathology in Australian children: a normative study. *Australian and New Zealand Journal of Psychiatry*, **40**, 581–586.

Del Bove, G. D., Caprara, G. V., Pastorelli, C., *et al* (2008) Juvenile firesetting in Italy: relationship to aggression, psychopathology, personality, self-efficacy, and school functioning. *European Journal of Child and Adolescent Psychiatry*, **17**, 235–244.

DiMillo, J. (1996) *Children and Fire: 'A Bad Match'. A Juvenile Firesetter Intervention Program Developed for the State of Maine*. Portland Fire Department.

Estrada, A. U. & Pinsof, W. M. (1995) The effectiveness of family therapies for selected behavioural disorders of childhood. *Journal of Marital and Family Therapy*, **21**, 403–440.

Farrington, D. P. & Welsh, B. C. (2007) *Saving Children from a Life of Crime: Early Risk Factors and Effective Interventions*. Oxford University Press.

Federal Emergency Management Agency (1979) *Interviewing and Counseling Juvenile Firesetters*. US Government Printing Office.

Federal Emergency Management Agency (1983) *Juvenile Firesetter Intervention Handbook: Dealing with Children Ages 7–14*. US Government Printing Office.

Federal Emergency Management Agency (2002) *Juvenile Firesetter Intervention Handbook*. US Government Printing Office.

Feinfeld, K. A. & Baker, B. L. (2004) Empirical support for a treatment program for families of young children with externalizing problems. *Journal of Clinical Child and Adolescent Psychology*, **33**, 182–195.

Fineman, K. R. (1980) Firesetting in childhood and adolescence. *Psychiatric Clinics of North America*, **3**, 483–500.

Fineman, K. R. (1995) A model for the qualitative analysis of child and adult fire deviant behavior. *American Journal of Forensic Psychology*, **13**, 31–60.

Forehand, R., Wierson, M., Frame, C. L., *et al* (1991) Juvenile firesetting: a unique syndrome or an advanced level of antisocial behavior? *Behaviour Research and Therapy*, **29**, 125–128.

Freud, S. (1932) The acquisition of power over fire. *International Journal of Psychoanalysis*, **13**, 405–410.

Gallagher-Duffy, J., MacKay, S., Duffy, J., *et al* (2009) The Pictorial Fire Stroop: a measure of processing bias for fire-related stimuli. *Journal of Abnormal Child Psychology*, **37**, 1165–1176.

Gannon, T. A. & Pina, A. (2010) Firesetting: psychopathology, theory and treatment. *Aggression and Violent Behavior*, **15**, 224–238.

Gaynor, J. (1996) Firesetting. In *Child and Adolescent Psychiatry: A Comprehensive Textbook* (2nd edn) (ed. M. Lewis), pp. 591–603. Williams & Wilkins.

Gelhorn, H., Hartman, C., Sakai, J., *et al* (2009) An item response theory analysis of DSM-IV conduct disorder. *Journal of the American Academy of Child and Adolescent Psychiatry*, **48**, 42–50.

Grolnick, W., Cole, R., Laurentis, L., *et al* (1990) Playing with fire: a developmental assessment of children's fire understanding and experience. *Journal of Clinical Child Psychology*, **19**, 128–135.

Hall, J. R., Jr (2005) *Fire in the US and the United Kingdom*. National Fire Protection Association.

Hanson, M., MacKay-Soroka, S., Staley, S., *et al* (1994) Delinquent fire-setters: a comparative study of delinquency and fire-setting histories. *Canadian Journal of Psychiatry*, **39**, 230–232.

Hawkins, J. D., Herrenkohl, T., Farrington, D. P., *et al* (1998) A review of predictors of youth violence. In *Serious and Violent Juvenile Offenders: Risk Factors and Successful Interventions* (eds R. Loeber & D. P. Farrington), pp. 106–146. Sage.

Heath, G. A., Hardesty, V. A., Goldfine, P. E., *et al* (1983) Childhood firesetting: an empirical study. *Journal of the American Academy of Child Psychiatry*, **22**, 370–374.

Henderson, J. L., MacKay, S. & Peterson-Badali, M. (2006) Closing the research–practice gap: factors affecting adoption and implementation of a children's mental health program. *Journal of Clinical Child and Adolescent Psychology*, **35**, 2–12.

Jackson, H. F., Hope, S. & Glass, C. (1987) Why are arsonists not violent offenders? *International Journal of Offender Therapy and Comparative Criminology*, **31**, 143–151.

Jacobson, R. R. (1985) Child firesetters: a clinical investigation. *Journal of Child Psychology and Psychiatry and Allied Disciplines*, **26**, 759–768.

Johnstone, J., Gilbert, K., MacKay, S., *et al* (2004) *TAPP-C Fire Service Educator's Manual: A Guide for Stopping Juvenile Firesetting in the Community*. Centre for Addiction and Mental Health Press.

Jones, K. & Jackson, M. (1999) *Youth Firesetting Intervention Program 1996–1999 Overview*. Surrey Fire Service.

Kafry, D. (1978) *Fire Survival Skill: Who Plays With Matches?* US Department of Agriculture.

Kaufman, I., Heims, L. & Reiser, D. (1961) A re-evaluation of the psychodynamics of firesetting. *American Journal of Orthopsychiatry*, **31**, 123–136.

Kazdin, A. E. & Wassell, G. (2000) Therapeutic changes in children, parents and families resulting from treatment of children with conduct problems. *Journal of the American Academy of Child and Adolescent Psychiatry*, **39**, 414–420.

Kazdin, A. E., Siegel, T. C. & Bass, D. (1992) Cognitive problem-solving skills training and parent management training in the treatment of antisocial behavior in children. *Journal of Consulting and Clinical Psychology*, **60**, 733–747.

Kelso, J. & Stewart, M. A. (1986) Factors which predict the persistence of aggressive conduct disorder. *Journal of Child Psychology and Psychiatry*, **27**, 77–86.

Koles, M. & Jensen, W. (1985) Comprehensive treatment of chronic fire-setting in a severely disordered boy. *Journal of Behavioural Therapy and Experimental Psychiatry*, **16**, 81–85.

Kolko, D. J. (1985) Juvenile firesetting: a review and methodological critique. *Clinical Psychology Review*, **5**, 345–376.

Kolko, D. J. (1988) Community interventions for juvenile firesetters: a survey of two national programs. *Hospital and Community Psychiatry*, **39**, 973–979.

Kolko, D. J. (2001) Efficacy of cognitive–behavioral treatment and fire safety education for children who set fires: initial and follow-up outcomes. *Journal of Child Psychology and Psychiatry*, **42**, 359–369.

Kolko, D. J. (2002) *Handbook on Firesetting in Children and Youth*. Academic Press.

Kolko, D. J. & Kazdin, A. E. (1986) A conceptualization of firesetting in children and adolescents. *Journal of Abnormal Child Psychology*, **14**, 49–61.

Kolko, D. J. & Kazdin, A. E. (1988) Prevalence of firesetting and related behaviors among child psychiatric patients. *Journal of Consulting and Clinical Psychology*, **56**, 628–630.

Kolko, D. J. & Kazdin, A. E. (1989*a*) Assessment of dimensions of childhood firesetting among child psychiatric patients and nonpatients. *Journal of Abnormal Child Psychology*, **17**, 157–176.

Kolko, D. J. & Kazdin, A. E. (1989*b*) The Children's Firesetting Interview with psychiatrically referred and nonreferred children. *Journal of Abnormal Child Psychology*, **17**, 609–624.

Kolko, D. J. & Kazdin, A. E. (1991) Motives of childhood firesetters: firesetting characteristics and psychological correlates. *Journal of Child Psychology and Psychiatry*, **32**, 535–550.

Kolko, D. J. & Kazdin, A. E. (1992) The emergence and recurrence of child firesetting: a one-year prospective study. *Journal of Abnormal Child Psychology*, **20**, 17–37.

Kolko, D. J. & Kazdin, A. E. (1994) Children's descriptions of their firesetting incidents: characteristics and relationship to recidivism. *Journal of the American Academy of Child and Adolescent Psychiatry*, **33**, 114–122.

Kolko, D. J., Watson, S. & Faust, J. (1991) Fire safety/prevention skills training to reduce involvement with fire in young psychiatric inpatients: preliminary findings. *Behavior Therapy*, **22**, 269–284.

Kolko, D. J., Day, B. T., Bridge, J. A., *et al* (2001) Two-year prediction of children's firesetting in clinically referred and nonreferred samples. *Journal of Child Psychology and Psychiatry and Allied Disciplines*, **42**, 371–380.

Kolko, D. J., Herschell, A. D. & Scharf, D. M. (2006) Education and treatment for boys who set fires: specificity, moderators, and predictors of recidivism. *Journal of Emotional and Behavioral Disorders*, **14**, 227–239.

Kolko, D. J., Scharf, D. M., Herschell, A. D., *et al* (2008) A survey of juvenile firesetter intervention programs in North America: overall description and comparison of independent vs. coalition-based programs. *American Journal of Forensic Psychology*, **26**, 41–66.

Lahey, B. B., Applegate, B., Barkley, R. A., *et al* (1994) DSM-IV field trials for oppositional defiant disorder and conduct disorder in children and adolescents. *American Journal of Psychiatry*, **151**, 1163–1171.

Lambie, I., McCardle, S. & Coleman, R. (2002) Where there's smoke there's fire: firesetting behaviour in children and adolescents. *New Zealand Journal of Psychology*, **31**, 73–78.

Leschied, A., Chiodo, D., Nowicki, E., *et al* (2008) Childhood predictors of adult criminality: a meta-analysis drawn from the prospective longitudinal literature. *Canadian Journal of Criminology and Criminal Justice*, **50**, 435–467.

Lewis, N. O. C. & Yarnell, H. (1951) *Pathological Firesetting (Pyromania)*. Nervous and Mental Disease Monographs no. 82. Coolidge Foundation.

Linnoila, M., De Jong, J. & Virkkunen, M. (1989) Family history of alcoholism in violent offenders and impulsive fire setters. *Archives of General Psychiatry*, **46**, 613–616.

Lipsey, M. W. & Derzon, J. H. (1998) Predictors of violent or serious delinquency in adolescence and early adulthood: a synthesis of longitudinal research. In *Serious and Violent Juvenile Offenders: Risk Factors and Successful Interventions* (eds R. Loeber & D. P. Farrington), pp. 86–105. Sage.

Loeber, R., Wung, P., Keenan, K., *et al* (1993) Developmental pathways in disruptive child behavior. *Development and Psychopathology*, **5**, 103–133.

MacKay, S. & Henderson, J. (2009) A brief actuarial tool to predict firesetting recidivism in youth. Poster presented at the annual meeting of the American Academy of Child and Adolescent Psychiatry, Honolulu, HI.

MacKay, S., Henderson, J., Root, C., *et al* (2004) *TAPP-C Clinician's Manual for Preventing and Treating Juvenile Fire Involvement*. Centre for Addiction and Mental Health Press.

MacKay, S., Henderson, J., Del Bove, G., *et al* (2006) Fire interest and antisociality as risk factors in the severity and persistence of juvenile firesetting. *Journal of the American Academy of Child and Adolescent Psychiatry*, **45**, 1077–1084.

MacKay, S., Paglia-Boak, A., Henderson, J., *et al* (2009) Epidemiology of firesetting in adolescents: mental health and substance use correlates. *Journal of Child Psychology and Psychiatry*, **50**, 1282–1290.

MacKay, S., Feldberg, A., Ward, A. K., *et al* (2011) Research and practice in adolescent firesetting. *Criminal Justice and Behavior* (in press).

Martin, G., Bergen, H. A., Richardson, A. S., *et al* (2004) Correlates of firesetting in a community sample of young adolescents. *Australian and New Zealand Journal of Psychiatry*, **38**, 148–154.

McCarty, C. A. & McMahon, R. J. (2005) Domains of risk in the developmental continuity of fire setting. *Behavior Therapy*, **36**, 185–195.

McGrath, P., Marshall, P. & Prior, K. (1979) A comprehensive treatment program for a fire setting child. *Journal of Behavioural Therapy and Experimental Psychiatry*, **10**, 69–72.

Moore, J. K., Thompson-Pope, S. K. & Whited, R. M. (1996) MMPI-A profile of adolescent boys with a history of firesetting. *Journal of Personality Assessment*, **67**, 116–126.

Nurcombe, B. (1964) Children who set fires. *Medical Journal of Australia*, **i**, 579–584.

Office of the Ontario Fire Marshal (2009) *Ontario Fire Incident Summary 2000–2009*. At http://www.ofm.gov.on.ca/en/Media%20Relations%20and%20Resources/Statistics/All%20Fire%20Incidents.asp (accessed 20 December 2010).

Palmer, E. J., Caulfield, L. S. & Hollin, C. R. (2007) Interventions with arsonists and young fire setters: a survey of the national picture in England and Wales. *Legal and Criminological Psychology*, **12**, 101–116.

Patterson, G. R. (1982) *A Social Learning Approach. Vol. 3: Coercive Family Process*. Castalia Publishing.

Patterson, G. R. & Dishion, T. J. (1985) Contribution of families and peers to delinquency. *Criminology*, **23**, 63–79.

Patterson, G. R., Reid, J. B. & Dishion, T. J. (1992) *A Social Learning Approach. Vol. 4: Antisocial Boys*. Castalia Publishing.

Perrin-Wallqvist, R. & Norlander, T. (2003) Firesetting and playing with fire during childhood and adolescence: interview studies of 18-year-old male draftees and 18–19-year-old female pupils. *Legal and Criminal Psychology*, **8**, 151–157.

Pollack-Nelson, C., Faranda, D. M., Porth, D., *et al* (2006) Parents of preschool fire setters: perceptions of the child-play fire hazard. *International Journal of Injury Control and Safety Promotion*, **13**, 171–177.

Pollinger, J., Samuels, L. & Stadolnik, R. (2005) A comparative study of the behavioral, personality, and fire history characteristics of residential and outpatient adolescents (ages 12–17) with firesetting behaviors. *Adolescence*, **40**, 345–353.

Putnam, C. T. & Kirkpatrick, J. T. (2005) Juvenile firesetting: a research overview. *Juvenile Justice Bulletin*, May, 1–7.

Ramsey, E., Patterson, G. R. & Walker, H. M. (1990) Generalization of the antisocial trait from home to school settings. *Journal of Applied Developmental Psychology*, **11**, 209–223.

Räsänen, P., Hirvenoja, R., Hakko, H., *et al* (1995) A portrait of the juvenile arsonist. *Forensic Science International*, **73**, 41–47.

Repo, E. & Virkkunen, M. (1997) Young arsonists: history of conduct disorder, psychiatric diagnoses and criminal recidivism. *Journal of Forensic Psychiatry*, **8**, 311–320.

Rice, M. E. & Harris, G. T. (1991) Firesetters admitted to a maximum security psychiatric institution: offenders and offenses. *Journal of Interpersonal Violence*, **6**, 461–475.

Ritvo, E., Shanok, S. S. & Lewis, D. O. (1983) Firesetting and nonfiresetting delinquents: a comparison of neuropsychiatric, psychoeducational, experiential and behavioural characteristics. *Child Psychiatry and Human Development*, **113**, 259–267.

Root, C., MacKay, S., Henderson, J., *et al* (2008) The link between maltreatment and juvenile firesetting: correlates and underlying mechanisms. *Child Abuse and Neglect*, **32**, 161–176.

Sakheim, G. A. & Osborn, E. (1999) Severe vs. nonsevere firesetters revisited. *Child Welfare*, **78**, 411–434.

Sakheim, G. A., Vigdor, M., Gordon, M., *et al* (1985) A psychological profile of juvenile firesetters in residential treatment. *Child Welfare*, **64**, 453–476.

Sharp, D. L., Blaakman, S. W., Cole, E. C., *et al* (2006) Evidence-based multidisciplinary strategies for working with children who set fires. *Journal of the American Psychiatric Nurses Association*, **11**, 329–337.

Showers, J. & Pickrell, E. (1987) Child firesetters: a study of three populations. *Hospital and Community Psychiatry*, **38**, 495–501.

Slavkin, M. (2001) Enuresis, firesetting, and cruelty to animals: does the ego triad show predictive validity? *Adolescence*, **36**, 461–466.

Snyder, H. N. (1999) *Juvenile Arrests 1999*. US Department of Justice.

Snyder, H. N. (2008) *Juvenile Arrests 2006*. US Department of Justice.

Sparber, A. (2005) Juvenile firesetters. *Journal of Child and Adolescent Psychiatric Nursing*, **18**, 93.

Stadolnik, R. (2010) *Firesetting Risk Assessment Tool for Youth (FRAT-Y): Professional Manual.* FirePsych, Inc.

Stewart, M. A. & Culver, K. W. (1982) Children who set fires: the clinical picture and a follow-up. *British Journal of Psychiatry*, **140**, 357–363.

Stickle, T. R. & Blechman, E. A. (2002) Aggression and fire: antisocial behavior in firesetting and nonfiresetting juvenile offenders. *Journal of Psychopathology and Behavioral Assessment*, **24**, 177–193.

Strachan, J. G. (1981) Conspicuous firesetting in children. *British Journal of Psychiatry*, **138**, 26–29.

Vreeland, R. G. & Levin, B. M. (1980) Psychological aspects of firesetting. In *Fires and Human Behaviour* (ed. D. Canter), pp. 31–46. Wiley.

Webb, N., Sakheim, G., Towns-Miranda, L., *et al* (1990) Collaborative treatment of juvenile firesetters: assessment and outreach. *American Journal of Orthopsychiatry*, **60**, 305–309.

World Health Organization (2007) *International Statistical Classification of Diseases and Related Health Problems* (10th edn). WHO. At http://apps.who.int/classifications/apps/icd/icd10online (accessed 20 December 2010).

CHAPTER 6

Intellectual disability and arson

John Devapriam and Sabyasachi Bhaumik

Arson and other offending behaviours by people with intellectual disability are recognised to be a significant problem for healthcare and social care services and the criminal justice system. There is a lack of robust research evidence and guidance for assessment and treatment procedures for this group of individuals. There has always been an uncertainty in defining who these individuals are and establishing what works for them. Few studies have examined the characteristics of offenders with intellectual disability, especially in relation to arson. The difficulties in attempting to study the characteristics of offenders in this population are due to changing definitions of the terms 'intellectual disability' and 'offending behaviour'. This is compounded by the shifting attitudes of society, the reactionary political agenda towards public safety (Thornicroft & Szmukler, 2005) and the reaction and tolerance levels of carers to the behaviour of people with intellectual disabilities (Lyall *et al*, 1995) which may be deemed to be challenging or criminal, depending on the context and seriousness of the behaviours concerned. There are also ongoing changes in the criminal justice system (CJS), highlighted below, and several other factors that affect those who are labelled as 'offenders with intellectual disability' (Barron *et al*, 2002). The other limitations in interpreting research findings are that the numbers of offenders with intellectual disability are small even in larger, general cohorts of offenders and that studies specifically of offenders with intellectual disability have small sample sizes (Johnston & Halstead, 2000).

Background

History has provided us with some useful insights into the association between the concepts of intellectual disability and offending and challenging behaviour. In the 14th century people who were subnormal were called 'idiots' and were considered not to blame for their crimes, and in the 17th century people were acquitted of crimes on the basis of their cognitive difficulties (Walker & McCabe, 1968). In the early 20th century, the eugenics movement resulted from scientific theories that were used to imply a causal link between 'feeble mindedness' and criminality. This resulted in distorting effects on the political agenda, prejudices and preconceptions, and eventually in social programmes like negative eugenics and voluntary sterilisation. This problem was compounded by the enactment of the Mental Deficiency Act 1913, which increased the segregation and isolation of those with intellectual disability. More recently, the changes to the mental health legislation for England and Wales (Mental Health Act 1983 (amended 2007)) have shown that lessons from history have not been learnt. First, the Act made powers available to ensure that patients continue to comply with treatment while in the community. Second, the Act made it easier to admit and detain those with psychopathic disorder and deemed 'untreatable'. Third, the Act provided safeguards for the detention and treatment of people who lack capacity as an alternative to compulsory admission under the Mental Health Act 1983. Critics of the draft Bill argued that the seeds for the process of reform which led to the 2007 amendments were sown by three main events, two of which were tragic homicides committed by people who suffered from mental disorder, and that the emphasis of the reform was on public protection and segregation in institutions, with mental health professionals 'suborned as agents of social control' (Mullen, 2005).

Terminology

Before we move on to defining arson in people with intellectual disability, it is important to highlight the difficulties of defining the terms 'intellectual disability' and 'offending behaviour'.

Intellectual disability

Intellectual disability is one of the terms (others are developmental disability, mental retardation, mental handicap and learning disability) used to refer to a group of individuals who have:

- significant impairment of intellectual functioning, defined as an IQ of less than 70 on an established test such as the Wechsler Adult Intelligence Scale (WAIS-IV; Wechsler, 2008), and
- significant impairment of social functioning which has been present from childhood (onset during the developmental period).

As there is no gold standard test to measure impairment of social functioning, clinicians tend to use scales like the Vineland Adaptive Behavior Scales (Sparrow *et al*, 1984) or the second edition of the Adaptive Behaviour Assessment System (ABAS-II; Harrison & Oakland, 2003).

The Mental Health Act 1983 (amended 2007) defines mental disorder as 'any disorder or disability of the mind' and defines intellectual disability in section 1(4) as 'a state of arrested or incomplete development of the mind which includes significant impairment of intelligence and social functioning'. The term 'learning difficulties', which has a broader remit and includes specific reading and writing difficulties, has also been used by local authorities, education systems and some advocacy groups to describe people with intellectual disability.

Even by the strictest possible definition, people with intellectual disabilities are a heterogeneous group with different degrees of ability, comorbidities and several other confounding factors, including those relating to communication, sensory impairments, mobility and other health problems. Compounded by the confusion of defining what is 'intellectual disability', historically there have been boundary disputes between services due to differing eligibility criteria developed by these services. This problem is more so for community learning disability services, and therefore, offenders with intellectual disability find themselves stuck in secure hospital settings due to the paucity of suitable community services to be discharged to (Brooke, 1998). In addition, because of the wide range of abilities in this group, therapeutic interventions cannot be uniform and must be tailored to individual need. This compounds the general lack of evidence base in this area.

Offending behaviour

The term 'offending behaviour' is also associated with problems when used in relation to people with intellectual disability. In England and Wales, a crime is defined by two components – actus reus (the act of crime) and mens rea (the intent to commit that crime). The latter is difficult to interpret in people with intellectual disability, especially where the degree of disability is moderate to profound. Mens rea is a key issue when it comes to the legal perception of the difference between challenging behaviour and criminal behaviour. Similarly, these factors influence any police decision to caution or to arrest and charge an individual with intellectual disability. A majority of illegal or antisocial behaviours involving people with an intellectual disability do not get reported (Hales & Stratford, 1996) because of the current community care system. Even if they are reported, the perceived seriousness of the offence may be downgraded by carers (Lyall *et al*, 1995) as they view the involvement of the CJS as punitive and draconian (Clare & Murphy, 1998). Moreover, the decision of the Crown Prosecution Service (CPS) to prosecute depends on the perceived likelihood of conviction and the extent to which this course of action is considered to be in the public interest (Holland *et al*, 2002). There has been a general shift towards attempting to rehabilitate these individuals either in open hospitals or in community settings rather than by sentencing them to prison terms. This in turn has an effect on prevalence studies of offending in this population, as these are usually conducted in prisons or secure hospital settings, where there would inevitably be an over-representation of people with intellectual disability who are more able (i.e., with mild or borderline levels of disability) and who have committed serious offences necessitating their commitment to such a setting.

Arsonists/firesetters

The distinction between the terms 'arsonist' and 'firesetter' is important when it comes to people with intellectual disability. Swaffer *et al* (2001) made a useful distinction between 'arsonists', defined as those who go through the CJS and are arrested, charged and convicted of starting serious fires, and 'firesetters', defined as those who have committed acts of starting serious fires that may or may not have resulted in contact with the CJS because of a perceived lack of malicious intent. It is the second group of individuals who come into contact with health and social services. There is also the dilemma of distinguishing challenging behaviour from offending behaviour. Ironically, in clinical practice, sometimes individuals with no malicious intent may be arrested and charged for an offence due to the unlawful nature of their challenging behaviour, whereas other individuals with repeated antisocial acts are never prosecuted. This shows again the lack of uniformity in approaching the issue of criminal and challenging behaviours in people with intellectual disability (Jones & Talbot, 2010).

Epidemiology

The prevalence of intellectual disability among offenders reported in the literature varies from 2.6% to 39.6% (MacEachron, 1979). This wide variability appears to be due to the use of different population bases (samples may, for example, come from community disability services, police stations, courts, prisons or secure hospitals) and to the way 'intellectual disability' and 'offending' are defined for research purposes (Holland *et al*, 2002).

It is generally assumed that offences that need meticulous planning, skills and opportunities, such as 'white collar crime' (e.g., fraud and deception), are less likely to be committed by people with intellectual disability. It is, however, also assumed that others, like sex offences and arson, are highly likely to be committed by them. The latter assumption was borne out by a study of people made subject to hospital orders under the Mental Health Act 1959 (Walker & McCabe, 1973) which showed that, although only one-third of the sample of men were classified as 'subnormal' or 'severely subnormal', they were responsible for more than half the sexual and arson offences of the entire group. However, in this study intellectual disability was not determined by any formal assessment.

It has been shown that the prevalence rates of arson in offenders with intellectual disability may be higher than those in the general population of offenders (Bradford & Dimock, 1986; Raesaenen *et al*, 1994) and that it is over-represented in people with borderline intellectual functioning (Day, 1993). Raesaenen *et al* (1994) and Rix (1994) both reported that around 11% of their samples of firesetters could be classified as having an intellectual disability. Leong & Silva (1999) reported that 15% of an out-patient sample of arsonists were classified as having intellectual disability. However, other studies have reported prevalence rates far lower. For example, Puri *et al* (1995) reported that only 3% of a sample of 36 firesetters who were referred to a forensic psychiatry service had intellectual disability. Holland *et al* (2002), in a mini-review of prevalence studies (Jackson *et al*, 1987; Lyall *et al*, 1995; Hodgins *et al*, 1996; Thompson, 1997; Lindsay & Smith, 1998; Marshall *et al*, 1999), suggested that although studies in the UK, the USA and Australia show that people who are significantly intellectually disadvantaged are over-represented throughout the CJS, it is uncertain whether these individuals would fulfil all the criteria for a diagnosis of intellectual disability. They also found from their review that there was little support for the view that people with intellectual disability are over-represented among sex offenders and firesetters.

Aetiology

Several attempts have been made over the years to explain why people with intellectual disability set fires. In his classification of the motives for arson Prins (1980) placed 'the dull and subnormal fire-raiser' under 'fire-raising for pathological reasons or for mixed motives'. Prins *et al* (1985) revised

---

Box 6.1 Reasons proposed for firesetting behaviour in people with intellectual disability

- Poor self-esteem/social isolation
- Poor ability to communicate one's needs to others
- General feelings of frustration
- A need for revenge against society/anger
- A need for some power or control
- A desire to be seen as a hero by peers
- Peer pressure (a desire to please, being highly suggestible/vulnerable)
- A need to be heard (a cry for help)
- An interest in watching fires
- Pyromania (an irresistible impulse to set fires)
- Mental disorder (affective disorders, psychotic illnesses and personality disorders)

this classification and 'mental subnormality (retardation)' was classified under 'arson due to the presence of an actual mental or associated disorder'. The classification is neither clinical nor adequate, as having an intellectual disability does not constitute a motive (Soothill, 1990).

Clinicians have proposed a number of reasons to attempt to understand firesetting in people with intellectual disability (see Box 6.1). It is also felt that treatment options are dictated very much by which of the reasons apply (Hall *et al*, 2005).

Functional analysis paradigm of recidivistic arson

Jackson *et al* (1987) provided a definition of a pathological arsonist and cited recidivism as a core feature. They developed a 'functional analysis paradigm' of recidivistic arson, which defines arson as a behaviour that has to be viewed in relation to its antecedents, including settings and stimuli, and its consequences, including reinforcers (see Fig. 6.1). Although not

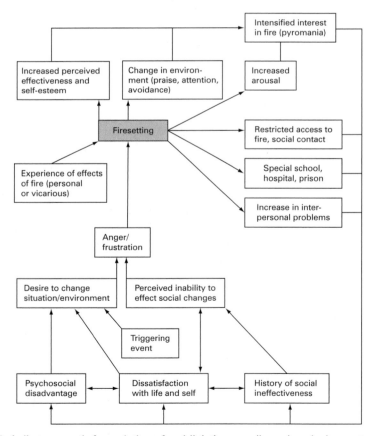

Fig. 6.1 A diagrammatic formulation of recidivistic arson (based on Jackson *et al*, 1987)

developed specifically to understand recidivistic arson among firesetters with intellectual disability, Jackson *et al*'s model has been used in research about this group (e.g. Kelly *et al*, 2009). Jackson's theory has been described as particularly applicable given the social and emotional problems that are associated with intellectual disability (Taylor *et al*, 2004). This model is also suited to analysis of the developmental aspects of firesetting. It remains one of the most significant models in the current literature and has been used to help guide treatment programmes (see under 'Treatment').

Antecedents

The antecedent events to firesetting include the general setting conditions, and the specific psychological stimuli and triggering events. General setting conditions include psychosocial disadvantage, dissatisfaction with life and the self, and ineffective social interaction. These apply especially to arsonists with intellectual disability, who are a psychosocially disadvantaged group and are impaired in their abilities to influence their environment. Specific psychological stimuli that precede firesetting may relate to the individual's personal experience of fire, and fire may have played a significant role in their life prior to any firesetting behaviour. The triggering events for people with intellectual disability are likely to be emotionally significant, like anger, frustration, stress, insult and disappointment (Bumpass *et al*, 1983).

Consequences

The consequences are an especially significant component of the model for this group of firesetters, as it has been shown that people with intellectual disability are usually able to understand the emotions (usually of anger and negative affect) and triggers for firesetting behaviour but have limited insight into its consequences (Murphy & Clare, 1996). The consequences of firesetting may be understood in terms of positive and negative reinforcement. For example, firesetting may be a way for the young, isolated and rejected individual to gain contact with parents, thereby positively reinforcing the behaviour. Alternatively, a young firesetter may be overprotected and sometimes even institutionalised in response to this behaviour. As a result, the person may not be able to cope with stressful situations and this may lead to further firesetting.

Firesetting: the 'only viable option' theory

The act of firesetting has been described by Jackson (1994) as the 'only viable option' theory. From this perspective, firesetting is seen as a behaviour which is solitary, involves no face-to-face contact or confrontation with others, and has the purpose of regaining control of the environment for the individual. The three basic tenets to the theory are as follows:

1   Arsonists are a disadvantaged group with little or no effective means of influencing their environment. This results in a perceived lack of

social effectiveness, perceived worthlessness and an increased need to resolve internal and external conflicts.

2   They do not have the means to solve these conflicts in a socially acceptable manner because of a lack of social skills and lack of opportunities to learn. They therefore resort to the socially unacceptable action of arson.

3   The act of arson itself is not intended to bring about specific changes but is a desperate attempt to effect *any* change in life circumstances.

This theory is particularly relevant to people with intellectual disability. Jackson (1994) explains that firesetting stems from childhood curiosity and experimentation with fire, but because people with intellectual disability often experience psychosocial deprivation from early childhood, their opportunities to learn social skills are impaired and fire can increasingly become a way of expressing emotions. The model suggests that a transition from firesetting in the company of others to setting fires alone constitutes a significant factor in the pathological process. Firesetting provides an opportunity, in fact the 'only viable option', for the socially deprived, underassertive individual to achieve internal and external conflict resolution without the need for face-to-face confrontation.

Characteristics

The typical characteristics of offenders (not specifically arsonists) with intellectual disability include concomitant mental illness, a background of psychosocial deprivation, a history of serious childhood behavioural problems, a family history of offending (Day, 1988) and homelessness (Lyall *et al*, 1995). Those with an intellectual disability are more likely to be arrested after an offence because of their lesser ability to conceal their actions or because of a desire to please (Moffitt & Silva, 1988). In an initial study they appeared to be susceptible to interrogative suggestibility (Gudjonsson, 1988) but this correlation was not supported in a subsequent study (Gudjonsson *et al*, 1993). Due to the increased prevalence of epilepsy in people with intellectual disability (Corbett & Pond, 1979), there is also a rare possibility that offences in this group may be committed as a consequence of an epileptic seizure, a post-ictal confusional state, or as a direct result of the underlying brain dysfunction predisposing to the epilepsy. Other factors associated with offending behaviour in this population are male gender (Thompson, 1997), unemployment (Murphy *et al*, 1995; Simons, 2000), younger age (although the actual peak may be delayed by several years in people with intellectual disability), low socioeconomic status and a history of behavioural problems or previous offending (Simpson & Hogg, 2001). The degree of intellectual disability is also a factor, with the association being strongest in the borderline range and tending to decline as the degree of disability increases. It may be argued that this is due to under-reporting of offending behaviours in individuals with more severe disabilities, or their interpretation as challenging behaviours. There is no substantial evidence to suggest that the profile of an offender with intellectual disability differs from that of a typical offender.

Firesetting in people with intellectual disability is predominantly found in the late adolescent or young adult male and often appears to be motiveless (Lewis & Yarnell, 1951). It may also be a result of anger, revenge or communication of distress (Jackson et al, 1987). Women with intellectual disability who set fires tend to have borderline levels of intelligence and a long-standing history of emotional difficulties, self-harm, criminal damage, promiscuity and sexual abuse at home (Tennent et al, 1971).

In a study of a sample of 1100 adults who were accessing intellectual disability health services over a 20-year period, Devapriam et al (2007) highlighted that the prevalence of firesetting could have been as low as 1.36% (based on identification of 15 people with a documented history of arson). However, this study was a retrospective case-note analysis study with the consequent problems of poor documentation in medical notes and clinical bias. Nonetheless, the authors found that the majority of people with intellectual disability who had set fires lived in the community (Table 6.1). Forty per cent of the incidents of arson occurred in residential homes, 27% in National Health Service hospitals, 20% in hostels and 13% in the person's home. All had contact with the intellectual disability psychiatric services. Following the incident, 47% were admitted to National Health Service hospitals, 13% were transferred to high-security units and 7% to a low-security unit, 20% were sent to prison and 13% were discharged back into the community. About 53% had set fire on more than one occasion and 73% had committed other offences. Whereas studies of firesetters in the general population report male:female ratios of up to 9:1, Devapriam et al (2007) reported a ratio of approximately 1:1. The majority of individuals in this study had a mild degree of intellectual disability. Additionally, a significant proportion had repeated episodes of firesetting behaviour and had committed other offences. This highlights the importance of identifying this high-risk group in order to prevent recidivism. None of the patients had epilepsy. All of the individuals in the sample had some form of behavioural problem. One individual had Klinefelter syndrome and one had Wilson's disease. The mean age of the first firesetting episode was 22 years in males and 30 years in females. In this study, the most common reason for firesetting appears to have been revenge, followed by peer pressure (see Table 6.1). A majority (60%) had a comorbid psychiatric diagnosis, but only in one was there a direct association between firesetting behaviour and underlying psychopathology (command hallucinations due to schizophrenia). In total, 80% had a personality disorder (borderline and antisocial types), suggesting lack of impulse control. Only one person had a diagnosis of pervasive developmental disorder. Only a minority had a family history of intellectual disability. Other findings, similar to findings in general population studies, included belonging to a large family, a history

Table 6.1 Characteristics of a community sample of firesetters with intellectual disability (Devapriam *et al*, 2007)

Characteristics	Proportion of sample ($n = 15$)
Gender	
Male	47%
Female	53%
Ethnicity	
White Caucasian	80%
Black African	7%
South Asian	13%
Residential status (current)	
Residential home	66%
National Health Service hospital	7%
Secure unit	13%
Own home	7%
Social services hostel	7%
Setting where arson took place	
Residential home	40%
National Health Service hospital	27%
Own home	13%
Social services hostel	20%
Degree of intellectual disability	
Borderline	7%
Mild	80%
Moderate	13%
Psychiatric diagnosis	
Schizophrenia	13%
Bipolar affective disorder	7%
Schizoaffective disorder	13%
Recurrent depressive disorder	20%
Pervasive developmental disorder	7%
No psychiatric diagnosis	40%
Comorbid personality disorder	
Borderline type	60%
Antisocial type	20%
No personality disorder	20%
Reasons for firesetting cited in the medical notes	
Revenge	60%
Mental illness	7%
Peer pressure	20%
Pyromania	13%

of childhood behavioural problems, childhood abuse and homelessness, unemployment and relationship difficulties.

Treatment

Holistic treatment strategies are required for firesetting behaviour in people with intellectual disability because there are multiple and complex issues to address. There are few validated treatment programmes for adults with intellectual disability who set fires (Fraser & Taylor, 2002). Most of the validated treatment programmes are for children and adolescents in the general population; they include family therapy (Eisler, 1974), implosion (Cowell, 1985) and aversion (Carstens, 1982) therapies, stimulus satiation (Wolff, 1984), covert sensitisation and combined approaches (McGrath *et al*, 1979). A report commissioned by the Arson Control Forum to establish good practice in interventions with arsonists and young firesetters acknowledged that further research needs to be carried out in this area as existing evidence for these treatment programmes is very sparse (Caulfield *et al*, 2005).

Functional analysis paradigm

The functional analysis paradigm (Jackson *et al*, 1987; see pp. 112–113 in this chapter) has been the building block of individualised and group treatment models. Central to this model is the concept that firesetters are a disadvantaged group with little or no effective means of influencing their environment and who find themselves in highly undesirable situations. The firesetting behaviour is thought to provide the individual with some means of influencing the environment and improving self-esteem. According to Jackson *et al* (1987), the therapeutic implications of this model are as follows:

- Simple education regarding the dangers of fire is unlikely to be useful unless it considers the antecedents and consequences in detail.
- Focusing on firesetting behaviour alone is unlikely to be effective.
- Punitive approaches are not only ineffective but may increase the likelihood of solitary firesetting behaviour.
- Exploration of alternative responses as well as the examination of situational factors is vital.

Murphy & Clare (1996) administered a Fire-Setting Assessment Schedule (FSAS), which was based on the functional analysis paradigm model, to ten individuals with mild intellectual disability who had set fire and had been admitted to a hospital facility. The participants were interviewed about their perceptions of events, feelings and cognitions prior to and after setting fire. They were also asked to rate their excitement/upset in a series of fire-related situations. These individuals could identify reliably the events, feelings and cognitions prior to firesetting but were less reliable at identifying the consequences. Most commonly, people had felt angry prior to setting fires, but it was also common for them to feel not listened to, sad or depressed. Multiple factors were relevant for most people. Some identified the excitement of setting fire as relevant, and these people gave the highest ratings on the FSAS. The findings of this study have been useful in developing group and individual treatment programmes.

Adapted or specialised treatment?

Given the fact that the degree of intellectual disability in the offending group falls in the mild to borderline range, there is a debate about whether firesetter treatment programmes need to be adapted for individuals with intellectual disability or whether mainstream forensic and prison programmes would be sufficient. It is quite clear that treatment programmes in prisons are targeted towards individuals with an IQ of 80 and above (Talbot, 2007). There is also a debate about whether offenders with intellectual disability require a forensic service that is different from that provided for the general population, with no definite conclusions. There is little evidence on what the special needs of this group are in treatment programmes. There is a general consensus among clinicians that there needs to be some adaptation, such as the use of simple language, pictures and symbols. Whether the content needs to be different is debatable. It may be useful for firesetters with intellectual disability to repeat the programme, to have more or longer sessions, and for the programme to be split into smaller components, with sufficient time for focused individual support to consolidate learning.

Individual versus group treatment approaches

The existing evidence can be broadly classified across two approaches – individual and group treatment.

Individual treatment programmes

Clare *et al* (1992) have presented a single case report of the successful treatment of firesetting in a young man with a mild intellectual disability and facial disfigurement. The comprehensive package of treatment included facial surgery, social skills and assertiveness training, alternative coping strategies and 'assisted' covert sensitisation. Significant clinical improvements were noted, with no reports of firesetting 30 months after discharge.

Clayton (2000) described the use of cognitive analytic therapy (CAT) with a firesetter with borderline intellectual functioning. It has been shown that CAT can be adapted and used for individuals with a mild degree of intellectual disability (King, 2000; Crowley, 2002). CAT is an integrative model of short-term psychotherapy delivered in 16–24 sessions; the therapist helps the client understand why things have gone wrong in the past and explores how to make sure things do not go wrong in the future. The conceptual framework is based on the step-by-step pragmatic model of cognitive–behaviour therapy and the analytical approach of psychodynamic psychotherapy. The main stages of the therapy programme are as follows:

1   *Developing the psychotherapy file*. This is based on the 'personal construct theory', whereby problem areas are identified in relation to self-perception and relationships with others. The problem areas are categorised under three main headings – traps, dilemmas and snags. In people with intellectual disability, simpler language and pictures may be used (King, 2000).

2   *Reformulation*. This consists of exploring past experiences and relationships and writing a reformulation letter, in which a tentative account of the origins of presenting problems and the factors that maintain them are made explicit. This is also presented in a diagrammatic form (sequential diagrammatic reformulation), which gives a client an overview of the problems and maintaining factors.

3   *Goodbye letter*. At the end of the treatment programme a goodbye letter is written by the therapist, summarising what happened during the therapy and recommendations.

Group treatment programmes

Rice & Chaplin (1979) reported good outcomes (no firesetting at 12-month post-discharge follow-up) for group therapy involving social skills training to two groups of five firesetters with mild intellectual disability in a maximum-security hospital. Similar good outcomes for social skills training have been reported by McGrath *et al* (1979).

Taylor *et al* (2004) developed a group treatment for arsonists with intellectual disability that is based on the functional analysis paradigm model (Jackson *et al*, 1987) and focuses on antecedents (including the settings and triggers), behaviours (including the associated cognitions and emotions) and consequences (both positive and negative) (see above). The programme runs for 31 sessions and the main components of the treatment package include a review of offence cycle, education and information, skills acquisition and development, and relapse prevention. A number of outcome measures were used before the programme and following its completion. Taylor *et al* (2004) reported a significant improvement in anger measures across the group and an increase in goal attainment scores, indicating improvements in acceptance of guilt, personal responsibility, victim issues, emotional expression, relationships and understanding of risks.

Hall *et al* (2005) have described a group treatment programme which is based on the FSAS and incorporated the outcome measures used in Taylor's programme described above, but was shorter in duration (16 sessions) and incorporated pictorial aids like the 'blame cake' and 'risk swamp'. The aims were to help firesetters to identify risk factors and learn alternative coping strategies. The programme consists of three sections:

1 *Introduction to fire*. This includes expectations of the group, dangers of fire, media portrayal of fire and so on.

2 *Personal firesetting*. This focuses on the individual's history of fire, antecedents, behaviours and consequences.

3 *Alternative ways of coping*.

The outcome was reported as generally good, with two out of six clients stepping down to lower-security provisions, but the authors stated there was a need for further research in this area.

The criminal justice system and intellectual disability

In recent years, the CJS has made significant efforts to identify individuals with intellectual disability in the system, to understand the needs of these individuals and to develop care pathways that facilitate their diversion into systems of care that are more suitable and appropriate. The 'No One Knows' programme was undertaken by the Prison Reform Trust (Talbot, 2008) to address concerns raised by prison staff, prisoners and their families regarding the unmet needs of people with intellectual disabilities. The programme review confirmed that decision-making by the police on enforcement, diversion and disposal for people with intellectual disabilities is inconsistent. Adults who are considered to be mentally vulnerable must have an 'appropriate adult' with them when they are interviewed by the police. This can be a family member, friend or is often a volunteer or social care or healthcare professional. However, the use of 'appropriate adults' during police interviews was reported by Talbot (2008) to be patchy, either because the need is not identified or because there are not enough individuals to perform this role. People with intellectual disabilities and their carers are often baffled by court proceedings, which are rarely adapted to enable them to participate appropriately (Talbot, 2008). It has also been reported that in prisons there is a lack of adequate staff skills to identify intellectual disability, or where such skills exist, there is a perverse disincentive to do so, as this brings statutory responsibilities which staff feel unable to fulfil (Loucks, 2007; Talbot, 2007, 2008). There is a scarcity of adapted treatment programmes for people with intellectual disabilities in prison, which has been raised as a human rights issue (Joint Committee on Human Rights, 2008).

Experience has indicated a lack of a joined-up approach between the CJS and the health and social care systems in dealing with offenders who have an intellectual disability (Fig. 6.2). The effectiveness and quality of court diversion schemes varies between regions, depending on awareness and available training. One study (Devapriam *et al*, 2007) demonstrated that the usual outcome after an incident of firesetting by an individual with an intellectual disability was treatment within National Health Service settings,

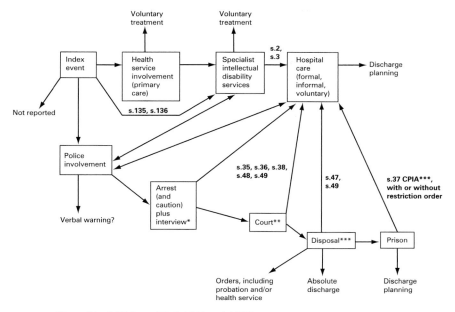

Fig. 6.2 Pathway of care through the health and the criminal justice systems for a person with intellectual disability

including low-, medium- and high-security facilities appropriate to the risks involved, as an alternative to prison custody. Therefore, it appears imperative that psychiatric services should be geared to manage this group. However, in clinical practice, service provision in the community is inadequate to deal with patients presenting with such problems. Awareness of disability-related issues on the part of police and prison officers is crucial for this pathway to be efficient, effective and useful for people with intellectual disability. Unfortunately, despite good local initiatives, most regions do not have a training programme in place for all staff concerned, and support for training and liaison work through the commissioning route is at times missing.

Conclusions and future directions

The topic of arson and intellectual disability is fraught with poor research evidence, both about its epidemiology and about treatment programmes. Moreover, confusion remains over terminology, classificatory systems and outcomes in relation to the CJS and social programmes. What is clearly well established through research is that firesetting is one of the offending behaviours seen in those with borderline intellectual functioning and in those with a mild degree of intellectual disability. A number of individuals with firesetting behaviours end up in secure care settings or prison. What is not yet clear is whether firesetting occurs as a behaviour in its own right or as a part of a cluster of offending behaviours. We do not know to what extent the cognitive and social impairment associated with intellectual disability *per se* contributes to such behaviours or to what extent other factors play a role, such as mental illness, personality disorder and social environment.

The CJS and the health and social care system are not linked up in a meaningful way to offer appropriate support and treatment programmes for this population. Services that have been developed for offenders with intellectual disability can at best be described as patchy, with little link-up with the wider system. The complexity of the problems presented by this group means that joint assessment and joint working arrangements are essential but this seldom takes place. The needs of these offenders are assessed by a wide range of professionals, depending both on the nature of the offending behaviour and on where in the health and social care system the individual is identified (see Fig. 6.2). Many of these professionals do not have any experience or training in intellectual disability. For instance forensic psychiatrists have the necessary set of skills in relation to risk assessment and management but do not necessarily have training in intellectual disability. The contrary is also true, in that intellectual disability psychiatrists who work with offenders may not have the formal training that forensic psychiatrists have, and hence may not possess the necessary competencies.

Another ongoing problem is that those with borderline intellectual functioning or mild intellectual disability who offend may be disowned by either or both the intellectual disability and the forensic psychiatry services. This also suggests the lack of an appropriate care pathway and clinical networks to aid joint working in most services. Similar problems are encountered in the step-down pathway for individuals with intellectual disability from high- and medium-security hospitals to lower-security facilities, locked rehabilitation facilities and eventually reintegration into the community, because the community teams lack the necessary skills and expertise to manage these individuals. The need for a joint approach, care pathways and clinical networking has been taken up by the Faculty of the Psychiatry of Learning Disability and the Faculty of Forensic Psychiatry of the Royal College of Psychiatrists, and a working group is also looking at multi-professional training needs.

Acknowledgement

The authors would like to thank Dr Glyn Jones for his contribution to this chapter.

References

Barron, P., Hassiotis, A. & Banes, J. (2002) Offenders with intellectual disability: the size of the problem and therapeutic outcomes. *Journal of Intellectual Disability Research*, **46**, 454–463.

Bradford, J. & Dimock, J. (1986) A comparative study of adolescents and adults who wilfully set fires. *Psychiatric Journal of the University of Ottowa*, **11**, 228–234.

Brooke, D. (1998) Patients with learning disability at Kneesworth House Hospital. The first five years. *Psychiatric Bulletin*, **22**, 29–32.

Bumpass, E. R., Fagelman, F. D. & Brix, R. J. (1983) Intervention with children who set fires. *American Journal of Psychotherapy*, **37**, 328–345.

Carstens, C. (1982) Application of a work penalty threat in the treatment of and care of juvenile firesetting. *Journal of Behaviour Therapy and Experimental Psychiatry*, **13**, 159–161.

Caulfield, L. S., Palmer, E. J. & Hollin, C. R. (2005) *Interventions with Arsonists and Young Fire Setters*. Arson Control Forum Research Bulletin no. 6. Office of the Deputy Prime Minister.

Clare, I. C. H. & Murphy, G. H. (1998) Working with offenders or alleged offenders with intellectual disabilities. In *Clinical Psychology and People with Intellectual Disabilities* (eds E. Emerson, C. Hatton, J. Bromley, *et al*), pp. 154–176. Wiley.

Clare, I. C. H., Murphy G. H., Cox, D., *et al* (1992) Assessment and treatment of fire-setting: a single-case investigation using a cognitive–behavioural model. *Criminal Behaviour and Mental Health*, **2**, 253–268.

Clayton, P. (2000) Cognitive analytic therapy: learning disability and fire-setting. In *Forensic Mental Health Care: A Case Study Approach* (eds D. Mercer, T. Mason, M. McKeown, *et al*). Churchill Livingstone.

Corbett, J. A. & Pond, D. A. (1979) Epilepsy and behavioural disorders in the mentally handicapped. In *Psychiatric Illness and Mental Handicap* (eds F. E. James & R. P. Snaith), pp. 37–44. Headley Bros.

Cowell, P. (1985) Implosion therapy in the counselling of a pupil who sets fires. *British Journal of Guidance and Counselling*, **13**, 157–165.

Crowley, V. (2002) CAT in various conditions and contexts. In *Introducing Cognitive Analytic Therapy* (eds I. B. Kerr & A. Ryle). Wiley.

Day, K. (1988) A hospital-based treatment programme for male mentally handicapped offenders. *British Journal of Psychiatry*, **153**, 635–644.

Day, K. (1993) Crime and mental retardation: a review. In *Clinical Approaches to the Mentally Disordered Offender* (eds K. Howells & C. R. Hollin), pp. 111–144. Wiley.

Devapriam J., Raju L. B., Singh N., *et al* (2007) Arson: characteristics and predisposing factors in offenders with intellectual disabilities. *British Journal of Forensic Practice*, **9**, 23–27.

Eisler, R. M. (1974) Crisis intervention in the family of a fire-setter. *Psychotherapy: Theory, Research and Practice*, **9**, 76–79.

Fraser, W. I. & Taylor, J. L. (eds) (2002) Forensic learning disabilities: the evidence base. *Journal of Intellectual Disability Research*, **46**, suppl. 1.

Gudjonsson, G. H. (1988) The relationship of intelligence and memory to interrogative suggestibility: the importance of range effects. *British Journal of Clinical Psychology*, **27**, 185–187.

Gudjonsson, G. H., Clare, I. C. H., Rutter, S., *et al* (1993) *Persons at Risk During Interviews in Police Custody: The Identification of Vulnerabilities*. Royal Commission on Criminal Justice Research Study no. 12. HMSO.

Hales, J. & Stratford, N. (1996) *British Crime Survey*. Social and Community Planning Research.

Hall, I., Clayton, P. & Johnson, P. (2005) Arson and learning disability. In *The Handbook of Forensic Learning Disabilities* (eds. T. Riding, C. Dale & B. Swann), pp. 51–72. Radcliffe Publishing.

Harrison, P. & Oakland, T. (2003) *Adaptive Behaviour Assessment System* (2nd edn) (ABAS-II). Psychological Corporation.

Hodgins, S., Mednick, S. A., Brennan, P. A., *et al* (1996) Mental disorder and crime. Evidence from a Danish cohort. *Archives of General Psychiatry*, **53**, 489–496.

Holland, T., Clare, I. C. H. & Mukhopadhyay, T. (2002) Prevalence of 'criminal offending' by men and women with intellectual disability and the characteristics of 'offenders': implications for research and service development. *Journal of Intellectual Disability Research*, **44**, 6–20.

Jackson, H. F. (1994) Assessment of fire-setters. In *The Assessment of Criminal Behaviours of Clients in Secure Settings* (eds M. McMurran & J. Hodge), pp. 94–126. Jessica Kingsley.

Jackson, H. F., Glass, C. & Hope, S. (1987) A functional analysis of recidivistic arson. *British Journal of Clinical Psychology*, **26**, 175–185.

Johnston, S. J. & Halstead, S. (2000) Forensic issues in intellectual disability. *Current Opinion in Psychiatry*, **13**, 475–480.

Joint Committee on Human Rights (2008) *A Life Like Any Other? Human Rights of Adults with Learning Disabilities*. Seventh report of session 2007–08. TSO.

Jones, G. & Talbot, J. (2010) No one knows: the bewildering passage of offenders with learning disability and learning difficulty through the criminal justice system. *Criminal Behaviour and Mental Health*, **20**, 1–7.

Kelly, J., Goodwill, A. M., Keene, N., *et al* (2009) A retrospective study of historical risk factors for pathological arson in adults with mild learning disabilities. *British Journal of Forensic Practice*, **11**, 17–23.

King, R. (2000) CAT and learning disability. *Association for Cognitive Analytic Therapy (ACAT) News*, spring, 3–4.

Leong, G. B. & Silva, J. A. (1999) Revisiting arson from an out-patient forensic perspective. *Journal of Forensic Science*, **44**, 558–563.

Lewis, N. O. C. & Yarnell, H. (1951) *Pathological Firesetting (Pyromania)*. Nervous and Mental Disease Monographs no. 82. Coolidge Foundation.

Lindsay, W. R. & Smith, A. H. W. (1998) Responses to treatment for sex offenders with a learning disability: a comparison of men with 1 and 2 year probation sentences. *Journal of Intellectual Disability Research*, **42**, 346–353.

Loucks, N. (2007) *Prisoners with Learning Difficulties and Disabilities – Review of Prevalence and Associated Needs*. Prison Reform Trust.

Lyall, I., Holland, A. J. & Collins, S. (1995) Offending by adults with learning disabilities: identifying need in one health district. *Mental Handicap Research*, **8**, 99–109.

MacEachron, A. E. (1979) Mentally retarded offenders: prevalence and characteristics. *American Journal of Mental Deficiency*, **84**, 165–176.

Marshall, W. L., Anderson, D. & Fernandez, Y. (1999) *Cognitive Behavioural Treatment of Sexual Offenders*. Wiley.

McGrath, P., Marshall, P. G. & Prior, K. (1979) A comprehensive treatment program for a fire setting child. *Journal of Behaviour Therapy and Experimental Psychiatry*, **10**, 69–72.

Moffitt, T. E. & Silva, P. A. (1988) IQ and delinquency: a direct test of the differential detection hypothesis. *Journal of Abnormal Psychology*, **97**, 330–333.

Mullen, P. E. (2005) Facing up to our responsibilities. *Psychiatric Bulletin*, **29**, 248–249.

Murphy, G. H. & Clare, I. C. H. (1996) Analysis of motivation in people with mild learning disabilities (mental handicap) who set fires. *Psychology, Crime and Law*, **2**, 153–164.

Murphy, G. H., Harnett, H. & Holland, A. J. (1995) A survey of intellectual disabilities amongst men on remand in prison. *Mental Handicap Research*, **8**, 81–98.

Prins, H. (1980) *Offenders, Deviants or Patients? An Introduction to the Study of Socio-Forensic Problems*. Tavistock Publications.

Prins, H., Tennant, G. & Trick, K. (1985) Motives for arson (fire raising). *Medicine, Science and the Law*, **25**, 275–278.

Puri, B. K., Baxter, R. & Cordess, C. C. (1995) Characteristics of firesetters: a study and proposed multi-axial psychiatric classification. *British Journal of Psychiatry*, **166**, 393–396.

Raesaenen, P., Hirvenoj, A., Hakko, H., *et al* (1994) Cognitive functioning ability of arsonists. *Journal of Forensic Psychiatry,* **5,** 615–620.

Rice, M. E. & Chaplin, T. (1979) Social skills training for hospitalized male arsonists. *Journal of Behavior Therapy and Experimental Psychiatry,* **10,** 105–108.

Rix, K. G. B. (1994) A psychiatric study of adult arsonists. *Medicine, Science and the Law,* **34,** 21–34.

Simons, K. (2000) *Life on the Edge. The Experiences of People with Learning Disability Who Do Not Use Specialist Services.* Pavilion Publishing/Joseph Rowntree Foundation.

Simpson, M. K. & Hogg, J. (2001) Patterns of offending among people with intellectual disability: a systematic review. Part I: methodology and prevalence data. *Journal of Intellectual Disability Research,* **45,** 384–396.

Soothill, K. (1990) Arson. In *Principles and Practice of Forensic Psychiatry* (eds R. Bluglass & P. Bowden), pp. 779–786. Churchill Livingstone.

Sparrow, S. S., Balla, D. A. & Cicchetti, D. V. (1984) *Vineland Adaptive Behavior Scales (Interview Edition).* American Guidance Service.

Swaffer, T., Haggett, M & Oxley, T. (2001) Mentally disordered firesetters: a structured intervention programme. *Clinical Psychology and Psychotherapy,* **8,** 468–475.

Talbot, J. (2007) *Identifying and Supporting Prisoners with Learning Difficulties and Learning Disabilities: The Views of Prison Staff.* Prison Reform Trust.

Talbot, J. (2008) *Prisoner's Voices: No One Knows Report and Final Recommendations.* Prison Reform Trust.

Taylor, J. L., Thorne, I. & Slavkin, M. L. (2004) Treatment of fire-setting behaviour. In *Offenders with Developmental Disabilities* (eds W. R. Lindsay, J. L. Taylor & P. Strumey), pp. 221–240. Wiley.

Tennent, T. G., McQuaid, A., Loughnane, T., *et al* (1971) Female arsonists. *British Journal of Psychiatry,* **119,** 497–502.

Thompson, D. (1997) Profiling the sexually abusive behaviour of men with intellectual disabilities. *Journal of Applied Research in Intellectual Disabilities,* **10,** 125–139.

Thornicroft, G. & Szmukler, G. (2005) The draft Mental Health Bill in England: without principles. *Psychiatric Bulletin,* **29,** 244–247.

Walker, N. & McCabe, S. (1968) Hospital orders. In *The Mentally Abnormal Offender* (eds A. V. S. de Reuck & R. Porter). Churchill.

Walker, N. & McCabe, S. (1973) *Crime and Insanity in England, Vol. 2.* Edinburgh University Press.

Wechsler, D. (2008) *Wechsler Adult Intelligence Scale – Fourth Edition (WAIS–IV).* Pearson.

Wolff, R. (1984) Satiation in the treatment of inappropriate fire setting. *Journal of Behaviour Therapy and Experimental Psychiatry,* **15,** 337–340.

CHAPTER 7

Female arsonists and firesetters

Theresa A. Gannon, Nichola Tyler, Magali Barnoux
and Afroditi Pina

Understanding the aetiology of arson and firesetting and how to assess and treat individuals who deliberately set fires is a complex process that is still very much 'work in progress'. However, as with most forensic issues, the research literature examining *male* individuals who set fires is substantially more developed than that focusing on females. To date, for example, review articles examining the concept of arson and firesetting either focus very little attention on females (e.g., Barnett & Spitzer, 1994; Smith & Short, 1995) or focus solely on males (Gannon & Pina, 2010). The main aim of this chapter is to provide a summary overview of what is currently known regarding women who set fires. It focuses on outlining the key characteristics and features of women who set fires, the aetiology of female-perpetrated firesetting, and the key treatment and risk issues. Where possible, the reported findings on women are compared with what is currently known about males who set fires and women offenders who do not set fires. Throughout this chapter, we generally use the term 'firesetting' to refer to any intentional lighting of fires, since 'arson' is an arguably narrow and legally constructed term that is unable to account for those whose firesetting remains unapprehended (e.g., firesetting in forensic psychiatry settings). Using the term 'firesetter' in relation to women may be especially important, since women appear to be treated more leniently than men by criminal justice officials, perhaps due to childcare responsibilities or other stereotyped preconceptions around females' risk (Wilbanks, 1986; Steffensmeier & Demuth, 2006). Thus, many females who set a fire may not hold a conviction for 'arson' on record. However, taking into account clinical figures, professionals estimate that male firesetters outnumber females at a figure of around 6:1 (Stewart, 1993).

Key characteristics and features

Sociodemographic features

Many of the sociodemographic features noted in male firesetters who come to professional attention (see Gannon & Pina, 2010, for a review) are similar to those noted for females. For example, research suggests that female firesetters who come to professional attention – like other female offenders – are typically of low-average IQ (Tennent *et al*, 1971; Stewart, 1993; Noblett & Nelson, 2001), have low socioeconomic status and are poorly educated (Tennent *et al*, 1971; Harmon *et al*, 1985; Stewart, 1993; Wachi *et al*, 2007). Female firesetters are also generally noted as being primarily of Caucasian ethnicity (Puri *et al*, 1995; Noblett & Nelson, 2001) and in their mid-20s (Bourget & Bradford, 1989) to late 30s (Wachi *et al*, 2007).

Developmental context

Female firesetters appear to experience developmental backgrounds that are characterised by negative and labile features, including physical, sexual and emotional abuse, negligent parenting and separation from one or other genetic parent (Lewis & Yarnell, 1951; Harmon *et al*, 1985; Puri *et al*, 1995; Dickens *et al*, 2007; Hickle & Roe-Sepowitz, 2010). These features appear similar to those observed in male firesetters and other female offenders (Lewis & Yarnell, 1951; Bradford, 1982; Bennett & Hess, 1984; Puri *et al*, 1995; Blanchette & Brown, 2006). However, of the small number of studies that have compared female firesetters' childhoods with those of other female offenders, two discrepancies have been noted (see Gannon, 2010): (1) female firesetters appear more likely to have been separated from one or both genetic parents (Tennent *et al*, 1971; Stewart, 1993); and (2) female firesetters appear more likely to have experienced sexual abuse or premature sexual interactions (Tennent *et al*, 1971; Stewart, 1993; Noblett & Nelson, 2001). There is very little research directly comparing female and male firesetters. Some research does, however, suggest that female firesetters are more likely to have been sexually abused as children (Dickens *et al*, 2007). The wider research literature also suggests that female offenders – relative to males – are likely to have had more pervasive developmental experiences of abuse (Blanchette & Brown, 2006).

Clinical features

Psychopathology associated with fire

A key psychopathology often used interchangeably with firesetting is *pyromania*. Pyromania is defined by DSM-IV-TR (American Psychiatric Association, 2000) under the category of impulse control disorders not otherwise specified and is dependent upon establishing the following criteria:

- deliberate and repeated firesetting
- tension or arousal prior to firesetting
- fascination with fire, its consequences and fire paraphernalia

- enjoyment, satisfaction or relief following partaking in, or witnessing, firesetting events.

Furthermore, the firesetting must not be motivated by economic gain, sociopolitical ideology, crime concealment, anger or revenge, or intended enhancement of residential conditions. Neither should the firesetting be associated with impaired judgement (e.g., delusions, intoxication, dementia) or be explained by the psychiatric diagnoses of conduct disorder, mania or antisocial personality disorder. Thus, a diagnosis of pyromania is reserved for individuals who set fires out of intense preoccupation with fire, to the exclusion of all other motivating factors.

Perhaps unsurprisingly, given the specificity of the criteria, pyromania is rarely diagnosed in either male or female firesetters (O'Sullivan & Kelleher, 1987; Leong, 1992; Ritchie & Huff, 1999; Dickens *et al*, 2007). For example, Bourget & Bradford (1989) reported finding only one female and two male pyromaniacs in their groups of 15 female and 77 male psychiatrically referred firesetters. However, commentators in the area (e.g., Mavromatis, 2000; Moore & Jefferson, 2004) and DSM-IV-TR itself describe pyromania as being less prevalent in females relative to males, at a ratio of around 1:2 (American Psychiatric Association, 2000; Howell & Watson, 2005). Nevertheless, it is unclear how such conclusions have been drawn, since a variety of published studies highlight rather variable findings regarding pyromania diagnoses or features: no evidence of pyromania in males and females (Geller & Bertsch, 1985; Leong, 1992); higher rates of pyromania among females than among males (Grant *et al*, 2007); and higher rates of pyromania among males than among females (Lochner *et al*, 2004; Dickens *et al*, 2007). However, such studies typically operationalise pyromania in differing ways and use arguably unrepresentative sampling techniques, making it very difficult to draw definitive conclusions.

Other psychopathology

It is not unusual for professionals and psychiatrists to document general psychopathological diagnoses in female firesetters (Harmon *et al*, 1985; Bourget & Bradford, 1989; Barnett & Spitzer, 1994). Common diagnoses include affective disorders (Bourget & Bradford, 1989; Stewart, 1993; Dickens *et al*, 2007), schizophrenia (Tennent *et al*, 1971; Harmon *et al*, 1985; Leong, 1992) and substance misuse (Harmon *et al*, 1985; Bourget & Bradford, 1989). Unfortunately, however, very few researchers appear to have compared such psychopathology with that exhibited by relevant comparison groups (e.g., male firesetters or female offenders in general), although there are some exceptions (Tennent *et al*, 1971; Bourget & Bradford, 1989; Stewart, 1993; Dickens *et al*, 2007; Enayati *et al*, 2008; Anwar *et al*, 2011). In an early study, Tennent *et al* (1971) examined psychopathologies recorded over a 5-year period for in-patient female firesetters and a comparison group of female in-patients. The two groups displayed similar rates of schizophrenia (approximately 30%) and depression (approximately 9%). Finally, although psychosis appeared to be more prevalent in the firesetting group than in the comparison group (52% v. 39%), this difference was not statistically significant.

In a recent study, Enayati et al (2008) examined 214 psychiatrically referred male and female firesetters (28% of whom were female) and compared them with violent offender referrals on psychiatric diagnoses using DSM-IV criteria (American Psychiatric Association, 1994). Male and female firesetters could not be differentiated on Axis I or II diagnoses. However, relative to female violent offenders, female firesetters were found to exhibit higher rates of intellectual disability (8.5% of firesetters v. 2.6% of controls) and alcohol use disorder (25.4% of firesetters v. 14.4% of controls).

In a comparatively rare prison study, Stewart (1993) compared psychiatric diagnoses acquired via file and self-report interview for female firesetters and a comparison group of female offenders. In this study, both groups were found to exhibit similarly high rates of substance misuse (44.4% of firesetters and 46.4% of comparisons), depression (37.0% of firesetters and 28.6% of comparisons) and schizophrenia (33.3% of firesetters and 25.0% of comparisons). In this study, then, it was not possible to discriminate female firesetters from other female offenders on psychiatric diagnoses.

Finally, in a Swedish study, Anwar et al (2011) examined 1689 individuals in Sweden convicted of firesetting (349 of whom were women) and sought to establish the prevalence of schizophrenia. When these individuals were compared with a large group of general population controls, it was found that, after controlling for confounding factors, diagnoses of schizophrenia were greatly over-represented in those convicted of firesetting (i.e., the diagnosis was more than 20 times more likely). Furthermore, it was women firesetters who exhibited the highest prevalence of schizophrenia; they appeared to be nearly 40 times more likely than the general population to have a diagnosis of schizophrenia. Nevertheless, as the authors themselves noted, this finding appears to mirror a gender difference found for other violent offences (see Fazel et al, 2009).

Personality disorder

Similarly to general psychopathology, it is common for professionals to document the presence of personality disorder in female firesetters (Tennent et al, 1971; Harmon et al, 1985; Rix, 1994; Coid et al, 1999). In particular, both borderline personality disorder and antisocial personality disorder appear to be commonly associated with female firesetters (Harmon et al, 1985; Coid et al, 1999). Furthermore, research suggests that, for females diagnosed with borderline personality disorder, firesetting and self-harm may share an aetiological link (Coid, 1993; Miller & Fritzon, 2007).

129

Unfortunately, however, research comparing the prevalence of personality disorder in female firesetters and other relevant subgroups is scant and underdeveloped. Bourget & Bradford (1989), for example, described findings suggesting that over half of a sample of female firesetter psychiatric referrals (58%; 7 out of 12) held diagnoses of personality disorder, compared with only 40.8% of male firesetter psychiatric referrals (*n* = 31). Nevertheless, although Bourget & Bradford appear to stress the importance of personality disorder in the aetiology of female-perpetrated firesetting, it remains unclear as to whether or not these differences were statistically significant. Furthermore, no information is provided regarding the specific subtypes of personality disorder characterising either male or female firesetters. Similarly, Rix (1994) found that approximately half of his male and female firesetter referrals held a diagnosis of personality disorder. However, it is unclear how firesetters compare statistically on diagnostic subtypes. In a study of UK female prisoners who had self-harmed, Coid *et al* (1999) reported that those who had been involved in firesetting had similar levels of borderline personality disorder to non-firesetters. What was notable, however, was that female firesetters – relative to non-firesetters – were significantly more likely to have a diagnosis of antisocial personality disorder (76%, *n* = 19, *v.* 24%, *n* = 12, respectively).

In terms of general interpersonal traits, research shows that female firesetters tend to be characterised by passive personality traits and low self-worth relative to female offender comparisons (Noblett & Nelson, 2001). Female firesetters also appear to have more traits of neuroticism relative to female offender and non-offender comparisons (Tennent *et al,* 1971) but do not appear differentially to endorse aggressive personality traits (Noblett & Nelson, 2001).

Neurobiological deficits

Both low cerebrospinal fluid monoamine metabolite concentrates – specifically 5-hydroxyindoleacetic acid (5-HIAA) and 3-methoxy-4-hydroxyphenylglycol (MHPG) – and irregularities in glucose metabolism have been linked to male convictions for firesetting and firesetting recidivism (Virkkunen, 1984; Roy *et al,* 1986; Virkkunen *et al,* 1987, 1989). However, these links are not yet totally understood, although researchers suggest that serotonin reductions, for example, may generally increase impulsivity and risk-taking (Moore *et al,* 2002). Although female firesetters have not yet been specifically examined in studies of glucose metabolism, they have been included in some studies examining the general link between 5-HIAA concentrations and antisocial behaviour in general. In a meta-analysis of such studies, Moore *et al* have shown that although the link is significant, the effect size is reduced substantially when females are included with men in study samples. Thus, it may be that low 5-HIAA concentrations exhibit different effects for female firesetters and this is something that clearly warrants further investigation.

Sexual pathology

Interestingly, in the 19th century the onset of menstruation was linked not only to criminal behaviour but also to firesetting (Harry & Balcer, 1987; Barker, 1994). However, there does not appear to be any substantial empirical evidence supporting this link (see Lewis & Yarnell, 1951; Harry & Balcer, 1987). Tennent *et al* (1971) appear to be the only researchers to have examined the presence of menstruation abnormalities in female psychiatric in-patient firesetters. They found that female firesetters – relative to female offender comparisons – were significantly more likely to experience acute dysmenorrhoea (43% of the firesetters *v*. 14% of the comparisons). However, given the lack of empirical work in this area it is unclear whether or not menstruation problems play a role in firesetting aetiology for women.

Finally, firesetting has been linked to sexual fetishism (Freud, 1932) and a small number of researchers have noted that some males set fires in order to fulfil such sexual fetishes (Lewis & Yarnell, 1951; Kocsis & Cooksey, 2002). However, the literature examining female firesetters has not generally highlighted such sexual pathology as an issue linked to their firesetting (Lewis & Yarnell, 1951).

Aetiology

The aetiological underpinnings of female firesetting are poorly understood. To illustrate, there are no comprehensive theories available specifically to describe female firesetting (although see Chapter 2 for Fineman's 1995 or Jackson *et al*'s 1987 theoretical accounts of *male* firesetting) and our understanding of the motives underlying female firesetting are based on only a small number of studies, some of which do not employ adequate controls (i.e., male firesetters). In the absence of a comprehensive theory of female firesetting, we turn our attention to studies examining the possible factors motivating female firesetting.

Motives underlying female firesetting

Studies with a comparison group

In studies that have included a male firesetter comparison group (e.g., Lewis & Yarnell, 1951; Icove & Estepp, 1987; Rix, 1994; Dickens *et al*, 2007), there appear to be some small differences in the motivators underlying female and male firesetting. For example, Rix (1994) examined the motives of 153 firesetters who were referred for psychiatric evaluation (24 of whom were female; 16%). Overall, 15 categories were found to accommodate all of the firesetters' motivations. The three most popular motivators for females were revenge (21%, $n = 5$), rehousing (i.e., setting a fire to promote residential relocation; 21%, $n = 5$) and attention-seeking (i.e., firesetting to elicit help or attract attention; 17%, $n = 4$). The three most popular motivations for males were revenge (33%, $n = 42$), excitement (12%, $n = 16$) and vandalism (10%, $n = 13$). Thus, revenge appeared to be the most popular motive for both male- and female-perpetrated firesetting.

Icove & Estepp (1987) examined 1016 arrest interviews (50% male, 8% female, remainder unspecified) for crimes involving fire or firesetting and reported that motivators for males could be categorised under the following themes: excitement (40%, $n = 200$), vandalism (27%, $n = 136$), revenge (18%, $n = 91$), crime concealment (3%, $n = 13$) and profit (<1%, $n = 4$). However, females did not fit into the crime concealment or profit categories and instead were classified into the themes of revenge (28%, $n = 40$), vandalism (21%, $n = 21$) and excitement (17%, $n = 14$). Although gender differences are not discussed in detail by Icove & Estepp, they do note the preference for females to use firesetting as a form of revenge.

More recently, Dickens *et al* (2007) studied the motives of 167 firesetters referred for psychiatric evaluation, 38 of whom were female (22.8%). They reported that females, relative to males, were significantly more likely to set fires as a cry for help (36.8% of females v. 17.8% of males). Females also appeared to be significantly less likely than males to set fires due to traits associated with pyromania (13.2% of females v. 32.6% of males). A novel aspect of this study is the statistical comparison of motivators across female and male firesetters.

Studies without a comparison group

The vast majority of researchers – even recently – have examined the motivators of female firesetters in the *absence* of any male firesetting control group (Tennent *et al*, 1971; Harmon *et al*, 1985; Stewart, 1993; Noblett & Nelson, 2001; Wachi *et al*, 2007; Cunningham *et al*, 2011). For example, Harmon *et al* (1985) examined the case files of 27 US female firesetters referred for psychiatric evaluation and reported two overarching categories that appeared to account for the motivators underlying female firesetting: *anger* (i.e., firesetting motivated by anger, with or without a target, and sometimes associated with delusions; $n = 17$); and *a cry for help* (i.e., firesetting motivated by the desire to draw attention to one's circumstances or issues, often associated with mental health issues; $n = 7$). A small number of women also appeared to have engaged in firesetting that was accidental or motiveless ($n = 3$). Interestingly, Harmon *et al* noted that planned firesetting was associated with anger-related motivators.

Stewart (1993) found that just over a third of her female firesetter prisoners had multiple motives for their firesetting (e.g., revenge and mental_illness). The most common motives characterising the sample, however, fell into the categories *revenge* (33%, $n = 13$), *attention-seeking* (20%, $n = 8$) and *instrumental* (i.e., firesetting as a way of achieving another goal such as crime concealment; 20%, $n = 8$). Far less prevalent motivators were also noted, however, in the categories *mental illness* (10%, $n = 4$), *suicide* (8%, $n = 4$) and *pyromania traits* (5%, $n = 2$). Although specific examples of each of the motives are not discussed, Stewart's study is unusual since she provides readers with interrater reliability figures for her motive classification (84.6% agreement).

Tennent *et al* (1971) examined 56 UK female firesetter in-patients who were associated with 111 instances of firesetting. The most prevalent motivator was reported to be *conflict with authority* (hospital, prison or work; 39%, $n = 43$). Other noted motivators were *revenge* (directed at non-authority targets; 24%, $n = 27$), *attention-seeking* (15%, $n = 17$) and *self-harm/ destruction* (6%, $n = 7$). Unfortunately, however, more specific examples of each motive are not provided.

In a more recent UK study, designed to examine the personal reflections of nine female in-patient firesetters, Cunningham *et al* (2011) found that females tended to report firesetting in the context of *distressing life experiences* and in an attempt to *manage* such experiences. For example, the majority of these firesetters described experiencing a period of constant stress – as a result of myriad factors – prior to their firesetting, and themes of isolation were also highly evident. Some female participants appeared to use firesetting as a way of promoting change in these stressful or lonely circumstances (i.e., being taken to hospital or prison, where they would be looked after); others, however, appeared to use firesetting as a means of obtaining personal satisfaction and control (e.g., a sense of achievement and pride). Some women reported setting fires with no real thought as to the consequences of their actions (seemingly as the result of impaired reasoning). This study provides an insight into the personal reflections of female firesetters. However, because the aim of the study was simply to examine firesetting reflections and not motivators *per se*, it is unclear how many of the participants were motivated by each individual factor.

Some very preliminary observations have been made regarding the *targets* of firesetting committed by females. For example, Lewis & Yarnell (1951) commented that females tended not to set fires 'beyond the limits of their own circumscribed world' (p. 347). Put simply, females appear to set fires to property related to themselves in some way rather than unknown targets. Other research appears to support this basic premise (Tennent *et al*, 1971; Harmon *et al*, 1985; Bourget & Bradford, 1989; Stewart, 1993; Wachi *et al*, 2007). To illustrate, Bourget & Bradford (1989, p. 298) found that Canadian female firesetter psychiatric referrals selected a target 'invested with emotional meaning' and Wachi *et al* (2007) found that Japanese female firesetters committed their offences in or close to their place of residence.

Summary

The literature examining the reasons for female-perpetrated firesetting is scant and underdeveloped. There are no comprehensive female-specific theories designed to explain the onset or maintenance of firesetting, and in their absence, we have examined the range of studies investigating the possible motivators underlying female-perpetrated firesetting. Overall, our examination of the literature shows that there do not appear to be large differences across female and male firesetters. Nevertheless, in studies that include a male firesetter comparison group, a cry for help as a motivator appears to be much more prevalent among female firesetters.

Risk and treatment issues

There appear to be few treatment programmes for adult firesetters generally (see Palmer *et al*, 2007) and although attempts are now being made to develop standardised programmes for males (see Chapter 12), there are no standardised programmes for females. There appear to be two main issues underlying the lack of treatment for firesetters generally and these issues appear to be exacerbated for females. First, there is very little information examining recidivism in relation to apprehended firesetters. Thus, knowledge of how such recidivism may vary as a function of gender is conspicuously absent. Second, very little is known about risk factors for firesetting in males or females and so it is unclear which factors require targeting to reduce future acts of this nature. There are three highly relevant questions in relation to risk:

1 Do females recidivate at a rate that warrants specific assessment and treatment of their firesetting?
2 Is this recidivism notably different from that reported for males?
3 What types of risk factors are specifically related to firesetting?

Recidivism

Rice & Harris (1996) reported a base rate of firesetting reoffending of about 16% in males ($n = 208$) with a mental disorder over a 7.8-year follow-up. However, other studies – notably those that have been critiqued methodologically (see Brett, 2004) – have suggested higher figures, in the region of 28% (Lewis & Yarnell, 1951; Geller *et al*, 1992). Thus, the yardstick with which to compare figures for female firesetting recidivism is extremely poor. In the few studies that have examined this issue, the low numbers of females examined relative to males (e.g., Soothill & Pope, 1973) make it almost impossible to compare female recidivism rates adequately. Furthermore, the only study to examine the recidivism of females *prospectively* (Lewis & Yarnell, 1951) is extremely old and used such poor recidivism criteria that the result (a rate of 13% over 15 years) may be unreliable.

In the absence of rigorously derived prospective measures of female firesetting recidivism, an examination of the proportions of females who engage in multiple firesetting behaviours may be somewhat informative. However, an examination of such studies reveals significant variation across samples (i.e., around 11% to 79%; see Brett, 2004). To illustrate, Harmon *et al* (1985) found that just 3 (or 11%) of their psychiatric referrals for firesetting had previous firesetting convictions on file. At the other extreme, Tennent *et al* (1971) found that the majority of their female firesetter psychiatric in-patients (79%) reported multiple firesetting acts. Undoubtedly, the various sampling sources, methods and differing criteria used to define and record firesetting behaviours lead to wildly differing estimates across studies. In a more recent retrospective study, however, Dickens *et al* (2009) examined the criminal histories and files of 167 UK firesetter psychiatric referrals, 38 of whom were female (23%). Dickens *et al* reported findings suggesting that gender was not a variable that predicted repeat firesetting. Nevertheless, of interest was the finding that repeat firesetting occurred in nearly half of the sample overall (49%, $n = 81$). Other studies have compared male and female firesetters' previous acts of firesetting and found that multiple firesetting appears to be comparable across the genders, with approximately one in five of both males and females likely to have a history of firesetting (Geller & Bertsch, 1985; Rix, 1994; Puri *et al*, 1995).

To summarise, we know very little about the recidivism of females in relation to firesetting. However, the existing research that we have examined suggests that: (1) the figure may be quite substantial and (2) the figure is likely to be comparable with the figures suggested for males. Thus, the recidivism of females in relation to firesetting is an issue likely to warrant specialist treatment. Nevertheless, until more rigorous studies have examined this issue it is impossible to ascertain exactly the extent of the problem regarding female firesetter recidivism.

Risk factors

An issue highly associated with recidivism is knowing the exact risk factors to pinpoint in order to reduce the future risk of firesetting offences. As noted in the literature (Dickens *et al*, 2009; Gannon & Pina, 2010), there is little information available for professionals regarding how to predict or establish severity of risk for males or females who have engaged in firesetting. For example, there are no published risk assessment tools for firesetting, although some schedules of risk for violence include such offences within a general assessment (e.g., the HCR-20; Webster *et al*, 1997). In addition, most of the research examining factors predictive of firesetting has focused on either male children and adolescents (e.g., Kolko *et al*, 2006) or adult males in psychiatric services (e.g., Rice & Harris, 1996). In a recent exception, Dickens *et al* (2009) used predictive regression analyses to examine the key characteristics of male and female firesetter recidivists. Dickens *et al* reported that recidivist firesetters are characterised by features such as: being *young, single,* having some developmental history of *family violence* or *substance misuse, early onset of criminal convictions, lengthier prison stays, relationship troubles* and *previous convictions for property offences.* Dickens *et al* also discovered that male and female firesetters who were coded as having lit a dangerous fire (i.e., one that would likely cause significant harm or damage) appeared no more likely to recidivate than seemingly less dangerous firesetters. Dickens *et al*'s overall findings are valuable, since they not only contravene intuitively appealing assumptions about firesetters (i.e., that those who light the most dangerous fires will be those most likely to reoffend) but also suggest that those most likely to recidivate are property offenders who experience developmental adversity and problems with later relationships. Dickens *et al* also report that more recidivist firesetters experienced anxiety or excitement associated with their firesetting. Consequently, it appears that interest in, sensory reinforcement from, or excitement around fire is likely to be one type of risk factor for both male and female firesetters (see also Rice & Harris, 1996).

In summary, there is a distinct lack of research examining the risk factors and associated treatment needs of either male or female firesetters. In order for effective risk assessments and treatment programmes to be developed, further research needs to explore both static and dynamic risk factors for repeat firesetting. Furthermore, in addition to the paucity of work in this general area, there is little attention paid to females *specifically* in relation to these issues. Nevertheless, based on our review of the literature, we would suggest that developmental adversity might represent one set of stable risk factors for female firesetting. Furthermore, in relation to dynamic risk factors, or factors directly amenable to treatment, general mental illness and factors relating to the motivators underlying firesetting (e.g., poor communication) would appear to be suitable variables for future study in relation to female firesetting more generally.

Treatment initiatives

Given the paucity of research examining the recidivism rates or risk factors associated with female firesetting, it is perhaps unsurprising that there is no standardised treatment programme for either male or female firesetters. The only published descriptions of treatment for female firesetters have concerned either tailored treatment for unusual cases (e.g., Awad & Harrison, 1976) or treatment of women in psychiatric facilities using cognitive–behavioural frameworks (e.g., Swaffer *et al*, 2001; Taylor *et al*, 2002, 2006). For example, Swaffer *et al* (2001) describe their group treatment for firesetting with patients with a variety of mental disorders ($n = 10$, six of whom were female). This comprised 62 sessions covering:

- fire danger
- coping skills (e.g., social skills, assertiveness, conflict resolution)
- reflective insight (e.g., self-esteem and self-concept)
- relapse prevention work.

In addition to the group work, Swaffer *et al* (2001) describe individualised treatment for the patients and also individualised psychometric treatment needs assessment, examining fire interest, anger, depression, self-esteem and assertiveness. A detailed case study description of one of the female patients is provided to illustrate the overall effectiveness of the intervention. Nevertheless, a detailed analysis of clinical change is not provided, due to the small numbers of patients within the programme.

A group programme for patients with intellectual disability in the UK has been described by Taylor *et al* (2002). This programme appears to have been implemented separately for male and female patients, although the treatment appears to have examined the same basic content over 40 sessions. This content included fire education, analysis of offending patterns, a focus on coping skills and family adversity, and general relapse prevention. Nevertheless, although Taylor *et al* report some encouraging post-treatment progress using psychometric measures, males and females are not compared and it would perhaps be misleading to do so given the small numbers of patients involved in the intervention ($n = 14$).

In a more recent study, Taylor *et al* (2006) describe a very similar treatment programme to that outlined by Taylor *et al* (2002). In this case, however, the treatment clients were six female psychiatric in-patients with intellectual disability. Following treatment completion, Taylor *et al* (2006) reported post-treatment progress on self-esteem (measured via the Culture-Free Self-Esteem Inventory; Battle, 1992), anger (measured via the Novaco Anger Scale; Novaco, 1994), depression (measured via the Beck Depression Inventory – Short Form; Beck & Beck, 1972) and goal attainment in relation to treatment needs (measured via the Goal Attainment Scales; Kiresuk & Sherman, 1968). However, of note was the fact that the only *significant* treatment progress related to goal attainment in relation to treatment needs. Nonetheless, overall treatment did look promising as described via individual case reports and it is possible that the small number of patients involved precluded meaningful statistical significance testing.

To summarise, there is evidence of encouraging individual treatment initiatives for female firesetters in the UK. However, to date, these initiatives appear to relate only to women in psychiatric settings and very small sample sizes preclude meaningful interpretation of the overall success of each treatment programme. Clearly, it will take larger sample sizes and more sophisticated designs and follow-up methods (i.e., the addition of a matched comparison group) in order for us better to understand what actually *works* regarding the treatment of female firesetters.

Future research and treatment initiatives

The overview of female arson and firesetting research provided in this chapter highlights a number of areas in need of research. A prominent need is to gain more understanding of the overall features and characteristics of females who start fires in relation to (1) their male firesetting counterparts and (2) females who do not start fires. Furthering our understanding of the factors associated with female-perpetrated firesetting will inevitably lead to better interventions. Particularly pertinent areas for future investigation are the specific and general psychopathologies associated with female firesetters (e.g., the prevalence and nature of pyromania and other mental disorders in female firesetters relative to appropriate comparison groups). Also required are prospective studies of firesetting recidivism that examine the base rates of firesetting for females relative to males. Establishing these base rates will enable researchers to ascertain more effectively the range of factors predicting female-perpetrated firesetting so that they may be utilised in effective and gender-responsive treatment programmes.

In terms of treatment needs, our overview of the research literature suggests that male and female firesetters may share similar factors (e.g., childhood adversity, personal characteristics and motivators for firesetting). Thus, it may be reasonable to suggest that male and female firesetters would both benefit from flexible treatment that emphasises:

- analysis of offending behaviour
- the links between childhood experiences and adult functioning (e.g., coping, conflict resolution, communication)
- attitudes supporting firesetting
- preoccupation or interest in fire
- general relapse prevention work.

However, based upon the treatment targets established for female offenders more generally (see Koons *et al*, 1997; Covington & Bloom, 2006) it could be hypothesised that in order for firesetter treatment to be responsive to the needs of females, it needs to address previous victimisation (particularly in relation to men) and the effect of such victimisation on communication skills, self-esteem and coping. Based on our review of the motivators underlying female-perpetrated firesetting, it may also be the case that females require specific work examining the development of personally satisfying and supportive relationships that enable women to gain attention in a pro-social manner. A particularly appealing rehabilitation model to use in this respect would be the 'good lives' model (Ward & Stewart, 2003), which conceptualises risk factors or treatment needs as obstructions (due to either lack of skills or lack of external supports) that limit people's abilities to obtain the human experiences essential for psychological well-being (e.g., satisfactory relationships).

Another topic that may be particularly relevant for female firesetters in treatment is an exploration of the link between self-harm and firesetting. Given that self-harm and firesetting may have similar aetiologies – including an inability to communicate trauma and needs successfully (see Coid *et al*, 1999) – exploring and learning new communication styles may be essential for any form of comprehensive rehabilitation for female firesetters who also have evidence of self-harm in their history. In relation to trauma, it is worth noting that treatment effectiveness for female offenders generally is believed to be optimised in all-female groups (see Lex, 1995; Ashley *et al*, 2003); in particular, women who have experienced abuse at the hands of men are likely to feel safer exploring their past in an all-female treatment group.

Conclusions

In this chapter, we have explored the main features, characteristics, psycho-pathologies and treatment needs of female firesetters. Our examination of the empirical literature suggests that female firesetters are typically neglected in research and are rarely studied within their own right or are included in large, general, mixed-sex cohorts and are not analysed or discussed separately. Thus, few studies have made adequate comparisons between male and female firesetters or female firesetters and the general female offender population. Because of this it is almost impossible to draw definitive conclusions regarding the features and characteristics of female firesetters. This in turn hinders professionals' abilities to assess and treat female firesetters in an empirically informed manner. We urge researchers to carefully consider the design of any study that includes female firesetters. In particular, in studies with a sole focus on female firesetters, relevant comparison groups should be included where possible to help ascertain which features are unique to female firesetters. Furthermore, in larger cohort studies of male and female firesetters, time should be taken to include gender-based analyses and comparison. Only by making such comparisons will the research field begin to hold a more empirically informed and rigorous understanding of female-perpetrated firesetting.

References

American Psychiatric Association (1994) *Diagnostic and Statistical Manual of Mental Disorders* (4th edn) (DSM-IV). APA.

American Psychiatric Association (2000) *Diagnostic and Statistical Manual of Mental Disorders* (4th edn, text revision) (DSM-IV-TR). APA.

Anwar, S., Långström, N., Grann, M., *et al* (2011) Is arson the crime most strongly associated with psychosis? A national case–control study of arson risk in schizophrenia and other psychoses. *Schizophrenia Bulletin*, **37**, 580–586 .

Ashley, O. S., Marsden, M. E. & Brady, T. M. (2003) Effectiveness of substance abuse treatment programming for women: a review. *American Journal of Drug and Alcohol Abuse*, **29**, 19–53.

Awad, G. A. & Harrison, S. I. (1976) A female fire-setter: a case report. *Journal of Nervous and Mental Disease*, **163**, 432–437.

Barker, A. F. (1994) *Arson: A Review of the Psychiatric Literature*. Oxford University Press.

Barnett, W. & Spitzer, M. (1994) Pathological fire-setting 1951–1991: a review. *Medicine, Science and the Law*, **34**, 2–3.

Battle, J. (1992) *Culture-Free Self-Esteem Inventory*. Pro-Ed.

Beck, A. T. & Beck, R. W. (1972) Screening depressed patients in family practice. A rapid technique. *Postgraduate Medicine*, **52**, 81–85.

Bennett, W. M. & Hess, K. M. (1984) *The Arsonist: A Closer Look*. Charles C. Thomas.

Blanchette, K. & Brown, S. (2006) *The Assessment and Treatment of Women Offenders: An Integrative Perspective*. Chichester, UK: Wiley.

Bourget, D. & Bradford, J. M. W. (1989) Female arsonists: a clinical study. *Bulletin of the American Academy of Psychiatry and Law*, **17**, 293–300.

Bradford, J. M. (1982) Arson: a clinical study. *Canadian Journal of Psychiatry*, **27**, 188–193.

Brett, A. (2004) 'Kindling theory' in arson: how dangerous are firesetters? *Australian and New Zealand Journal of Psychiatry*, **38**, 419–425.

Coid, J. W. (1993) An affective syndrome in psychopaths with borderline personality disorder. *British Journal of Psychiatry*, **162**, 641–650.

Coid, J., Wilkins, J. & Coid, B. (1999) Fire-setting, pyromania and self-mutilation in female remanded prisoners. *Journal of Forensic Psychiatry*, **10**, 119–130.

Covington, S. S. & Bloom, B. E. (2006) Gender-responsive treatment and services in correctional settings. *Women and Therapy*, **29**, 9–33.

Cunningham, E. M., Timms, J., Holloway, G., *et al* (2011) Women and firesetting: a qualitative analysis of context, meaning and development. *Psychology and Psychotherapy: Theory, Research and Practice*, **82**, 128–140.

Dickens, G., Sugarman, P., Ahmad, F., *et al* (2007) Gender differences amongst adult arsonists at psychiatric assessment. *Medcine, Science and the Law*, **47**, 233–238.

Dickens, G., Sugarman, P., Ahmad, F., *et al* (2009) Recidivism and dangerousness in arsonists. *Journal of Forensic Psychiatry and Psychology*, **20**, 621–639.

Enayati, J., Grann, M., Lubbe, S., *et al* (2008) Psychiatric morbidity in arsonists referred for forensic psychiatric assessment in Sweden. *Journal of Forensic Psychiatry and Psychology*, **19**, 139–147.

Fazel, S., Gulati, G., Linsell, L., *et al* (2009) Schizophrenia and violence: systematic review and meta-analysis. *Plos Medicine*, **6**, 1–15. At http://www.ncbi.nlm.nih.gov/pmc/articles/PMC2718581/pdf/pmed.1000120.pdf (accessed 17 December 2010).

Freud, S. (1932) The acquisition of power over fire. *International Journal of Psychoanalysis*, **13**, 405–410.

Gannon, T. (2010) Female arsonists: key features, psychopathologies and treatment needs. *Psychiatry: Interpersonal and Biological Processes*, **73**, 173–187.

Gannon, T. A. & Pina, A. (2010) Firesetting: psychopathology theory and treatment. *Aggression and Violent Behavior*, **15**, 224–238.

Geller, J. L. & Bertsch, G. (1985) Fire-setting behavior in the histories of a state hospital population. *American Journal of Psychiatry*, **142**, 464–468.

Geller, J. L., Fisher, W. H. & Bertsch, G. (1992) Who repeats? A follow up study of state hospital patients' firesetting behavior. *Psychiatric Quarterly*, **63**, 143–157.

Grant, J. E., Williams, K. A. & Potenza, M. N. (2007) Impulse control disorders in adolescent psychiatric inpatients: co-occurring disorders and sex differences. *Journal of Clinical Psychiatry*, **68**, 1584–1592.

Harmon, R. B., Rosner, R. & Wiederlight, M. (1985) Women and arson: a demographic study. *Journal of Forensic Sciences*, **30**, 467–477.

Harry, B. & Balcer, C. M. (1987) Menstruation and crime: a critical review of the literature from the clinical criminology perspective. *Behavioral Sciences and the Law*, **5**, 307–321.

Hickle, K. E. & Roe-Sepowitz, D. E. (2010) Female juvenile arsonists: an exploratory look at characteristics and solo and group arson offences. *Legal and Criminological Psychology*, **15**, 385–399.

Howell, A. J. & Watson, D. C. (2005) Impairment and distress associated with symptoms of male-typed and female-typed DSM-IV axis-I disorders. *Journal of Clinical Psychology*, **61**, 389–400.

Icove, D. J. & Estepp, M. H. (1987) Motive-based offender profiles of arson and fire-related crimes. *FBI Law Enforcement Bulletin*, **56**, 17–23.

Jackson, H., Glass, C. & Hope, S. (1987) A functional analysis of recidivistic arson. *British Journal of Clinical Psychology*, **26**, 175–185.

Kiresuk, T. & Sherman, R. (1968) Goal attainment scaling: a general method of evaluating comprehensive mental health programmes. *Community Mental Health Journal*, **4**, 443–453.

Kocsis, R. N. & Cooksey, R. W. (2002) Criminal psychological profiling of serial arson crimes. *International Journal of Offender Therapy and Comparative Criminology*, **46**, 631–656.

Kolko, D. J., Herschell, A. D. & Scharf, D.M. (2006) Education and treatment for boys who set fires: specificity, moderators, and predictors of recidivism. *Journal of Emotional and Behavioral Disorders*, **14**, 227–239.

Koons, B. A., Burrow, J. D., Morash, M., *et al* (1997) Expert and offender perceptions of program elements linked to successful outcomes for incarcerated women. *Crime and Delinquency*, **43**, 512–532.

Leong, G. B. (1992) A psychiatric study of persons charged with arson. *Journal of Forensic Science*, **37**, 1319–1326.

Lewis, N. O. C. & Yarnell, H. (1951) *Pathological Firesetting (Pyromania)*. Nervous and Mental Disease Monographs no. 82. Coolidge Foundation.

Lex, B. W. (1995) Alcohol and other psychoactive substances dependence in women and men. In *Gender and Psychopathology* (ed. M. V. Seeman), pp. 311–357. American Psychiatric Press.

Lochner, C., Hemmings, S. M., Kinnear, C. J., *et al* (2004) Corrigendum to 'Gender in obsessive–compulsive disorder: clinical and genetic findings'. *European Neuropsychopharmacology*, **14**, 437–445.

Mavromatis, M. (2000) Serial arson: repetitive firesetting and pyromania. In *Serial Offenders: Current Thought, Recent Findings* (ed. L. B. Schlesinger), pp. 67–102. CRC Press.

Miller, S. & Fritzon, K. (2007) Functional consistency across two behavioural modalities: firesetting and self-harm in female special hospital patients. *Criminal Behaviour and Mental Health*, **17**, 31–44.

Moore, D. P. & Jefferson, J. W. (2004) *Handbook of Medical Psychiatry* (2nd edn). Elsevier-Mosby.

Moore, T. M., Scarpa, A. & Raine, A. (2002) A meta-analysis of serotonin metabolite 5-HIAA and antisocial behaviour. *Aggressive Behavior*, **28**, 299–316.

Noblett, S. & Nelson, B. (2001) A psychosocial approach to arson – a case controlled study of female offenders. *Medicine, Science and the Law*, **41**, 325–330.

Novaco, R. W. (1994) Anger as a risk factor for violence among the mentally disordered. In *Violence and Mental Disorder: Developments in Risk Assessment* (eds J. Monahan & H. J. Steadman), pp. 21–59. University of Chicago Press.

O'Sullivan, G. H. & Kelleher, M. J. (1987) A study of firesetters in the south-west of Ireland. *British Journal of Psychiatry*, **151**, 818–823.

Palmer, E. J., Caulfield, L. S. & Hollin, C. R. (2007) Interventions with arsonists and young firesetters: a survey of the national picture in England and Wales. *Legal and Criminological Psychology*, **12**, 101–116.

Puri, B. K., Baxter, R. & Cordess, C. C. (1995) Characteristics of fire-setters: a study and proposed multiaxial psychiatric classification. *British Journal of Psychiatry*, **166**, 393–396.

Rice, M. E. & Harris, G. T. (1996) Predicting the recidivism of mentally disordered firesetters. *Journal of Interpersonal Violence*, **11**, 364–375.

Ritchie, E. C. & Huff, T. G. (1999) Psychiatric aspects of arsonists. *Journal of Forensic Science*, **44**, 733–740.

Rix, K. J. B. (1994) A psychiatric study of adult arsonists. *Medicine, Science and the Law,* **34**, 21–34.

Roy, A., Virkkunen, M., Guthrie, S., *et al* (1986) Indices of serotonin and glucose metabolism in violent offenders, arsonists and alcoholics. In *Psychology of Suicidal Behavior* (eds J. J. Mann & M. Stanley), pp. 202–220. New York Academy of Sciences.

Smith, J. & Short, J. (1995) Mentally disordered firesetters. *British Journal of Hospital Medicine,* **53**, 136–140.

Soothill, K. L. & Pope, P. J. (1973) Arson: a twenty-year cohort study. *Medicine, Science and the Law,* **13**, 127–138.

Steffensmeier, D. & Demuth, S. (2006) Does gender modify the effects of race – ethnicity on criminal sanctions? Sentences for male and female, White, Black, and Hispanic defendants. *Journal of Quantitative Criminology,* **22**, 241–261.

Stewart, L. A. (1993) Profile of female firesetters: implications for treatment. *British Journal of Psychiatry,* **163**, 248–256.

Swaffer, T., Hagget, M. & Oxley, T. (2001) Mentally disordered firesetters: a structured intervention programme. *Clinical Psychology and Psychotherapy,* **8**, 468–475.

Taylor, J. L., Thorne, I., Robertson, A., *et al* (2002) Evaluation of a group intervention for convicted arsonists with mild and borderline intellectual disabilities. *Criminal Behaviour and Mental Health,* **12**, 282–293.

Taylor, J. L., Robertson, A., Thorne, I., *et al* (2006) Responses of female fire-setters with mild and borderline intellectual disabilities to a group intervention. *Journal of Applied Research in Intellectual Disabilities,* **19**, 179–190.

Tennent, T. G., McQuaid, A., Loughnane, T., *et al* (1971) Female arsonists. *British Journal of Psychiatry,* **119**, 497–502.

Virkkunen, M. (1984) Reactive hypoglycaemia tendency among arsonists. *Acta Psychiatrica Scandanavica,* **69**, 445–452.

Virkkunen, M., Nuutila, A., Goodwin, F. K., *et al* (1987) Cerebrospinal fluid monoamine metabolite levels in male arsonists. *Archives of General Psychiatry,* **44**, 241–247.

Virkkunen, M., DeJong, J., Bartko, J., *et al* (1989) Relationship of psychobiological variables to recidivism in violent offenders and impulsive fire setters. A follow-up study. *Archives of General Psychiatry,* **46**, 600–603.

Wachi, T., Watanabe, K., Yokota, K., *et al* (2007) Offender and crime characteristics of female serial arsonists in Japan. *Journal of Investigative Psychology and Offender Profiling,* **4**, 29–52.

Ward, T. & Stewart, C. A. (2003) Treatment of sex offenders: Risk management and good lives. *Professional Psychology, Research, and Practice,* **34**, 4, 353–360.

Webster, C. D., Douglas, K. S., Eaves, D., *et al* (1997) *HCR-20: Assessing Risk for Violence* (version 2). Simon Fraser University.

Wilbanks, W. (1986) Are female felons treated more leniently by the criminal justice system? *Justice Quarterly,* **3**, 517–552.

CHAPTER 8

Power and excitement in arson: the case of firefighter arson

Rebekah M. Doley and Kenneth R. Fineman

Perhaps more than most crimes, the crime of arson is often shrouded in anecdotal descriptions concerning what actually motivates the offender. Arson in any form is repugnant, but even more so when the individual involved is a serving member of the fire service. Fire department personnel and the community alike abhor incidents of this nature. Although the incidence of firefighter arson is low in comparison with the total number of currently serving firefighters, the impact on community faith and fire service morale is disproportionately great. The integrity of the service is demonstrated in the performance of its personnel. While the service operates with full accountability, the very public nature of its business and the high visibility of its staff create unique problems for management. One of these is the amount of media attention (representing the 'public's right to know') the activities of the service and its individual members can expect, especially when something particularly newsworthy occurs, such as the detection of a firefigher arsonist within the ranks of current serving officers. On these occasions it is safe to assume that much of the good work that preceded the incident, and certainly some of it that follows, will be lost in the media frenzy to focus on the one case in which someone did something they should not have done.

This chapter focuses on the notion of power and excitement as mediators of firesetting in the context of a special case of arson: firesetting firefighters. The discussion opens with an overview of the common typology of motives and an explanation of where firefighter arson fits within this classification. Subsequently, the concept of power, and sometimes excitement, as driving the behaviour is addressed and examples from case studies are provided to illustrate the core concepts. The chapter concludes with consideration of implications of this proposal for the selection and screening of firefighters.

Motives for firefighter arson

Most convicted firefighter arsonists have refused to admit their guilt or to state their reason for their actions. However, the nature of the offences (usually targeting derelict buildings, scrub or rubbish skips) suggests it may be for the excitement in attending the fire, to feel part of a well-functioning team that is involved in playing an important role in society, or even to create enough work to justify the resources allocated to the fire department (particularly in rural areas). In their comprehensive study, Lewis & Yarnell (1951) speculated that the following reasons may apply:

- wanting to pose as heroes
- seeking the opportunity to operate new or upgraded equipment
- competition with other fire brigades in the area to be first at the scene
- wanting to justify their jobs
- trying to keep funding or to generate funding for their brigade.

In some countries a financial incentive may be more relevant. In Australia, for instance, volunteer firefighters are not generally paid per fire attendance. However, in the USA, while there is no pay for the volunteers, some departments will provide a stipend, which is usually based upon the percentages of fires the firefighter attends.

The National Center for the Analysis of Violent Crime (NCAVC) provides specialist research and operational support to the US Federal Bureau of Investigation (FBI). Its widely used classification of motives for arson has six major categories (Douglas *et al*, 1992):

1   profit (or fraud)
2   revenge
3   excitement
4   vandalism
5   crime concealment
6   extremism.

In its report, the United States Fire Administration (2003) provided examples of cases of firefighter arson for each of these motive types. These explanations are useful to the extent that each case of firefighter arson can be classified into one or the other of the chosen motive categories. It is assumed that the specification of motive category will provide more information, upon which recidivism and dangerousness can be better predicted. But this is not always the case. In fact, frequently an offender's reason for lighting fires is more complex than can be neatly articulated into one or other category. Fineman (1995) created eight motivational categories with 25 subcategories. His assumption was that the provision of multiple motive categories would help in the analysis and especially the recidivism prediction of those arsonists whose motive pattern bridges multiple categories. Not all of these motivational factors are implicated in the reinforcement pattern of firefighter arsonists, yet some stand out as factors to be considered in an assessment of these offenders. These are discussed below in more detail.

Profit (or fraud)

The profit (or fraud) category is equivalent to category 4 of Fineman's (1995) dynamic–behavioural typology, which focuses upon the antisocial firesetter. Fineman's typology deals with the profit motive and also includes in this category the 'cover another crime' situation, vandalism, hate and revenge. Fineman considered that many firefighters who set fires (along with other 'would-be heroes') fall into his antisocial category.

Revenge

This category also appears in Fineman's (1995) category 4. Revenge-motivated arsonists focus on personal retaliation, societal retaliation, institutional retaliation or group retaliation, with intent to intimidate. The present authors acknowledge the dangerousness of the revenge-focused arsonist. We find, however, that few of the firefighters who set fires whom we have studied fall into this category or its subtypes.

Excitement

This category is consistent with Fineman's (1995) category 6, which describes the severely disturbed firesetter. With regard to sensation-seeking or excitement, Fineman focuses on those firesetters who obtain significant sensory (physiological) reinforcement from their firesetting. This category would also include the pyromaniac who appears to obtain significant sensory reinforcement when a fire is set. Fineman also considers in this category the paranoid, overtly psychotic and self-harming firesetter. Fineman's (1995) category 6 has specific reference to sensory reinforcement.

Douglas *et al* (1992) included under this 'excitement' category thrill-seekers, attention-seekers and recognition-seekers, and those with fire-related sexual perversions. Fineman's dynamic–behavioural categories differ from Douglas *et al*'s categories with regard to recognition-seekers. Fineman perceives this group as receiving less sensory reinforcement for their firesetting and more cognitive reinforcement, in the sense of perceiving themselves to be exceptionally empowered and in control, as a function of their firesetting. We note that arsonists seeking thrills and excitement often put themselves in a position to observe the fire that they have started.

Fineman (2003) posits three reinforcement situations that help one understand the reinforcement process in firesetting. As applied to sensory reinforcement, the first refers to the reinforcement that may occur when a firesetter looks at and is reinforced by the flame itself, and what the flame does. The second reinforcement situation occurs as a function of the specific target that is set on fire. The third situation looks at the reinforcement that is obtained from the chaos that ensues from a fire *vis-à-vis* the confluence of all the protective agencies coming together to put the fire out. Both the first and the third situations can generate significant sensory reinforcement (e.g., excitement) in the firesetter. Those situations may be perceived by the arsonist not only at a sensory level, but also at a cognitive level relative to the feeling of power and control. It might be reasonable to assume that firefighters who are able to control both firesetting and fire suppression situations can obtain significant levels of sensory reinforcement and cognitive reinforcement, especially if they, by circumstances, perceive themselves to be empowered and in control. Additional feelings of power and control are generated when the firefighter arsonist receives kudos for discovering and/or putting out a fire.

Reinforcement

There is growing evidence to support the integration of biologically based reinforcers within a discussion of firefighter arson. Though aspects of sensation-seeking (excitement) may be reinforced by a biochemical mechanism, this type of reinforcement may be quite rare. Information on its base rate in the population of arsonists would be a relevant research topic. The reinforcement (i.e., excitement generated *vis-à-vis* firesetting) obtained through sensation-seeking may be quite powerful and may interact with other motivational variables. Strong biochemical factors may help reinforce aspects of the excitement motive. These biochemical reinforcers may also reinforce aspects of the sensory reinforcement quality described in Fineman's (1995) category 6.

A mechanism by which some firesetters obtain sensory reinforcement for setting fires may be understood by looking at Zuckerman's analysis (1994, 2007) of reinforcement for sensation-seeking. Zuckerman (1994) talks about sensation-seeking as a 'trait defined by the seeking of varied, novel, complex, and intense sensations and experiences, and the willingness to take physical, social, legal, and financial risks for the sake of such experiences' (p. 27). Zuckerman's sensation-seeking traits are partitioned into four dimensions: thrill- and adventure-seeking; experience-seeking; disinhibition; and boredom susceptibility. This model of sensation-seeking suggests that an underlying trait is created by biological changes in the sensation-seeker. Zuckerman's (1994, 2007) theories appear to answer questions concerning what it is that motivates people to override their natural protection mechanism when they take risks. Some individuals choose to override their fight-or-flight response signals and participate in dangerous or risky situations. Zuckerman (2007) believes that the biochemical reinforcers that the body is capable of producing are powerful enough to overcome what some might consider a more sensible response to a dangerous or risky situation. He associates sensation-seeking with 'strong dopaminergic reactivity and weak serotonergic and noradrenergic reactivities' (p. 27).

Zuckerman (2007) states in essence that there are some who seek dangerous situations in order to obtain the biochemical reinforcement that is produced when one anticipates or is exposed to dangerous/risky situations. An implication of Zuckerman's work is that sensation-seekers may require this internal biochemical reinforcer at a higher level than most others. This might suggest that the non-sensation-seeker might be able to obtain the types of biochemical reinforcers suggested by Zuckerman through acts that are not significantly dangerous or risky, or that the non-sensation-seeker may not require an extensive amount of this biochemical reinforcer to reach a level of satisfaction. In contrast, sensation-seekers may require participation in these acts in order to obtain what they consider to be a necessary level of biochemical reinforcement. As an example, when Zuckerman discusses parachuters he notes, 'it could be that impulsive sensation seekers are hyperarousable in many situations and that the arousal that they experience in risky sensations is therefore more enjoyable because it brings them up to their optimal levels' (Zuckerman, 2007, p. 97). This theory may have implications for those firesetters who obtain significant sensory reinforcement from setting fires or who enjoy the activity and chaos-laden aftermath of a fire that they have caused.

Few studies pairing sensation-seeking models and fire-related issues have been reported. Slovic *et al* (2000) had participants rate the perceived risk of death and the perceived benefits of a variety of activities on a scale of 0–100. Out of 18 activities, firefighting was rated eighth in terms of risk. Yet, it was rated highest in terms of perceived benefits. In a study of risky vocations, Musolino & Hershenson (1977) asked personnel specialists to rank ten occupations according to the degree of risk involved with the job. 'Fireman' was rated fourth, after 'test pilot', 'air traffic controller' and 'police officer'. Firefighting was rated in the top 5% of risky professions by this sample. Thus it was noted, in both of these samples, that 'firefighter' was perceived as a significantly risky profession.

Zuckerman (2007) reported that Goma-i-Freixanet *et al* (1988) compared Spanish firefighters and students using a Sensation Seeking Scale. It was noted that firefighters had significantly higher total scores on that scale, as well as on the 'Thrill and adventure' and 'Experience-seeking' subscales, than the student controls. This finding would suggest that professional firefighters, at least in Spain, look for thrills, excitement and novelty. The fact that they look for these types of reinforcement at a higher level than students in general is likely consistent with the general perception that firefighting will provide them.

Zuckerman (2007) comments on issues of boredom with firefighters as well as police officers when he states that lower boredom susceptibility would almost have to be a requirement for a job that requires long periods of inactivity. He notes that some people may be attracted to a profession because of its image as a provider of thrills and adventure, but then feel condemned to a life of boring routine. Are firefighter arsonists more susceptible than other firefighters to boredom? The issue of boredom appears a paradox for firefighters both in the USA and in Australia.

Fineman's clinical experience finds examples of individual firefighters also complaining of boredom. Volunteer firefighters who have disclosed their history of arson, or those who have been convicted of arson, have frequently spoken about boredom being a motive for their fires. Zuckerman (2007), when talking about boredom susceptibility and the monotony of long-distance driving, states that monotonous conditions are particularly aversive to sensation-seekers. A reasonable hypothesis may be that some firefighters who become arsonists are sensation-seekers and perhaps are exceptionally susceptible to boredom.

If in fact some firefighter arsonists set a fire to obtain a biochemical 'rush', one might still ponder their willingness to take personal risks when setting a fire and their willingness to risk the safety of their community. Earlier in this chapter, we discussed firefighters' ability to manifest significant control over both fire lighting and fire suppression if they chose to do so. Firefighter arsonists may not perceive safety to the community to be a realistic risk if they feel significantly empowered and in control of a fire. There appears to be an interaction between sensory reinforcement (especially excitement) and the power motive when setting certain illegal fires. It is noteworthy that, in Fineman's clinical experience, volunteer firefighters have talked of their abilities to control a fire in spite of the fact that these same volunteer fire-fighters have often received little training in fire safety, fire control and fire suppression compared with firefighting professionals in their communities.

Zuckerman (2007), when discussing sexual interactions, states that sensation-seekers may be among those who are willing to take risks for the sake of intensified sensations in unplanned encounters. Could the same be true for some firefighters, who, bored while sitting around the fire station, or while at home waiting for a call from the fire department, eventually and impulsively set a fire for the sensation produced? Assuming that firefighter arsonists are sensation-seekers, perhaps exceptionally inclined to boredom, and joined the fire service to obtain this specific form of reinforcement, it is reasonable to assume that they may be so reinforced by the thrill of the fire that they engage in this behaviour in a serial fashion.

An alternative approach: the role of power in arson

While excitement seems to be at the heart of much deliberate firesetting, albeit not always as the primary identified motive, arguably there is a more common reinforcer, power, that is particularly relevant to understanding the special case of firefighter arson.

The main tenet of a power-focused model is that firesetting arises from an individual sense of anger and frustration at times when a person perceives an inability to effect change in the environment. An essential assumption underlying this explanation is that the behaviour is associated with a limited repertoire of alternative responses, due to a combination of personal inadequacies and psychosocial disadvantages that inhibit the development of more appropriate reactions. This can set up a pattern of failure and punishment, leading to feelings of low self-esteem and inadequacy (Sakheim *et al*, 1986; Gaynor, 1996; Repo *et al*, 1997).

A plausible explanation for why firefighters set arson fires focuses on power as the underlying drive. Arsonists are generally disenfranchised members of society. Through bad luck or bad choices they have found themselves disadvantaged across a range of life domains – educationally, socially and economically at the very least. They experience a sense of helplessness in the face of adversity, an inability to make changes effectively in their world, which leads to anger and frustration. Firesetting, in this scenario, could be seen as a bid for power: the individual uses fire to *acquire power* over the environment.

Characteristics of firefighter arsonists from New Zealand ($n = 17$) and Australia ($n = 14$) were examined (unpublished data; further details available from the first author). The data were gleaned from interviews with senior fire officers and with convicted firefighter arsonists, questionnaires completed by fire service personnel who worked with convicted arsonists, as well as local media reports. Within the sample, two individuals were paid firefighters and the remainder were volunteers. All were male and their ages ranged from 18 to 42 years. The number of fires set varied from 2 to 55; however, this is likely to be an underestimation, given that these figures represent fires the individual was charged with, and exclude any which were undetected or for which there was insufficient evidence for charges to be laid. With few exceptions, most individuals were singly responsible for more than 12 fires. The desire to acquire power in this group was illustrated by arsonists in the study admitting that part of their reason for lighting fires was to demonstrate control over the fire, regardless of how big it became. That the majority of firefighter arsonists came from the volunteer ranks as opposed to the professional firefighting ranks is additional evidence of the demographics and dynamics of many individuals who join the volunteer firefighter ranks.

Having acquired power, arsonists are motivated to *demonstrate power* – after all, what is the use of having power if no one else knows you have it? Many of the arsonists in the Australasian study were first on the scene to fight the fire. Quite often they fought to have a prominent role in the firefighting effort – monopolising radio air space and ensuring they were seen at the front of the firefighting forces. The second author, from his American clinical sample, confirms the focus of the firefighter arsonist as well as older teen Explorer Scouts in putting themselves in the forefront of the fire-discovery/firefighting effort, acquiring acclaim from fire service colleagues as well as the public at large.

Once demonstrated, there is a need to *maintain power*. Arsonists may enjoy the kudos they receive from peers or the media attention devoted to a series of fires and this in itself can be a motivating factor. Certainly there is evidence to suggest that a copycat phenomenon exists for arson (Hitchens & Doley, 2006). This effect describes when arsonists are motivated either to start lighting fires or to refine their technique following media reporting of fire. The reinforcement provided by the media adds to the perceived sense of power by providing mass attention and excitement to the clinical picture. The notion of maintaining power may explain the trend for firefighter arsonists not to desist of their own accord. Not one of the individuals reviewed for a study by Doley (unpublished data; further details available from the first author), for instance, spontaneously desisted in their firesetting activities prior to detection.

But with the acquisition of power comes the inevitable loss of power at some point. In the arsonists' world this may occur through restrictions on their firesetting freedoms arising from increased surveillance, patrols or coming under police suspicion, which effectively curtails their behaviour for a while. Having experienced a threat to their power, arsonists may well be motivated to *regain power* by escalating their activities, perhaps in terms of magnitude of fire or frequency of firesetting.

While this is a relatively simplistic model, it can be applied to virtually all of the common reasons given for firesetting. Certainly, the firesetting pattern of firefighter arsonists fits this model, as most (in both the Australasian and the American samples) demonstrate an escalation in terms of magnitude of offence as well as potential to endanger life.

Self-esteem and justice sensitivity

Other factors that have yet to be explored in relation to recidivistic arson are discussed in Chapter 10. However, two additional variables of particular relevance potentially for investigators of firefighter arson are self-esteem and justice sensitivity. Doley (2009) has addressed the issue of self-esteem as a variable relevant to adult serial firesetting generally. However, it may be particularly pertinent to a discussion of firefighter arson, due to the hypothesised significant main effect of a drive for power and dominance over their environmental setting underlying this behaviour. Low self-esteem is often mentioned in association with firesetting but rarely has it been effectively operationalised and measured in arson studies, although it has prominence in studies of other types of crime (Marshall *et al*, 1997). Stewart (1993), in the only study of firesetters that explicitly defined and measured self-esteem, reported that female incarcerated arsonists had lower self-esteem than a sample of non-arsonists matched for age and length of time incarcerated. Other authors writing of clinical treatment options for arsonists report that interventions targeting self-esteem are useful as part of an overall treatment package (Hall, 1995; Taylor *et al*, 2002).

Along with the influence of self-esteem is a hypothesised interaction with justice sensitivity. Doley (2009) raises the idea that arsonists may be particularly prone to experiencing maladaptive vengeance, resulting in a high number of fires lit for motives defined as revenge-based. Revenge often follows from feelings of injustice, that is, feeling wrongly offended against. Gabriel & Monaco (1994) distinguish between adaptive and maladaptive vengeance, where adaptive vengeance is the driving desire to get even in response to a perceived injury, but which does not develop into a compulsion for destructive action and which diminishes in intensity over time. Maladaptive vengeance is aligned to narcissistic rage and serves as a specific form of aggression arising from a perceived injury to one's sense of self or self-concept (Horney, 1948; Kohut, 1972; Bushman & Baumeister, 1998). According to Gabriel & Monaco (1994), maladaptive vengeance is a compulsive desire to get even, which becomes an overriding and all-consuming force in the individual, resulting in dangerous or harmful behaviours expressed towards others or the self.

The field of justice sensitivity research specifically investigates people's perceptions of what is fair with regard to the distribution of scarce resources, as well as the decision-making process involved in that distribution and the psychological effects of injustice (Schmitt et al, 1995). It is postulated that individuals may differ not only in terms of what they perceive as unjust, but also in how often they perceive injustice and in the magnitude of their emotional response to perceived injustice (Schmitt et al, 1995; Schmitt, 1996). Clearly there is a strong potential association with firefighter arsonists who claim to have engaged in firesetting to 'support' brigade activities or to generate more fire events (and subsequently more allocated resources) for their region.

Screening for a propensity to arson

Work is just starting on the development of offence-specific assessments for arsonists (see Chapter 10). Due to the relatively infrequent occurrence of firefighter arson, it seems unlikely that progress in identifying appropriate tools specific to this context will be rapid. Nevertheless, on the basis of the limited clinical indicators available, some efforts have been made to develop a specific assessment process aimed at identifying arson propensity among potential firefighters (Doley, 2000) and this work is being extended by the current authors. The recommended approach focuses on exploring those factors that have been linked to characteristics of firefighter arsonists as well as considering a range of behavioural characteristics that may indicate the potential to adjust successfully to an operational role within the fire service. While not an absolute predictor of propensity to light fires, it provides for a more structured and formalised step in the screening process than has traditionally been applied. In addition, in the past decade more fire services worldwide have chosen to utilise mandatory criminal record checks as part of their screening process. Of course, the difficulty with this approach on its own is the under-representation of arson in official records. That is, crime-type clusters are more likely to prove fruitful as an indicator of potential firesetting than arson convictions alone.

The remainder of the chapter is devoted to providing case examples to illustrate key components of the discussion so far. A general overview of firefighter arson is provided, followed by specific illustrations of firefighter arson highlighting the notion of excitement as a reinforcer and power as the central underlying theme of all activity of this nature. To conclude, implications for future research are canvassed.

Who is the firefighter arsonist?

There is limited information about the characteristics of firefighters who light fires. This may be partly because these individuals are frequently not inclined to admit their guilt after detection. Further, offenders are not categorised by occupation and therefore it is difficult to gather information through official records unless the circumstances of a particular offender are known personally to the researcher, for example through a pre-trial assessment order or treatment programme. Two published studies originating in the USA provide an insight into the profile of firefighter arsonists.

The first was undertaken by the FBI (Huff, 1994). This study examined 25 solved cases of firefighter arson, involving 75 offenders responsible for 182 fires. While over half (16; 64%) of these cases involved lone offenders who lit multiple fires, nine (36%) cases involved multiple offenders, often from the same fire department, working together. The general profile was of a White, younger male (average age 23 years). There was a history of occupational instability, with frequent job changes due to poor work performance. A prior criminal record comprising minor offences such as theft, traffic violations or other misdemeanours was found, along with poor academic performance. Those in the sample who lit fires as part of a group were found to be younger (average age 19 years) but essentially similar in profile, with the exception of being less likely to have a criminal record and more likely to be still in school. The predominant motives for the arsonists in this study were excitement or wanting to appear heroic to peers, family and the community generally (Huff, 1994). Other motives were profit (such as being paid overtime) and revenge. Most set their fires with material at the scene, using accelerant and a lighter or matches. There was evidence of escalation in their fire offending pattern, starting with nuisance fires (piles of rubbish, rubbish skips) and progressing to abandoned vehicles, unoccupied structures and, later, occupied structures in some cases.

The second study was conducted by the South Carolina Forestry Commission (Cabe, 1996). A review of existing psychological research was conducted, resulting in a profile of the firefighter arsonist. Although specific details of the background to the profile have not been provided, the profile has apparently been endorsed by law-enforcement officers in the region (Cabe, 1996). This sample included a higher proportion of offenders working in teams. Most were relatively junior in the fire service, with less than 2 years' experience. The primary motive was excitement and these individuals were described as eager and lacking in maturity. There is significant similarity between the Cabe and Huff profiles, despite the fact that one sample was exclusively of forestry workers while the other included a spectrum of paid and volunteer firefighters covering rural and urban sectors.

The only other study to focus exclusively on firefighter arsonists is the pilot research conducted by the first author (unpublished data; further details available from Doley). Predominantly, the individuals in this sample set fires while alone. However, there were three groups, comprising three offenders each, who set fires together; in these, it appeared that one individual instigated the firesetting series and secured the support of the co-offenders primarily through intimidation. A summary of the profile is provided in Box 8.1. The second author points to the similarity between many of the characteristics noted in Box 8.1 and risk factors for recidivism noted with the juvenile firesetter (Fineman, 1980, 1995; Dolan *et al*, 2011), perhaps justifying the assumption that while few juvenile firesetters mature into adult arsonists, many adult arsonists have a history of juvenile firesetting.

Information about the family background for the Australasian firefighter arsonists was limited (unpublished data; further details available from the first author). Some instability was evident in numerous residential locations throughout childhood, although a stable, apparently supportive family was noted for several offenders in the study. Contrary to typical arsonists,

---

Box 8.1 Profile of the Australasian firefighter arsonist

- Male, aged 18–42 years (average age 25 years)
- Volunteer firefighter
- Stable family background but regular relocation during childhood
- High-school education; average to above average intelligence
- Unskilled or semi-skilled employment; self-employed; frequent job changes
- No prior criminal record
- Single, or if married usually not first marriage
- No significant stressors at time of firesetting
- Either very junior or very senior in fire service
- No remorse but aware of consequence of firesetting actions; unlikely to confess even when confronted
- Escalating pattern of fire offending, starting with rubbish bins and piles or bushland, progressing to unoccupied structures and abandoned vehicles then commercial property
- Materials at the scene used; accelerant
- Fires set close to home or work route or destination; area familiar to the offender

(Unpublished data; further details available from the first author)

these offenders appeared to have average to above average intelligence; many of them had completed high school and were undertaking further trade training or studies. Generally there was no prior criminal record, although if previous crimes were indicated they were usually theft or dishonesty offences. Many of these volunteers were employed at the time of their offences, usually in unskilled or semi-skilled occupations such as labourer, mill worker, or running a small business such as a laundrette. Their reasons for joining the fire service included: wanting to contribute to the community in a positive way; seeking status and recognition from peers, family and the wider community that they perceived would come through wearing the fire service uniform; and wanting to be part of a highly functioning, well-respected team.

In some cases the individual had left another fire service under doubtful circumstances, for example involving antisocial behaviour, disciplinary problems or suspected offences (theft or arson) (unpublished data; further details available from the first author). In the majority of these cases no formal action had been taken against the person but they were effectively 'frozen out' of that particular department. In the main, the subsequent fire service was aware of pre-existing difficulties but allowed the individual to join as 'a second chance' or because there was no clear evidence supporting the previous service allegations.

Their arson activity appeared not to commence immediately for many but usually started within 12 months of joining (unpublished data; further details available from the first author). Consistent with previous findings, the offenders in the Australasian sample evidenced a pattern of escalation in their firesetting – starting with rubbish bins and piles and small scrub fires and progressing to vehicles and abandoned or unoccupied structures. Commercial properties were also targeted. Bushfires and other wildfires were particularly prevalent in this sample, partly due to the fact that many of these offenders came from rurally based fire services and therefore surrounding bushland was their obvious and most accessible target. The second author notes a similar progression in his primarily American clinical sample. In one case the arsonist graduated from bushfires to abandoned homes; within the homes he changed from a single site for setting the fire to multiple sites.

The focus of the first author's research was on discovering characteristics about offenders, particularly as they present in a fire service environment (unpublished data; further details available from Doley). While less attention was given to the specific firesetting techniques these individuals employed, the research contributed to what was known previously about the psychology and personal characteristics of these offenders. For instance, the distinction first noted by Huff (1994) of a younger and older group of firefighter arsonists was very apparent in the Australasian study, where two distinct categories of firefighter arsonist were identified, each with two clear subgroups (see Box 8.2).

Box 8.2 Subgroups of Australasian firefighter arsonists

Younger firefighter: followers

- Age 17–20 years
- Less than 12 months with fire service
- Overeager; enthusiastic
- Co-offender (rather than instigator)
- Respectful of hierarchy
- Likely to confess when questioned

Younger firefighter: instigators

- Age 17–20 years
- Less than 12 months with fire service
- Overconfident; brash
- Instigator
- History of disciplinary action
- Unlikely to confess

Older firefighters: team leader

- Age 30–45 years
- Experienced firefighter
- Position of responsibility/authority in fire service
- Self-employed
- Team player; well liked; respected
- Unlikely to confess

Older firefighters: dictator

- Age 30–45 years
- Experienced firefighter
- Position of responsibility/authority in fire service
- Self-employed
- Autocratic; dictatorial; arrogant
- Unlikely to confess

(Unpublished data; further details available from the first author)

The first category is of younger firefighters (aged approximately 17–20 years) who are relatively junior to the fire service (less than 12 months' service). Within this category is one group who are described as 'followers'. These individuals present as shy, quiet and unassuming. They are often on the edges of the team, tending to be considered 'hangers-on' rather than being included in the main core of the group. They are eager, enthusiastic and overly helpful. When firesetting was conducted as part of a group, this type of individual was frequently one of the co-offenders. They would be more likely to have been pressured into the offending by a more dominant personality in the group (i.e., who instigated the firesetting). Interestingly, whereas most arsonists tend not to admit guilt, even once they have been detected, individuals in this category almost always confessed under questioning. Descriptions of individuals in this category include:

- 'he was a helpful, friendly sort of guy. He wasn't pushy but he was a ... good young fella. You can't explain why it [the firesetting] happened.'
- 'he was very happy to oblige. He was keen to learn and keen to do things ... if there was a course he could go to he would be wanting to go on it. No trouble with authority, done [sic] what he was asked, good as gold.'

The other group in this younger category are described as arrogant and cocky. These adolescents are considered immature, brash and difficult to train because they appear to think they are more capable and knowledgeable about fires and firefighting than their experience would suggest. Some senior fire service members spoke indignantly of the frequency with which these individuals would challenge the decisions made by other, more experienced members of the team. Disciplinary action may have been taken to curb insubordination or reckless behaviour during training. Colleagues might refer to instances when the behaviour of the young firefighter was abusive or disrespectful to peers and colleagues (particularly to female members). Senior fire officers made the following comments when describing individuals in this category:

- (when asked about conflict at the fire service) 'yes he did'; 'because he was inclined to be a bit lazy he had sort of run up against some of the other firemen off and on'
- 'he is probably the only one who has ever challenged me [about a disciplinary rebuke delivered during training] like that. I've been a Chief now for 24 years.'

The second category comprises older, more experienced firefighters (aged approximately 30–45 years). These individuals often have been with the fire department for several years and now held a position of responsibility within the service. One subgroup seems to comprise individuals who are well respected within the service and the community as hard workers. They may be self-employed business people, married with children, and community leaders. They are respected as leaders in the fire service and devote considerable time and energy to ensuring the functioning of the team. They may be summarised in the words of one fire officer:

- 'he was such a ... keen firefighter – a model – he really was. Down to earth, good fun. He was a model and a very special one.'
- 'his attendance record was outstanding. In fact he was going to get a trophy for the best attendance. I had to hurriedly change that. You can't give it to a bloke who has just been arrested for arson...'

The other group is similar in characteristics generally, but less well liked. These individuals are described as overbearing, arrogant, lacking in social skills, aggressive and prone to using bully tactics to ensure they get their own way. They are often self-employed in a series of small-scale business ventures, usually involving unskilled or semi-skilled work. In the fire service environment they were considered to be overly controlling and micro-managers, although some were willing to overlook these attributes in favour of their exceptional work performance and attendance rate. As their colleagues said about individuals in this category:

- 'you loved him or you hated him. He was one of those people who had an incredible ability to rub people up the wrong way or to make them absolute devoted best friends. ... I would say half the brigade celebrated when he got sent down and half wept.'
- 'people complained about [him], people left the brigade and voted with their feet.'
- 'he was not the sort of guy to take orders very easily.'

These individuals rarely confessed of their own accord. Any admission of guilt was made only under formal questioning and then only by the younger and less dominant individuals described above. Detection of their crime occurred through a pattern of their behaviour being noticed, including regularly being first at scene or first to report a fire, or being very knowledgeable about the location of the fire following a call; or having more knowledge of a fire series than had been made publicly available; or by being seen leaving the scene on multiple occasions.

Implications

All areas of arson research seem equally deficient at this stage in the field's development. Issues associated with the assessment of arsonists generally have been canvassed throughout this book. The current chapter has focused on the particular, and peculiar, case of firefighter arson. Perhaps even more so than the act of arson itself, firefighter arson seems an anathema because it betrays the trust of a community. As with corruption in public service officials, firefighter arson speaks to all of our fears and concerns for safety. Little is known about this phenomenon because those who commit the crime appear less willing (or less able) than other arsonists to discuss their actions.

As with arson generally, interest in exploring this process has waxed and waned, with public concern driven by the recency or otherwise of incidents of this nature affecting the community. For meaningful progress in this field to be made, there needs to be a commitment to sustained research into the psychosocial and behavioural variables associated with firefighter arson. Particular attention on a functional analysis of the act is warranted to identify triggers and emotions temporally close to the firesetting that are relevant in maintaining the behaviour. A model of firefighter arson then could be developed to inform the efforts of those concerned primarily with the selection and recruitment of firefighters to serve in our community either as paid or as volunteer officers. The utility of criminal history checks as they are currently employed in this context also requires scrutiny. Finally, attention should be devoted to developing appropriate and targeted campaigns within fire services to identify those individuals lighting fires. From the research reviewed in this chapter, it is evident that in many cases the identity of the firefighter arsonist was probably known long before official action was taken and in the meantime fires continued to be lit and lives and property lost as a consequence.

Conclusion

Many who have worked with a firefighter who has subsequently been convicted of lighting fires express anger at how they were duped. They describe a fire service member who was keen, enthusiastic and always willing to be involved in training and other fire service activities. These individuals seem to be committed members of the team, giving freely of their time to further the interests of the brigade. It is difficult to reconcile the evidence with the person they know, and often even after a guilty conviction has been recorded, colleagues may find it hard to accept. The feelings of anger and betrayal are heightened as firefighter arsonists, consistent with arsonists generally, rarely express remorse for their actions, although they admit to understanding the potential consequences and inherent dangerousness (perhaps more than most, given their training) of their firesetting. The betrayal of fire service colleagues is reason enough to suggest that some form of psychological crisis debriefing or some form of psychological intervention should be offered to the arsonist's team members.

Evidenced by their usual unwillingness to admit their guilt, it seems these arsonists will rarely 'burn out' but will continue to set fires while they remain undetected and unchecked. We suggest that this dangerous phenomenon of allowing an arsonist into the ranks of the fire service can be significantly reduced through a preventive approach, involving the application of relevant and comprehensive background and psychological evaluations, especially if the individual is applying for a position as a volunteer.

In this chapter we have elaborated upon many of the common background characteristics of the firefighter arsonist. This information could form the basis of a screening or comprehensive evaluation instrument for those who wish to gain entry into the ranks of the fire service. Such an instrument would be of value to reduce the opportunity for potential arsonists to become firefighters. Through a process of analysis one can use the information available concerning motivational themes to acquire additional information that will help in the selection of firefighters. This same analysis and the information subsequently acquired can help in the treatment of those convicted of arson. To guide the development of such a comprehensive and culture-sensitive assessment, we have developed four theorems and associated corollaries.

Theorem 1

- The specification of motives associated with firefighter arsonists will help identify those who might become arsonists.
- Present information suggests a focus on profit, excitement, power, control, boredom, attention and a desire for heroism.

Corollary 1

- It will be beneficial to identify the base rates of motives manifested by firefighter arsonists.

Theorem 2

- The specification of demographic and personality risk factors will help identify those fire service candidates who are more likely to offend.

Corollary 2a

- Motives identified will suggest demographic and personality risk factors. To illustrate, the 'profit' motive suggests financial need; 'excitement' suggests sensation-seeking; 'power' suggests low self-esteem; 'control' suggests low self-esteem; 'boredom' suggests susceptibility to boredom; 'attention' suggests peer relationship issues; 'would-be heroism' suggests peer-related issues.

Corollary 2b

- Demographic and personality risk factors suggest areas to question candidates about, areas to investigate and areas for focused psychological testing.

Theorem 3

- There may be present in the fire service candidate personality factors unrelated to motive that increase the risk of fire deviant behavior.

Corollary 3

- Available data suggest a focus is wanted on: lack of empathy with regard to risk to both community and fire service colleagues; the candidate's job history, especially ability to keep a job; a history of even minor criminal offences; whether there were any attitudinal or behavioural difficulties in past fire service jobs; whether a candidate's family of origin were unable to provide stable guidance and care, including disclosures concerning a problematic relationship between the candidate and father; whether the candidate has a stable interpersonal relationship presently or is still living at home with parents; whether the candidate has the skills to navigate the social network; whether the candidate shows an obsessive fascination with the fire service and fire paraphernalia; a history of significant academic problems at school; and whether the candidate is under exceptional environmental stress or perhaps capable of being described with a DSM Axis I or Axis II diagnosis.

Theorem 4

- Sensitivity to cultural differences may suggest factors other than those set out above. It is noteworthy, for example, that the theorem 3 examples may relate more to the US population (*per* Huff, 1994; Cabe, 1996) than to the Australasian sample (*per* Doley, unpublished data; further details available from the first author). Research should focus not only on the characteristics of the firefighter arsonist but on the determination of whether cultural factors differentiate these arsonists. The same may be said for arsonists in general.

These theorems and corollaries provide a methodology for the development of an assessment tool to help in the selection of firefighter candidates. This methodology may also be used to develop assessment tools for other identifiable subpopulations of those who commit arson. If one is able to look closely at specific motives, demographic and personality risk factors, and risk factors unrelated to motive, it is likely that one may identify a cluster of variables that form a new construct specific to the personality of the arsonist (i.e., personal inadequacies and reinforcement history).

The acceptance of these theorems and corollaries necessitates a continued commitment to an empirical approach to the acquisition of firesetting-related data concerning motives, base rates and risk factors. If one accepts that motive analysis is an important component of the assessment and treatment process, then research must focus on the development of assessment tools to measure these variables.

Acknowledgement

The authors appreciate the input of Dr Allen Sapp, criminologist, and Timothy Huff, former FBI analyst, during the development of the 'role of power in arson' model.

References

Bushman, B. & Baumeister, R. (1998) Threatened egotism, narcissism, self-esteem, and direct and displaced aggression: does self-love or self-hate lead to violence? *Journal of Personality and Social Psychology*, **75**, 219–229.

Cabe, K. (1996) Firefighter arson: local alarm. *Fire Management Notes*, **56**, 7–9.

Dolan, M., McEwan, T., Doley, R., *et al* (2011) Risk factors and risk assessment in juvenile firesetting. *Psychology, Psychiatry and Law*, **18**, 378–394.

Doley, R. (2000) Screening for arson: is it imminent? Is it possible? *Firepoint*, **11**, 17–20.

Doley, R. (2009) *A Snapshot of Serial Arson in Australia*. Lambert Academic Publishing.

Douglas, J. E., Burgess, A. W., Burgess, A. G., *et al* (1992) *Crime Classification Manual: A Standard System for Investigating and Classifying Violent Crimes*. Lexington.

Fineman, K. R. (1980) Firesetting in children and adolescents. In *Psychiatric Clinics of North America, Vol. 3. Child Psychiatry: Contributions to Diagnosis, Treatment, and Research* (ed. B. J. Blinder), pp. 483–500. W. B. Saunders.

Fineman, K. R. (1995) A model for the qualitative analysis of child and adult fire deviant behavior. *American Journal of Forensic Psychology*, **13**, 31–60.

Fineman, K. R. (2003) Arson/arsonists. *Encyclopedia of Murder and Violent Crime* (ed. E. W. Hickey), pp. 26–32. Sage.

Gabriel, M. & Monaco, G. (1994) 'Getting even': clinical considerations of adaptive and maladaptive vengeance. *Clinical Social Work Journal*, **22**, 165–178.

Gaynor, J. (1996) Firesetting. *Child and Adolescent Psychiatry: A Comprehensive Textbook* (2nd edn) (ed. M. Lewis), pp. 591–603. Williams & Wilkins.

Goma-i-Freixanet, M., Perez, J. & Torrubia, R. (1988) Personality variables in antisocial and prosocial disinhibitory behavior. *Biological Contributions to Crime Causation* (eds T. E. Moffitt & S. A. Mednick), pp. 211–222. Nijhoff.

Hall, G. (1995) Using group work to understand arsonists. *Nursing Standard*, **9**(23), 25–28.

Hitchens, K. & Doley, R. (2006) Copycat arson: a closer look. *Fire and Arson Investigator* (April), 22–24.

Horney, K. (1948) The value of vindictiveness. *American Journal of Psychoanalysis*, **8**, 3–12.

Huff, T. G. (1994) Fire-setting fire fighters: identifying and preventing arsonists in fire departments. *IAFC On Scene*, **8**, 6–7.

Kohut, H. (1972) Thoughts on narcissism and narcissistic rage. *Psychoanalytic Study of the Child*, **27**, 360–400.

Lewis, N. O. C. & Yarnell, H. (1951) *Pathological Firesetting (Pyromania)*. Nervous and Mental Disease Monographs no. 82. Coolidge Foundation.

Marshall, W., Anderson, D. & Champagne, F. (1997) Self-esteem and its relationship to sexual offending. *Psychology, Crime and Law*, **3**, 161–186.

Musolino, R. F. & Hershenson, D. B. (1977) Avocational sensation seeking in high and low risk-taking occupations. *Journal of Vocational Behavior*, **10**, 358–365.

Repo, E., Virkkunen, M., Rawlings, R., *et al* (1997) Criminal and psychiatric histories of Finnish arsonists. *Acta Psychiatrica Scandinavica*, **95**, 318–323.

Sakheim, G., Vigdor, M., Gordon, M., *et al* (1986) A psychological profile of juvenile firesetters in residential treatment. In *Juvenile Firesetters in Residential Treatment* (eds G. Sakheim, M. Vigdor, M. Gordon, *et al*), pp. 1–33. Child Welfare League of America.

Schmitt, M. (1996) Individual differences in sensitivity to befallen injustice (SBI). *Personality and Individual Differences*, **21**, 3–20.

Schmitt, M., Neumann, R. & Montada, L. (1995) Dispositional sensitivity to befallen injustice. *Social Justice Research*, **8**, 385–407.

Slovic, P., Fischhoff, B. & Lichtenstein, S. (2000) Facts and fears: understanding perceived risk. In *The Perception of Risk* (ed. P. Slovic), pp. 137–153. Earthscan.

Stewart, L. (1993) Profile of female firesetters: implications for treatment. *British Journal of Psychiatry*, **163**, 248–256.

Taylor, J., Thorne, I., Robertson, A., *et al* (2002) Evaluation of a group intervention for convicted arsonists with mild and borderline intellectual disabilities. *Criminal Behaviour and Mental Health*, **12**, 282–293.

United States Fire Administration (USFA) (2003) *Firefighter Arson: A Special Report.* Department of Homeland Security. At http://www.usfa.fema.gov/downloads/pdf/ publications/tr-141.pdf (accessed 17 December 2010).

Zuckerman, M. (1994) *Behavioral Expressions and the Biosocial Bases of Sensation Seeking.* Cambridge University Press.

Zuckerman, M. (2007) *Sensation Seeking and Risky Behaviour.* American Psychological Association.

Part II: Practice and law

CHAPTER 9

Legal perspectives on arson

Sally Averill

This chapter outlines the development of the law regarding arson in England and Wales, and discusses the application of the current legislation from the decision to prosecute through to sentence. It sets out statistics showing the conviction rate for offences of arson and sentences passed. It includes guidance to mental health professionals on the criminal court processes and their role in proceedings involving offenders with a mental disorder who have been charged with offences of arson.

Development of the law

Sir William Blackstone's *Commentaries on the Laws of England* records arson as 'the malicious and wilful burning of a house or outhouse of another man' (Blackstone, 1765–69). It was listed as a public wrong against property, but was considered an offence of 'great malignity and more pernicious than theft' because it threatened a man's right of habitation, not just his property. It could be more destructive than murder, because it frequently caused terror and injury that spread beyond the intended victim(s). The punishment was the death penalty without the benefit of clergy (i.e., it could not be commuted to a lesser sentence). 'Malicious mischief or damage', including damage by fire, to other property is recorded as an offence punishable by death, although transportation was an alternative. 'Malicious' meant a 'spirit of wanton cruelty or black and diabolical revenge'.

The Malicious Damage Act (MDA) 1861 consolidated the existing law and set out various offences of 'unlawfully and maliciously' setting fire to property. The distinction between burning buildings (arson) and other property (malicious burning) was maintained. It introduced specific offences of setting fire to an occupied dwelling and of setting fire to any building with intent to injure or defraud any person. Penal servitude for life could be imposed following conviction for these offences and for setting fire to a church or railway station. Penal servitude of up to 14 years, imprisonment or whipping for males under the age of 16 were available on conviction for setting fire to other buildings, chattels or crops. 'Maliciously' meant a wrongful act done intentionally and without just cause or excuse or done recklessly with a result that the offender foresaw or ought to have foreseen.

Current law: Criminal Damage Act 1971

The Criminal Damage Act (CDA) 1971 simplified the legislation in England and Wales concerning all forms of criminal damage, including damage by fire. It repealed almost all of the MDA 1861, removing the distinctions between the type of property damaged and the method of so doing. It creates two principal offences:

- Simple criminal damage is set out in section 1(1), in the following terms: 'a person who without lawful excuse destroys or damages any property belonging to another intending to destroy or damage any such property, or being reckless as to whether any such property would be destroyed or damaged shall be guilty of an offence'.
- The 'aggravated offence' is set out in section 1(2), in the following terms: 'a person who without lawful excuse destroys or damages any property, whether belonging to himself or another (a) intending to destroy or damage any property or being reckless as to whether any property would be destroyed or damaged; and (b) intending by the destruction or damage to endanger the life of another or being reckless as to whether the life of another would be thereby endangered; shall be guilty of an offence.'

There is no separate offence of arson nor is arson defined in the CDA 1971. Section 1(3) requires that an offence of criminal damage occasioned by fire shall be charged as arson. An offence of 'simple' criminal damage caused by fire will be charged as an offence contrary to section 1(1) and (3) CDA 1971, and the aggravated offence as contrary to sections 1(2) and (3) CDA 1971.

Arson continues to be classified as an offence against property, but the harm to human life as well as to property that can result from arson is regarded as so serious that all offences of arson carry a maximum sentence of life imprisonment. Despite its status as an offence against property, it is included in the schedule of violent offences in section 15 of the Criminal Justice Act (CJA) 2003. This enables a longer sentence to be passed if an offender convicted of such an offence is found to be dangerous. This is discussed in greater detail under 'Sentencing', below.

Elements of the offences of arson

All criminal offences comprise a physical act or omission (the actus reus) and a mental state of mind (mens rea). The actus reus for both forms of arson is that the defendant has damaged or destroyed property. For offences of simple arson, the property must belong to another person.

Mens rea

The mens rea for simple arson is that the defendant must intend to damage or destroy property that belongs to another or is reckless as to whether property belonging to another is damaged or destroyed. People lack mens rea if they damage property in the honest but mistaken belief that they own it.

The mens rea for the aggravated offence is that defendants must *intend* to destroy or damage property or are *reckless* as to whether it is destroyed or damaged. They must also have intended that the destruction or damage of the property should endanger someone's life or were reckless as to whether a human life might be endangered (*R v. Caldwell* [1982] AC 341 HL).

Intent

It should not be presumed that a person intended or foresaw the result of their actions just because it was a natural and probable result of those actions. Their actual intention or foresight of the result must be decided on all of the evidence, drawing such inferences from the evidence as appear proper in the circumstances (section 8 of the Criminal Justice Act 1967).

Recklessness

People act recklessly within the meaning of section 1 of the CDA 1971 with respect to a circumstance when they are aware that a risk exists or will exist; and are reckless with respect to a result when they are aware that a risk may occur; and it is, in the circumstances known to them, unreasonable to take the risk *(R v. G* [2004] 1 AC 1034 HL).

Defences

Defendants should be acquitted if they have a lawful excuse for damaging or destroying the property. 'Lawful excuse' is not defined in section 1(1) or 1(2) of the CDA 1971, but there is a partial definition in section 5, which applies only to the simple offence of arson set out in section 1(1). Section 5(2) of the CDA 1971 provides that people charged with simple arson will have a lawful excuse for damaging or destroying the property if:

- at the time of the act or acts alleged to constitute the offence, they believed that the person or persons whom they believed to be entitled to consent to the destruction of or damage to the property had consented or would have consented had they known of the damage or destruction and its circumstances; or
- they destroyed or damaged the property in order to protect property belonging to themselves or another or a right or interest in the property which was vested in themselves or another or which the offender

believed to be so vested, and at the time they destroyed the property they believed that the property, right or interest was in immediate need of protection and the means of protection was reasonable having regard to all of the circumstances.

It does not matter whether the defendant's belief was justified, provided that it was honestly held (section 5(3) of the CDA 1971). This includes an honest belief that was mistaken and the mistake was attributable to the defendant being intoxicated by alcohol or by drugs.

It is difficult to think of a situation in which the defence in section 5(2)(b) could apply to a charge of arson. However, wherever the defence is raised and there is any evidence of lawful excuse, the jury should be left to decide (*R v. Wang* [2005] 2 Cr App R). A genuine belief that the defendant was carrying out God's instructions is not a lawful excuse (*Blake v. DPP* [1993] CLR 586 DC). In *R v. Hunt* [1977] 66 Cr App R 105 CA, the defendant's conviction for setting fire to a bed in an old people's home was upheld. His defence that he wished to demonstrate the inadequacy of the fire alarm system was rejected.

Criminal proceedings

In 2009/10, a total of 32 579 offences of arson were recorded by the police (Home Office, 2010). The statistics are supplied with the caveat that although every effort is made to ensure that the figures presented are accurate and complete, they have been extracted from large administrative data systems generated by the police forces and courts. As a consequence, care should be taken to ensure data-collection processes and their inevitable limitations are taken into account when these figures are used.

This total comprised 28 954 offences of arson not endangering life (simple arson) and 3625 offences of arson endangering life (aggravated offence). From 1 April 2008, there was a new offence classification, of arson endangering life and of arson not endangering life. Only 9% of all cases – 1028 cases (28%) of the aggravated offence and 1894 cases (7%) of simple arson – resulted in a 'sanction detection', that is, the offender was charged with or summonsed for the offence or asked for it to be taken into consideration when sentenced for another offence, or the offender was cautioned or issued with a penalty notice for the offence. Not all detections by charge or summons will result in a conviction. The Crown Prosecution Service (CPS) may not continue the prosecution or the offender might be acquitted after trial. The sanction detection rate for arson is lower than for all offences of criminal damage (13%) and for all offences of property crime (17%). These rates are much lower than the total rate for offences of violence against the person (44%), homicide (86%) and all drugs offences (94%). This may be explained by the absence of witnesses to damage to property, which, in the absence of forensic evidence or a confession, prevents an offender being identified and brought to justice.

Diversion from prosecution

The police will submit the evidence they collect during the arson investigation to the CPS, which will decide whether a person should be charged with an offence. Decisions are taken in accordance with the *Code for Crown Prosecutors* (Crown Prosecution Service, 2010*a*) ('the Code') and the Director of Public Prosecutions' *Guidance on Charging* (Crown Prosecution Service, 2011). A prosecution will proceed to court only if the 'full Code test' is satisfied. It has two stages: the evidential stage and the public interest stage. The evidential stage requires sufficient evidence to provide a realistic prospect of conviction against each defendant on each charge. This means that a court is more likely than not to convict. It is a lower standard than is actually applied in court, as defendants can be convicted only if the court is sure of their guilt. A case which does not satisfy the evidential stage cannot proceed. Where there is sufficient evidence, the public interest stage will be considered. A prosecution usually takes place unless the prosecutor is sure that there are public interest factors tending against prosecution which outweigh those tending in favour, or that an out-of-court disposal is more suitable considering all of the circumstances of the case. The more serious the offence or the offender's record of criminal behaviour, the more likely it is that the public interest requires a prosecution. Some common public interest factors tending in favour of and against prosecution are listed in the Code. One of the factors tending against prosecution is that:

the suspect is, or was at the time of the offence, suffering from significant mental or physical ill health, unless the offence is serious or there is a real possibility that it may be repeated. Prosecutors apply Home Office guidelines about how to deal with mentally disordered offenders and must balance a suspect's mental or physical ill health with the need to safeguard the public or those providing care services to such persons.

The CPS legal guidance on offenders with a mental disorder (Crown Prosecution Service, 2010*b*) explains that:

there is no presumption either in favour of or against the prosecution of a mentally disordered offender. Each case must be considered on its merits, taking into account any information about the disorder and its relevance to the offence.

The CPS must consider whether the public interest can be satisfied by a disposal other than prosecution. A simple caution may be appropriate in cases of simple arson, if there is sufficient evidence to provide a realistic prospect of conviction and the offender admits the offence. The CPS may offer a conditional caution for an offence of simple arson where the full Code test is met and it is proportionate to the seriousness and the consequences of the offending. The offender must admit the offence and agree to accept the caution and carry out the conditions, which may be rehabilitative, reparative or restrictive. If any of the conditions are breached, the offender will usually be prosecuted for the original offence.

A caution or conditional caution cannot be given if there is any doubt about the reliability of the defendant's admissions or if their cognitive ability prevents them from understanding the significance of the caution or conditional caution or giving informed consent.

Where the public interest cannot be satisfied by a caution or conditional caution, it will usually be in the public interest to prosecute for an offence of arson. However, a prosecution may not be necessary if the offender is already receiving treatment that might be ordered by a court on conviction. The existence of a mental disorder is only one of the factors to be taken into account and will be balanced with the seriousness or the persistence of the offending behaviour; the views of the victim and any responsible clinician should also be considered.

Court proceedings

Simple arson can be tried summarily in the magistrates' court or by a judge and jury in the Crown Court (section 17(1) and Schedule 1 of the Magistrates' Courts Act 1980). It will be tried summarily if the court has sufficient sentencing powers to pass an appropriate sentence and the defendant consents. The maximum penalty on conviction in the magistrates' court is a fine of up to £5000 and up to 6 months' imprisonment. Compensation of up to £5000 can also be ordered. The Sentencing Guidelines Council (2008) identifies the appropriate starting points for offences of arson, which are based on the seriousness of the offence (i.e., the culpability of the offender and the harm he or she has caused). The starting points are based on a first-time offender who pleads not guilty and is convicted after trial. The starting point for such an offender who causes minor damage by fire is a high-level Community Order, with an indicated range from a medium-level Community Order to 12 weeks' custody. Moderate damage by fire attracts a sentencing range of 6–26 weeks' custody, with a starting point of 12 weeks' custody. Significant damage by fire requires the Crown Court sentencing powers of an unlimited fine, compensation and life imprisonment.

The court will then consider the aggravating and mitigating factors, in particular whether the arson was a revenge attack, which indicates higher culpability, and factors indicating a greater degree of harm, such as damage to emergency equipment or public amenity and significant public or private fear caused. Damage caused intentionally indicates higher culpability than damage caused recklessly.

If the offence is so serious that a sentence in excess of 6 months' custody is required, then the magistrates may commit an offender for trial or sentence in the Crown Court. The defendant may elect jury trial, irrespective of the likely sentence.

The aggravated offence is so serious that it can only be tried by a Crown Court. It is common for both forms of the aggravated offence to be charged, so that the jury can decide whether the offender intended to endanger life or was reckless as to whether life was endangered. The jury's decision will enable the judge to pass a sentence commensurate with the seriousness of the offence (*R v. Hoof* [1980] 2 Cr App R) (S) 299).

Expert witnesses

The role of the expert witness is to provide independent and impartial evidence on an issue that is outside the experience and knowledge of the judge and jury. This involves giving an opinion, including an opinion on the 'ultimate issue in a case'. The judge will decide whether expert evidence is necessary and whether a witness is qualified to provide that evidence. The court is not bound by an expert opinion and will reach its own decision based on all of the evidence in the case.

In cases of arson, expert evidence from a fire investigator regarding the causes, seats and spread of fire may be needed. Where the defendant is or appears to be mentally disordered, courts may require expert evidence from a mental health professional for various reasons, such as the impact of the disorder on a defendant's ability to form the necessary mens rea, to determine whether the defendant is fit to plead, to determine eligibility for a hospital order and to assess the risk of future harm that the offender poses.

The purpose of the report and the questions on which expert opinion is sought should be clearly set out in instructions. The General Medical Council (2008) publication *Acting as an Expert Witness: Guidance to Doctors* recommends that where instructions are unclear, inadequate or conflicting, clarification from those instructing should be sought. A report should not be provided if instructions are not sufficiently clear or if the advice or opinion sought is outside the area of expertise.

Experts' first duty is to the court and overrides any obligation to the person instructing or paying them. It includes an obligation to inform all parties and the court if their opinion changes from that contained in a report served as evidence or given in a statement.

Expert report

The Criminal Procedure Rules 2011 apply to all experts giving or preparing expert evidence for the purpose of criminal proceedings, including evidence needed to determine fitness to plead or for the purposes of sentencing (TSO, 2011). Rule 33.3 states that the expert's report must:

- give details of the expert's qualifications, relevant experience and accreditation
- give details of any literature or other information which the expert has relied on in making the report
- contain a statement setting out the substance of all facts given to the expert which are material to the opinions expressed in the report, or upon which those opinions are based

- make clear which of the facts stated in the report are within the expert's own knowledge
- say who has carried out any examination, measurement, test or experiment which the expert has used for the report and
  - give the qualifications, relevant experience and accreditation of that person
  - say whether or not the examination, measurement, test or experiment was carried out under the expert's supervision
  - summarise the findings on which the expert relies
- where there is a range of opinion on the matters dealt with in the report
  - summarise the range of opinion
  - give reasons for their own opinion
- if the expert is not able to give an opinion without qualification, state the qualification
- contain a summary of the conclusions reached
- contain a statement that the expert understands their duty to the court, and has complied and will continue to comply with that duty
- contain the same statement of truth as a witness statement.

Disclosure

When instructed by the CPS or by the police as an expert in the investigation of a crime or the prosecution of an offence, experts must comply with the disclosure duties set out in *Disclosure: Experts' Evidence and Unused Material* (Association of Chief Police Officers & Crown Prosecution Service, 2010). The three key duties are to retain, record and reveal:

- The expert should retain all material obtained in the course of the case until instructed otherwise by the prosecution team.
- Records should be kept from the time of instruction to show the date and means of the receipt and delivery of all materials, all notes made by the expert and any assistants, notes of all meetings and telephone calls, including points of agreement, dispute and agreed actions, and all emails.
- All recorded material must be revealed to the prosecution team.

Failure to comply with the duties of disclosure can have serious consequences, such as an unsafe conviction or a prosecution being terminated, and adverse professional consequences for the expert.

Giving evidence

There is a general principle that witnesses in criminal proceedings should not be trained or coached in giving evidence. This reduces the risk of witnesses adapting their evidence and any perception that they might have done so. It does not prevent expert witnesses from receiving training in general techniques such as presenting and explaining technical evidence and staying within the bounds of expertise. Professional bodies, including the Royal College of Psychiatrists, General Medical Council and British Psychological Society, offer guidance and training to equip their members to give expert evidence (see for example British Psychological Society, 2007).

Experts should confirm the time, date and place that they should attend to give evidence. They may be required to arrive before court begins, to attend a conference with lawyers to clarify evidence or to advise on issues which have recently arisen, such as a report from another expert. They may be required to attend for the whole case (experts are usually permitted to sit in court and listen to the evidence of other witnesses, including expert witnesses).

The British Psychological Society (2007) suggests that experts should prepare for oral testimony by listing the issues that are likely to be raised and then considering the established facts and their stated expert opinions in relation to each issue. When giving evidence, experts should answer all questions asked with courtesy but should stay within their area of expertise. They should avoid verbosity and explain any technical terms or jargon as succinctly as possible. It is essential to remain objective and not to tell untruths. Attacks on their report and evidence should be addressed without arrogance or anger. The main issues should be addressed without digressing and good use should be made of facts to support opinion, referring to the report. The expert is there to assist the court and is not expected to be an advocate.

Fitness to plead

The fitness-to-plead procedure seeks to strike a balance between: fairness to a defendant who is unable to stand trial but may be entitled to be acquitted of the charges; and protecting the public.

The issue of fitness to plead can be raised at any stage of the proceedings after the defendant is charged. The court must decide whether the defendant 'is of sufficient intellect to comprehend the course of the proceedings of the trial, so as to make a proper defence, to challenge any juror to whom he might wish to object, and to understand the details of the evidence' (*R v. Pritchard* [1836] 7 C&P 303).

Practice Direction (Criminal Proceedings: Consolidation), para. III.30 [2007] 1 WLR 1790) requires that all possible steps are taken to assist a vulnerable defendant (one with a mental disorder within the meaning of the Mental Health Act 1983 or any other significant impairment of intelligence) to understand and participate in criminal proceedings. The ordinary trial process should, so far as necessary, be adapted to meet those ends, including the use of an intermediary to assist a defendant to prepare for and participate in the trial (*C v. Sevenoaks Youth Court* [2009] EWHC 3088 Admin).

If defendants are likely to respond to medical treatment and can be tried within a reasonable period, they may be remanded to hospital for a report on their medical condition (under section 35 of the Mental Health Act 1983) or for treatment (section 36). Where the disorder is serious or enduring, the issue of fitness to plead should be determined. It may be postponed until after the close of the prosecution case, so that the defendant may be acquitted if there is no case to answer.

Crown Court

The fitness-to-plead procedure has two stages. First, the judge decides whether the defendant is unfit to be tried, on the basis of written or oral evidence from two or more registered medical practitioners. According to subsection 4(5) of the Criminal Procedure (Insanity) Act (CPIA) 1964, as amended by the Criminal Procedure (Insanity and Unfitness to Plead) Act 1991, at least one practitioner must be approved under section 12 of the Mental Health Act 1983. If the judge decides that a defendant is unfit to plead, a trial will not take place or continue. A jury will decide whether the defendant did the relevant act or made the omission, without considering mental state. They must acquit the defendant if they are not satisfied that the actus reus was complete. If they make a finding that the defendant did the act or made the omission, this does not amount to a conviction, but the court must make a hospital order, with or without a restriction order, a supervision order or an order for the offender's absolute discharge (section 5(2) of the CPIA 1964).

Magistrates' courts

Subsection 11(1) of the Powers of Criminal Courts (Sentencing) Act 2000 and subsection 37(3) of the Mental Health Act 1983, as amended by Mental Health Act 2007 (henceforth MHA), allows a magistrates' court to make a hospital order or guardianship order without convicting the offender. The court must be satisfied that the defendant did the act or made the omission with which he or she is charged. This procedure is to be used to determine fitness to plead in magistrates' courts and youth courts (*R (on the application of P) v. Barking Youth Court* [2002] EWHC 734 Admin).

Sentencing

Table 9.1 uses data from the Ministry of Justice (2010), supplied with the same caveat that accompanied the Home Office statistics on arson (see above). These statistics show that, despite a low sanction detection rate, when a case satisfies the evidential and public interest stages of the CPS full Code test, and proceeds to prosecution, the conviction rate is approximately 75%. This is lower than the conviction rate of 93% for drugs offences but compares favourably with the conviction rate of 69% for offences against the person and 61% for sexual offences.

Table 9.1 Sentencing data for all offenders (aged 10 and over) convicted of arson in all courts in 2008

	Male	Female	Not specified	Total
Total prosecuted	1749	378	6	2133
Total convicted	1212	263	3	1478
Total sentenced	1196	260	3	1459
Absolute discharge	3	4	0	7
Conditional discharge	27	9	0	36
Fine	13	3	0	16
Community sentences				
Community rehabilitation order*	4	0	0	4
Supervision order*	18	9	0	27
Community punishment order*	0	0	0	0
Attendance centre order*	1	0	0	1
Community punishment and rehabilitation order*	4	0	0	4
Curfew order	10	4	0	14
Reparation order**	5	1	0	6
Action plan order*	2	0	0	2
Drug treatment and testing order*	0	0	0	0
Referral order**	163	25	2	190
Community Order	200	67	1	268
Youth rehabilitation order***	71	17	0	88
Total number of community sentences	478	123	3	604
Custodial sentences				
Suspended sentence of imprisonment	106	31	0	137
Detention under sections 90–92 of the Powers of Criminal Courts** (Sentencing) Act (long-term detention for offenders up to 21 years)	4	1	0	5
Detention and training order (detention of up to 2 years for offenders aged 12–17 years)**	22	1	0	23
Detention in a young-offender institute (offenders aged 18–20 years inclusive)	83	5	0	88
Unsuspended imprisonment (21 years plus)	392	51	0	443
Total sentences of immediate custody	501	58	0	559
Otherwise dealt with				
Hospital order	0	0	46	46
Restriction order	0	0	18	18
Guardianship order	0	0	0	0
Hospital and limitation direction	0	0	0	0
Other	0	0	36	36
Total otherwise dealt with	68	32	0	100

*Sentences available only for youth offenders (aged 10–17 inclusive) for offences committed before 30 November 2009.
**Sentences available only for youth offenders (aged 10–17 inclusive) for offences committed any time.
***Sentences available only for youth offenders (aged 10–17 inclusive) for offences committed on or after 30 November 2009.
Data from Ministry of Justice (2010).

Psychiatric reports before sentencing

The court should always obtain a psychiatric report before passing sentence on any person convicted of arson, so that the court can judge the mental element in the perpetration of the offence (*R v. Calladine* [25 November 1975] *The Times* Law Reports). A medical report must be obtained and considered before passing a custodial sentence for any offence where the offender is or appears to be mentally disordered (section 157 of the Criminal Justice Act 2003). The local primary care trust (in England) or local health board (in Wales) has a duty to provide the court with information about the availability of facilities for diverting an offender to hospital for sentence in the area in which the offender was last resident (section 39 of the MHA).

Approach to sentencing offenders with a mental disorder

In *R v. Birch* [1990] 11 Cr App R (S) 202, the Court of Appeal identified the sentencing options in respect of an offender with a mental disorder and suggested the following approach to sentencing, which has been adapted here to reflect the legislative changes since 1990.

The first step is to decide whether a period of compulsory detention is necessary. If the offence is not sufficiently serious to justify custody or if the offender does not meet the criteria for a hospital order, a community sentence should be considered.

Community Order

A Community Order (with a mental health treatment requirement) can be made in the magistrates' court or the Crown Court. It lasts for up to 3 years and includes one or more of 12 requirements that are intended to restrict the liberty of the offender and provide punishment in the community rehabilitation of the offender and reparation or restoration. The requirements include unpaid work, specified activity, supervision, drug rehabilitation, alcohol treatment, mental health treatment and residence (section 177 of the Criminal Justice Act 2003).

In *R v. Dalton* [2009] EWCA Crim 1855, a 2-year Community Order with a specified activity requirement was passed after the offender pleaded guilty to one offence of arson. He turned on two rings of an electric cooker and placed items on top that caught fire. Smoke damage and damage to the cooker were caused. He had several previous convictions, including a conviction the previous year for an offence of causing minor criminal damage.

A mental health treatment requirement can be made only if the court is satisfied on the evidence of a practitioner approved under section 12 of the MHA that the offender has a mental condition that does not warrant the making of a hospital order but requires treatment. The offender must be susceptible to treatment and consent to it. Treatment must be available and can be provided by or under the care of a registered medical practitioner or psychologist, or as a resident patient in an independent hospital or care home within the meaning of the Care Standards Act 2000 or at a hospital within the meaning of the MHA, but not where high-security psychiatry services within the meaning of the MHA are provided, or as an out-patient at a facility specified in the order. All treatment will be for a finite period specified in the order and is given with a view to improving the offender's condition (Criminal Justice Act 2003).

In 2008, a total of 120 743 Community Orders were made and 739 of these included a mental health treatment requirement. The Criminal Justice Joint Inspection (2009) looked at work prior to sentence with offenders with mental disorders and considered the reasons why so few orders with such a requirement were made. It concluded that the requirement was unsuitable for offenders with low-level or untreatable conditions and for those who were already in contact with a treatment provider. Others were unwilling to engage with treatment or the treatment options were unsuitable for their chaotic lifestyles. Some treatment providers preferred to offer treatment via a voluntary route rather than through the enforcement culture of the criminal justice agencies.

If a Community Order is not suitable, the court should consider whether the criteria for making a hospital order are satisfied. If there is any doubt, the judge may make use of sections 38 and 39 of the MHA to make an interim hospital order while the offender's local primary care trust in England or the local health board in Wales provides information about the availability of hospital treatment for an offender.

Hospital order

The court must be satisfied on the written or oral evidence of two doctors, at least one of whom must be approved under section 12 of the MHA, that the defendant is suffering from a mental disorder of a nature or degree which makes it appropriate for the defendant to be detained in hospital for medical treatment. Appropriate medical treatment must be available and arrangements must be made for the offender's admission to hospital within 28 days (section 37 of the MHA).

There does not need to be a causal relationship between the mental disorder and the offence, but the court must be satisfied that, having regard to all of the circumstances, including the nature of the offence and the character and antecedents of the offender, and to the other available methods of dealing with the offender, that the most suitable method of disposing of the case is by way of a hospital order (section 37(2)(b)). If so satisfied, the judge should consider whether a restriction order running alongside the hospital order is necessary.

Restriction order

A restriction order can be made only by a Crown Court. A magistrates' court may commit for sentence any offender aged 14 or over if it considers that a hospital order coupled with a restriction order may be necessary (section 43(1)(b) of the MHA). The order will be added to the hospital order where restrictions on the offender's liberty are 'necessary for the protection of the public from serious harm' (section 43). It restricts the patient's discharge, transfer or leave of absence from hospital without the consent of the Lord Chancellor and Secretary of State for Justice and remains in force indefinitely. It can be discharged only with the agreement of the Secretary of State or by a mental health review tribunal.

The court will decide whether the order is necessary, after taking into account the nature of the offence, the defendant's antecedents and the risk of the defendant committing further offences. The court must hear oral evidence from one of the medical practitioners whose evidence was considered when the hospital order was made. Ideally this practitioner should be on the staff of the hospital to which the offender will be admitted pursuant to the hospital order (R v. Blackwood [1974] Cr App R 170). The decision to make the restriction order lies with the judge, who may make the order despite evidence from a medical practitioner that the order should not be made (R v. Royse [1981] 3 Cr App R (S) 58 CA).

Hospital and limitation direction

A hospital order is not always the most appropriate sentence. It is not wrong in principle to pass a custodial sentence on offenders with a mental disorder who are criminally responsible for their behaviour and are fit to be tried (R v. Drew [2003] UKHL 25). It may be more appropriate if there is an element of culpability in the offence that justifies punishment or where the offender's responsibility was reduced but not diminished (R v. IA [2005] EWCA Crim 2077).

The court should consider whether a 'hospital and limitation direction' is more appropriate than a custodial sentence. This can be made after conviction in a Crown Court. It allows the judge, when passing a prison sentence on an offender with a mental disorder, to give a direction for immediate admission to and detention in a specified hospital and a direction that the restrictions on liberty imposed in section 41 of the MHA apply.

The entire sentence may be served in hospital if the responsible clinician is satisfied that the offender is benefiting from treatment. The offender may be transferred to prison at any time during the sentence if the Secretary of State receives medical evidence that satisfies him or her that the patient is not suffering from a mental disorder, that the patient no longer requires hospital treatment or that no effective treatment can be given in hospital. Offenders transferred to prison may be considered for transfer back to hospital under section 47 of the MHA if they meet the criteria for a hospital order under section 37.

Custodial sentences

A custodial sentence may be passed if the offender is dangerous and there is no suitable secure accommodation available or where a hospital order is not suitable. In *R v. Wheeler* [1997] EWCA Crim 1032, the Court of Appeal had 'no doubt whatsoever that an offence of arson endangering life recklessly is one which, save in the most exceptional circumstances and/or in the case of mental trouble [*sic*], must attract an immediate prison sentence'. The length of the sentence was considered by the Court of Appeal in *R v. Myrie* [2009] 2 Cr App R (S) 48 CA. The starting point for an offender convicted after trial of arson with intent to endanger life is a sentence of imprisonment for 8–10 years. A lower range is appropriate for cases of reckless endangerment, but there is a fine line between the most serious cases of reckless endangerment and the least serious cases of intentional endangerment. A higher sentence is justified where there are aggravating features, such as:

- premeditation, especially where the arson is an act of revenge
- the offence is committed at night, at a time when occupants of a house are expected to be at home and asleep
- there is an increased risk of fire spreading to adjoining properties (e.g., where the fire is started in a terraced house)
- the fire is started at the main entry and exit point of the house
- the offender does nothing to raise the alarm after starting the fire.

Further aggravating features include: the use of accelerants or firebombs, causing injury, the extent of the damage, damage being caused to a dwelling, public building or school, significant fear being caused, the offence being a hate crime (i.e., motivated by hostility on the basis of race, religion, ethnicity, disability, gender, or sexuality) (Crown Prosecution Service, 2010c).

Life imprisonment is reserved for cases where the culpability of the offender is particularly high or the offence itself is particularly serious (*R v. Kehoe* [2009] Cr App R (S) (9) CA).

Sentences for public protection

A sentence for public protection is a custodial sentence that is greater than is justified by the seriousness of the offence alone. It can be passed only on an offender convicted of a violent or sexual offence that is 'specified' in Schedule 15 of the CJA 2003 and the court finds that the offender is 'dangerous' – that is, that there is a significant risk to members of the public of serious harm occasioned by the commission of further specified offences (section 229 of the CJA 2003). 'Serious harm' means death or serious personal injury, whether physical or psychological (section 224(3)). When assessing dangerousness, the court must take into account all available information about the nature and circumstances of the offence. It may also take into account any available information about the nature and circumstances of any other convictions and any pattern of behaviour of which the current offence and any previous offences form part. It can consider allegations of violence that have not resulted in a conviction or caution (*R v. Considine and Davis* [2007] EWCA Crim 1166). The court may also take into account any other information about the offender. This may include a psychiatric report, evidence of past behaviour and an assessment of future risk.

All offences of arson are 'serious specified offences', that is, specified offences that carry a maximum sentence of imprisonment of 10 years or more, so all of the following sentences for public protection can be passed, provided that the additional criteria are satisfied and the risk of harm posed by the offender cannot be addressed by any other sentence.

Life imprisonment

Where an adult offender is convicted of an offence that carries a maximum punishment of life imprisonment, and is assessed as dangerous by the court, he or she *must* be sentenced to life imprisonment, unless a life sentence cannot be justified by the seriousness of the offence (section 225(2) of the CJA 2003) or that a hospital order with a restriction order is the most suitable in all the circumstances of the case (*R v. Simpson* [2007] EWCA Crim 2666).

A life sentence was imposed in *R v. Bell* [2006] EWCA Crim 3028. The defendant, who was diagnosed with a personality disorder, pleaded guilty to two aggravated offences of arson. The first offence was committed by starting a fire in the basement of church premises, causing £530 damage. The offender helped to put out the fire. The second offence involved pushing lighted materials through the letterbox of an occupied flat at 3 a.m. The occupants were woken by thick smoke and managed to extinguish the fire. The offender had previous convictions, including an offence of arson for which he had been sentenced to 2 years' detention, and a caution for simple arson. The psychiatric report referred to a pattern of similar behaviour, including starting two fires at school, and assessed the offender as 'dangerous'. The Court of Appeal found that the offender was dangerous as his history showed him to be a person of unstable character and he was likely to commit further offences in the future. Those offences were deemed likely to be so serious that there was a grave risk that others might be severely injured.

Indeterminate imprisonment for public protection

Indeterminate imprisonment is available only if offenders would have served at least 2 years in custody if a standard sentence were passed or if they have a previous conviction for an offence listed in Schedule 15A of the CJA 2003(arson is not listed). The offender is not released automatically halfway through the sentence, as is the case with standard custodial sentences. The court will set a minimum term of at least 2 years, which must be served in full before the Parole Board can consider release. The minimum period to be served reflects the seriousness of the offence. The offender will not be released unless and until the Parole Board is satisfied that it is safe to do so. If released, the prisoner remains on licence for at least 10 years (section 225(4) of the CJA 2003 and Part 2, Chapter 2 of the Crime (Sentences) Act 1997) and for life if the Parole Board considers that supervision in the community remains necessary for public protection.

Extended sentence

An extended sentence comprises two parts: a period of custody and an extended licence period of up to 5 years for violent offences and 8 years for sexual offences. The total length of both must not exceed the maximum sentence available for the offence (sections 227 and 228 of the CJA 2003).

The custodial period must be fixed and will be for the shortest term warranted by the seriousness of the offence. If the offender has a previous conviction for an offence listed under Schedule 15A, the minimum custodial term must be set at 12 months; otherwise, the custodial term must be at least 4 years. The prisoner is released automatically after serving half the custodial sentence. The extended licence period commences at the end of the full sentence of imprisonment, not release from custody. The purpose of the extended licence period is neither punitive nor based on the seriousness of the offence. It is to provide public protection and is set at the length that the court considers necessary to protect the public from serious harm (section 227(2) of the CJA 2003). It may be set to coincide with a rehabilitation programme aimed at reducing the risk of reoffending.

Conclusion

All cases in which offenders with mental disorders are suspected of committing offences of arson require careful consideration, as the care and treatment needs of the offender must be balanced with the seriousness of the offence and the need for public protection. The provision of expert evidence is essential to understand the nature of a mental disorder, its impact on the culpability of the offender and the future risk he or she poses. The CPS needs this evidence when deciding whether the public interest requires a prosecution or whether an offender can be diverted from the court process. The courts must have expert evidence to fulfil their duty to pass the most suitable sentence, taking into account all of the evidence and circumstances of the case.

References

Association of Chief Police Officers & Crown Prosecution Service (2010) *Guidance Booklet for Experts. Disclosure: Experts' Evidence, Case Management and Unused Material*. TSO (The Stationery Office).

Blackstone, Sir W. (1765–69) *Commentaries on the Laws of England*. At Yale Law School, http://avalon.law.yale.edu/subject_menus/blackstone.asp (accessed 17 December 2010).

British Psychological Society (2007) *Report on Psychologists as Expert Witnesses: Guidelines and Procedure for England and Wales*. BPS. At http://www.bps.org.uk/document-download-area/document-download$.cfm?restart=true&file_uuid=3393E220-1143-DFD0-7EC1-94B653B296A6 (accessed 17 December 2010).

Criminal Justice Joint Inspection (2009) *Criminal Justice Joint Inspection Report on Work Prior to Sentence with Offenders with Mental Disorders*. HMI Probation, HMI Court Administration,

HMI Constabulary and HM Crown Prosecution Service Inspectorate. At http://www. justice.gov.uk/inspectorates/hmi-probation/docs/MDO_Joint_Report-rps.pdf (accessed 17 December 2010).

Crown Prosecution Service (2010a) *Code for Crown Prosecutors* (6th edn). CPS. At http:// www.cps.gov.uk/publications/code_for_crown_prosecutors/index.html (accessed 17 December 2010).

Crown Prosecution Service (2010b) *Legal Guidance on Mentally Disordered Offenders*. CPS. At http://www.cps.gov.uk/legal/l_to_o/mentally_disordered_offenders (accessed 17 December 2010).

Crown Prosecution Service (2010c) *Sentencing Manual*. CPS. At http://www.cps.gov.uk/ legal/s_to_u/sentencing_manual (accessed 17 December 2010).

Crown Prosecution Service (2011) *Director's Guidance on Charging* (4th edn). CPS. At http://www.cps.gov.uk/publications/directors_guidance/dpp_guidance_4.html (accessed 17 December 2010).

General Medical Council (2008) *Acting as an Expert Witness: Guidance to Doctors*. GMC. At http://www.gmc-uk.org/guidance/ethical_guidance/expert_witness_guidance.asp (accessed 17 December 2010).

Home Office (2010) *Home Office Statistical Bulletin: Crime in England and Wales 2009/10 Findings from the British Crime Survey and Police Recorded Crime* (eds J. Flatley, C. Kershaw, K. Smith, *et al*). Home Office. At http://rds.homeoffice.gov.uk/rds/pdfs10/hosb1210. pdf (accessed 17 December 2010).

Ministry of Justice (2010) *Criminal Statistics in England and Wales 2008 Statistics Report and Bulletin*. Ministry of Justice. At http://www.justice.gov.uk/publications/criminalannual-archive.htm (accessed 17 December 2010).

Sentencing Guidelines Council (2008) *The Magistrates Court Sentencing Guideline*. SGC. At http://www.sentencingcouncil.org.uk/professional/magistrates-guidelines.htm (accessed 17 December 2010).

TSO (2011) Criminal Procedure Rules 2011. Statutory Instrument no. 60 (L2). The Stationery Office. At http://www.legislation.gov.uk/uksi/2011/1709/contents/made (accessed 17 December 2010).

Practice directions and legal cases

Blake v. DPP [1993] CLR 586 DC

C v. Sevenoaks Youth Court [2009] EWHC 3088 Admin

Practice Direction (Criminal Proceedings: Consolidation), para. III.30 [2007] 1 WLR 1790

R (on the application of P) v Barking Youth Court [2002] EWHC 734 Admin

R v. Bell [2006] EWCA Crim 3028

R v. Birch [1990] 11 Cr App R (S) 202

R v. Blackwood [1974] Cr App R 170

R v. Caldwell [1982] AC 341 HL

R v. Calladine [25 November 1975] *The Times* Law Reports

R v. Considine and Davis [2007] EWCA Crim 1166

R v. Dalton [2009] EWCA Crim 1855

R v. Drew [2003] UKHL 25

R v. G [2004] 1 AC 1034 HL

R v. Hoof [1980] 2 Cr App R (S) 299

R v. Hunt [1977] 66 Cr App R 105 CA

R v. IA [2005] EWCA Crim 2077

R v. Kehoe [2009] Cr App R (S) 9 CA

R v. Myrie [2009] 2 Cr App R (S) 48 CA

R v. Pritchard [1836] 7 C & P 303

R v. Royse [1981] 3 Cr App R (S) 58 CA

R v. Simpson [2007] EWCA Crim 2666

R v. Wang [2005] 2 Cr App R
R v. Wheeler [1997] EWCA Crim 1032

Statutes

Care Standards Act (2000) c.14. London: The Stationery Office.
Crime (Sentences) Act (1997) c.43. London: The Stationery Office.
Criminal Damage Act (1971) c.48. London: HMSO.
Criminal Justice Act (1967) c.80. London: HMSO.
Criminal Justice Act (2003) c.44. London: TSO.
Criminal Procedure (Insanity) Act 1964 (as amended by Criminal Procedure (Insanity and Unfitness to Plead) Act 1991) c.84. London: HMSO.
Magistrates' Courts Act (1980) c.43. London: HMSO.
Malicious Damage Act (1861) 24 & 25 Vict. c.97. London: George Edward Eyre and William Spottiswoode.
Mental Health Act 1983 (as amended by Mental Health Act 2007) c.20. London: The Stationery Office.
Powers of Criminal Courts (Sentencing) Act (2000) c.6. London: The Stationery Office.

CHAPTER 10

Assessment of firesetters

Rebekah M. Doley and Bruce D. Watt

This chapter will equip readers with the information required to screen and assess arsonists effectively using a number of modalities. The appropriate tools are presented and discussed, along with the evidence base underlying them. The focus of the discussion is on risk assessment, recidivism and dangerousness. In particular, these issues are discussed with reference to mental health and psychiatric patients as arsonists. The terms 'arson' and 'firesetting' will be used interchangeably throughout this chapter; the term 'arson' is commonly acknowledged to have a legal definition, while firesetting describes the behaviour itself.

The process of assessing firesetters is tricky but perhaps not for the reason one might think initially. Firesetters are not especially distinct across many variables when compared with other types of offender. While they share more commonalities with property offenders than with violent offenders (Quinsey *et al*, 2006), the typical profile of an arsonist reveals a similar pattern of social and economic disadvantage to most criminals (Hurley & Monahan, 1969; Tennent *et al*, 1971; O'Sullivan & Kelleher, 1987; Barnett & Spitzer, 1994; Puri *et al*, 1995). However, unlike with some other types of offender (notably sex and violent offenders), the psychology of arsonists has not been the subject of extensive exploration, although interest is certainly growing. One of the consequences of this lack of attention is that arson-specific assessment protocols have not yet been fully developed. Work is progressing it seems more rapidly in the area of juvenile assessment (McEwan *et al*, in press; Fritzon *et al*, 2011) than in adult assessment (Gannon & Pina, 2010), but there remains a lack of empirical testing of any proposed protocols. The general principles of forensic mental health assessments are adequately addressed elsewhere (see Heilbrun *et al*, 2009). Accordingly, this chapter addresses those instruments currently available which may be useful for arson risk assessment. A key focus of the discussion is on exploring for inclusion in assessments aspects of risk of arson recidivism and level of harm, as well as issues relevant for assessing arsonists before treatment.

The chapter makes some of the same assumptions that have been criticised elsewhere. Specifically, in discussing the issue of assessment of firesetters we are treating the population as a homogeneous group. However, there is mounting evidence that, at least from a treatment perspective, it is important to consider the possibility of subgroups within the arsonist population, each with their own specific criminogenic needs. This issue is addressed in part by acknowledging it as a limitation of any discussion in this field because we simply do not know enough at this time to be able to speak knowledgeably about subgroups of firesetters. Furthermore, it is pertinent to acknowledge that the field is dynamic and by definition as soon as guidelines are published it is likely that they will be superseded by more recent information. Nevertheless, we do draw attention to variables for future consideration that may prove likely to be helpful in distinguishing subgroups of arsonists. Such variables are therefore priority targets for research and possible inclusion in assessment protocols.

Explaining recidivistic arson

In considering factors relevant for the assessment of risk of repeat arson as well as factors to inform treatment formulation, it is, naturally, important to base our enquiries on a sound theoretical formulation of recidivistic arson. A focus on serial firesetting can be found in the model proposed by Jackson and colleagues (Jackson et al, 1987a; Jackson, 1994). In this formulation, a functional analysis considering antecedent, behavioural and consequential variables hypothesised to be associated with serial firesetting is presented (see Chapter 6, especially Fig. 6.1, p. 112). Although not new to psychology (see Skinner, 1953; Ferster, 1965; Goren et al, 1977; Slade, 1982; Smith & Churchill, 2002; Hanley et al, 2003), a functional analytic type of approach has only relatively recently been applied to the problem of deliberate firesetting.

The model attempts to account for the function of firesetting for the individual by drawing attention to a background of psychosocial deprivations that stem from both individual-specific factors (e.g., low academic achievement, psychiatric disorder) and environmental conditions (e.g., family dysfunction, low socioeconomic status). These factors, it is suggested, result in individuals feeling dissatisfied with their lives or themselves. Further, it is postulated that these individuals tend to lack self-confidence, leading to a generally ineffective approach to interpersonal relations. Jackson et al (1987a) hypothesise that each of these three general firesetting conditions – psychosocial disadvantage, dissatisfaction with life and/or self, and a history of social ineffectiveness – interacts with and potentially exacerbates each of the others.

The consequence is a deficient repertoire of skills, which leaves individuals failing to effect change in their environment and developing a perception of themselves as being ineffective, resulting in feelings of anger and frustration. Jackson (1994) proposes that 'arson provides a highly effective means of escaping or changing difficult-to-tolerate circumstances where other means have proved impossible or excessively difficult, been inhibited, been ineffective or perceived as ineffective' (p. 107). This model of recidivistic firesetting devotes particular attention to the role of behaviours and emotions temporally close to the firesetting incident. Jackson (1994) argues that a clear pattern should be evident in the behaviour of serial arsonists, although this pattern may be specific to the individual.

Originally proposed by Fineman (1995), the dynamic behaviour model of firesetting is the only other multifactorial theory describing adult firesetting to have been widely discussed in the literature. That model, similar to the functional analysis model described above, explains firesetting as resulting from historical psychosocial influences shaped through early social learning. Fineman describes three major factors that, in combination, contribute to the initiation of firesetting in adults:

1   historical factors that predispose individuals to behave antisocially (e.g., social disadvantage, social ineffectiveness)
2   previous and existing environmental reinforcement contingencies promoting firesetting (e.g., childhood fire experiences, fire fascination)
3   instantaneous environmental reinforcement contingencies promoting firesetting (e.g., external, internal or sensory reinforcement).

Fineman identifies other potentially relevant factors, such as impulsivity triggers (e.g., rejection, victimisation or trauma), features of the crime scene that may provide clues as to the goal of the firesetting behaviour, cognitions before, accompanying and following firesetting, as well as affective influences, such as substance intoxication. Finally, Fineman suggests that the process of reinforcement of firesetting behaviours should be explored within this model.

Fineman's model views firesetting as resulting from unique and complex interactions between all of these factors and suggests that individual treatment should logically follow a careful assessment of each of these hypothesised risk factors. A notable strength of this model is that it describes firesetting as part of an offence chain and advocates an examination of offence-supportive cognitions in the offence sequence. Additionally, similar to the functional analysis model, key features of Fineman's model are well supported by the literature.

This chapter extends previous discussions (Doley *et al*, 2011) of risk and protective factors relevant to adult repeated firesetting. In the absence of arson-specific measures, our discussion highlights several core factors and tools relevant to the assessment of adult firesetting. The Fineman (1995) model remains empirically untested and fails specifically to address the issue of serial arson as clearly as the functional analysis model has attempted to do. Consequently, the functional analysis model will form the underlying framework for the current discussion.

Core factors relevant to the assessment of firesetters

Our premise is that a combination of clinical interview and an actuarial approach will produce the most comprehensive formulation and assessment of both treatment readiness and risk. The assessment considerations we highlight address variables relevant to the broadly defined antecedent, behavioural and consequential features of firesetting behaviour. For the treatment and assessment of firesetters, an understanding of the emotions and behaviours temporally close to the fire incident is vital to treatment formulation. It provides a window to the function of the behaviour, which subsequently then informs treatment targets. In this section, the core features critical for the assessment of firesetters are presented.

Demographics

While many offenders resemble each other across variables such as a history of dysfunctional family background, socioeconomic disadvantage and inadequate or nonexistent supervision as a child (Hurley & Monahan, 1969; Tennent *et al*, 1971; O'Sullivan & Kelleher, 1987; Barnett & Spitzer, 1994; Puri *et al*, 1995), arsonists tend to report less academic achievement, more problems at school, less skilled employment and earlier onset of psychosocial problems than other offenders (Bradford, 1982). The dysfunctional family backgrounds of arsonists has been highlighted (Blackburn, 1993; Hollin, 1989; Inciardi, 1970; Kolko & Kazdin, 1990, 1991, 1992; Rix, 1994), along with their tendency to a history of social deprivation, childhood adversity including physical and sexual abuse, and a high rate of behavioural disorders (Joukamaa & Tuovinen, 1983; Heath *et al*, 1985; Jackson *et al*, 1987b; Bourget & Bradford, 1989; Leong, 1992; Bland *et al*, 1999). Thus, specific attention to these factors will be relevant to any comprehensive assessment or formulation of firesetting behaviour.

Pyromania

The concept of an irresistible urge to light fires is gradually receiving less credence in the literature, particularly as a diagnosis of pyromania is relatively rare in arson samples (Geller *et al*, 1997; Huff *et al*, 1997; LeJoyeux *et al*, 2002; Doley, 2003). Pyromania as a clinical diagnostic term has had a chequered history. It appeared in the first edition of DSM (DSM-I, American Psychiatric Association, 1952) as a supplementary term but subsequently disappeared in DSM-II (American Psychiatric Association, 1968). When DSM-III (American Psychiatric Association, 1980) was published, pyromania featured under the category 'Impulse control disorders not otherwise specified' and has remained there in the current edition of DSM, DSM-IV-TR (American Psychiatric Association, 2000). An explanation for the gap between what is believed about pyromania and what is known has been provided elsewhere (Doley, 2003). The term is receiving less attention in clinical circles as although there appears to be quite an extensive range in the literature, on balance the reported incidence rate of true pyromania is reducing (Perr, 1979; Geller, 1987; Rice & Harris, 1991; McElroy et al, 1992; Soltys, 1992). Lindberg et al (2005), for example, reviewed the forensic psychiatric evaluations of 90 repeat firesetters. Only three were found to meet the diagnostic criteria for pyromania. Diagnoses of intellectual disability, psychosis, personality disorder and substance-related disorders were found to be the most prevalent. Nevertheless, while pyromania has been found to be a rare diagnosis, even among recidivist arson offenders, the term remains a favourite moniker for serial arsonists featured in the media.

An important question for any explanation of firesetting is why an individual would be drawn to fire as opposed to other tools or implements. In their formulation, Jackson et al (1987a) hypothesise that early exposure to fire leads to the arsonist identifying it as a potential means of asserting influence on the environment. It is important to note that, in this paradigm, fire *per se* has no special significance; rather, it is the effects of firesetting that attract the arsonist (Jackson, 1994). One of the strengths of the theory, therefore, is its attempt to reduce the complexity of the issue by not specifically differentiating between pyromaniacs and serial arsonists.

Mental disorder

Significant psychiatric disturbances have been noted in a number of arson samples (Geller, 1987, Geller et al, 1992; Leong, 1992; Puri et al, 1995; Repo, 1998). The reported prevalence rate of mental illness in firesetters varies from 10% to over 60% (Barnett & Spitzer, 1994). Chromosomal disorders such as Klinefelter syndrome, as well as conditions such as epilepsy and hypoglycaemia, have also been associated with firesetting (Pontius, 1999). Although there is limited evidence supporting a neuropsychological connection with firesetting, some authors have highlighted an association between firesetting and selected psychobiological variables (e.g., chromosomal abnormality) alone or in combination with certain behavioural variables, such as previous suicide attempts (Virkkunen et al, 1989a,b, 1996; DeJong et al, 1992; Volavka et al, 1992; Puri et al, 1995).

Although similar to other offenders across many domains, it appears that one of the main areas in which arsonists are distinct from other types of offender is in the severity of psychiatric disturbance (McKerracher & Dacre, 1966; Joukamaa & Tuovinen, 1983; Rice & Harris, 1991; Repo & Virkkunen, 1997; Coid et al, 1999). Enayati et al (2008) described the prevalence of mental health disorders among 214 convicted arsonists referred for psychiatric evaluation in Sweden between 1997 and 2001. Rates of mental health disorders among arsonists were compared with those among 2395 convicted non-arsonist violent offenders. The authors calculated that almost half of all convicted arson offenders would have been referred for forensic psychiatric evaluation, compared with approximately 2% of other offenders. Assessment of mental disorders involved comprehensive assessment conducted by a multidisciplinary team over a 4-week in-patient stay. Diagnoses were derived from a multidisciplinary team comprising a forensic psychiatrist, clinical psychologist and social worker, all of whom were involved in completing mental state examinations, as well as psychological and personality testing. Assessment information was integrated with ward observations, life history and collateral information obtained from multiple sources. Over the 5-year period, assessment information was available for 214 arsonists. The most common Axis I diagnoses were psychotic illnesses (29%) and substance use disorders (47%). Almost half of arsonists referred for assessment (46%) met diagnostic criteria for a personality disorder, primarily cluster B personality disorders (23%). Compared with violent offenders, arsonists were significantly more likely to meet diagnostic criteria for intellectual disability and Asperger syndrome. As the prevalence rates for mental disorders reported by Enayati *et al* (2008) were for arsonists referred for psychiatric evaluation, the calculated rates should be considered higher estimates than might be found for arsonists not referred for psychiatric evaluation (e.g., imprisoned arson offenders).

Clearly, with the elevated prevalence of mental health disorders, intellectual disability and developmental disorders in this population, clinicians need to utilise standardised and validated approaches to assessment. Mental health diagnoses assessed via non-standardised and unstructured procedures are notoriously unreliable (Groth-Marnat, 2009). We have recommended several tools below which we consider useful specifically to address assessment requirements for firesetters. Clinicians also need to evaluate the nexus between mental health disorders and firesetting. Quinsey *et al* (2006), for example, found that motives for firesetting among convicted arsonists diagnosed with schizophrenia and other psychotic disorders referred for psychiatric evaluation were often delusional in nature.

The Structured Clinical Interview for DSM-IV Axis I Disorders (SCID-I) is a semi-structured interview (First *et al*, 1996). It has better reliability for diagnoses than routine clinical assessments. Importantly, the SCID-I has been found to increase the accuracy and comprehensiveness of diagnosis in community mental health settings (Basco *et al*, 2000). For personality disorders, the Structured Clinical Interview for DSM-IV Axis II Personality Disorders (SCID-II) can be used (First *et al*, 1997). For clinicians conducting forensic assessments, the SCID-I and SCID-II are particularly useful when diagnosis has the potential to be questioned or challenged. Both versions of the SCID have been used with various offender populations in Malaysia (Zahari *et al*, 2010), Germany (Dudeck *et al*, 2009), Italy (Zoccali *et al*, 2008), Sweden (Fridell *et al*, 2007), England and Wales (Ullrich *et al*, 2008), as well as with US prisoners of diverse racial/ethnic groups (Duncan *et al*, 2008).

In relation to screening for mental disorders, the Brief Jail Mental Health Screen (BJMHS) has been found reliable and valid with US offender samples (Steadman *et al*, 2005). Consisting of only eight items, the BJMHS can be administered by non-mental health professionals who have attended a brief training programme. In relation to predicting diagnoses, the BJMHS achieved 74% accuracy in identifying arrested men who met diagnostic criteria for depression, bipolar disorder and schizophrenia, with a false negative rate of 15% (i.e., the proportion missed by the screening tool). The BJMHS, however, did not perform as well with female offenders: 62% were correctly classified and the false negative rate was 35%. A replication study with 10 258 jail detainees in four US jails reaffirmed the classification accuracy of the BJMHS, with 80% of males and 72% of females correctly classified in relation to mental disorder as assessed via the SCID-I (Steadman *et al*, 2007).

Intelligence

Whether or not arsonists have below average intellect and limited academic achievement is debatable. Some authors have found this to be the case for their samples (Lewis & Yarnell, 1951; Saunders & Awad, 1991; Alexander *et al*, 2002) but others have contested this conclusion (Räsänen *et al*, 1994; Lindsay & Macleod, 2001; Dolan *et al*, 2002). More recent work has suggested that lower IQs appear to be associated with different motives for arson offending (Quinsey *et al*, 2006). Assessment of intellectual functioning among arson offenders is important in relation to recidivism risk, potential motivation for firesetting and treatment responsivity. While revenge is frequently identified as the motivation for arson offenders with intellectual disability, Devapriam *et al* (2007) found a further 20% of these arsonists committed their offence 'motivated by suggestibility'. Unfortunately, the basis for coding arson as motivated by suggestibility was not clearly articulated by Devapriam *et al*. The potential relevance of suggestibility among offenders with an intellectual disability, however, highlights their potential vulnerability, exploitation and manipulation (Greenspan, 1999).

Firesetters who have an intellectual disability are not likely to respond well to interventions that require an understanding of abstract concepts, high-level reasoning abilities and content delivered primarily in verbal format, with considerable demands on memory processes. Consistent with the cognitive limitations of offenders with intellectual disability, modifications have been made to standard cognitive–behavioural interventions for offenders. Interventions incorporating greater use of concrete strategies, with an emphasis on demonstration and behavioural rehearsal, repetition of concepts and strategies to cue implementation are most relevant. Such modifications have been found to be helpful when treating offenders who have committed different types of offence, including arson (Lindsay, 2009).

Substance-related problems

A high prevalence of substance (especially alcohol) misuse has been found in different arson samples (Puri *et al*, 1995; Repo, 1998), especially samples of female firesetters (e.g., Raskind, 1986; Bourget & Bradford, 1989; Linaker, 2000). Lindberg *et al* (2005) found high rates of alcohol-related disorders among recidivist arsonists (61%), with two-thirds (68%) of recidivist arsonists being intoxicated with alcohol at the time of their index offence. Such findings highlight the need for screening and assessment for alcohol and other substance-related disorders.

The Global Appraisal of Individual Needs (GAIN; Dennis *et al*, 2007) is a semi-structured interview providing comprehensive coverage of alcohol/substance use, mental health, risk behaviours, physical health, environment, offending behaviours, vocational/financial circumstances and service history (mental health, substance-related service provision). The GAIN interview can be administered directly to clients, as well as via informant interview (e.g., with carer or significant other). Initial administration of the GAIN with clients requires approximately 120 minutes, but follow-up administration requires only around 45–60 minutes. The GAIN has support for reliability and validity with both juvenile and adult offenders (Rohesnow, 2008). A screening version of the GAIN is available – GAINS–Short screener – consisting of 20 self-report items. The GAINS–Short screener has excellent predictive validity for substance-related disorders, with sensitivity and specificity exceeding 0.90 (Dennis *et al*, 2007). Utilised with adolescents and adults in substance-related programmes, mental health settings and correctional programmes, the GAIN has been used throughout numerous counties and states across the USA.

Interpersonal characteristics

As with many offenders, arsonists exhibit limited social skills and difficulties in interpersonal relations, as well as maladjustment across a range of life domains such as education, employment, peer and personal relations (Sapsford *et al*, 1978; Vreeland & Levin, 1980; Bradford, 1982; O'Sullivan & Kelleher, 1987; Barker, 1994; Puri *et al*, 1995). Compared with other offenders, arsonists are also typically described as less self-confident and assertive (McKerracher & Dacre, 1966; Hurley & Monahan, 1969; Inciardi, 1970; Geller, 1987; Rice & Harris, 1991). In terms of serial arsonists specifically, the functional analysis model of recidivistic arson proposes that limited social skills reduce an individual's ability to create change in their life circumstances. The model does not explicitly indicate how fire in particular addresses this deficit for such an individual, but it does hypothesise that fire represents a powerful means of communication for people with limited alternative skill bases. As part of their overall findings, for instance, with no clear supporting evidence, Hurley & Monahan (1969) asserted that the serial arsonists in their sample 'had learned that fire solved their problems more efficiently and often more pleasurably than any other available means' (p. 19). In a similar vein, Stewart (1993) noted that firesetting behaviour is logical and adaptive because it provides 'an effective and powerful vehicle for disenfranchised individuals seeking attention, revenge, or excitement' (p. 254).

In spite of the lack of clarity concerning the specific mechanism by which fire may affect an individual's sense of self-efficacy, there is consistent evidence that the firesetting population is especially disadvantaged in terms of interpersonal skills. Various authors have noted among arsonists problems of shyness, social isolation, occupational maladjustment and difficulty in expressing anger verbally (Lewis & Yarnell, 1951; Inciardi, 1970; Tennent et al, 1971; Bradford, 1982; O'Sullivan & Kelleher, 1987; Leong, 1992; Rix, 1994; Puri et al, 1995).

Rice & Chaplin (1979) developed a rating system to evaluate inter-personal effectiveness in response to role-play scenarios and a multiple-choice questionnaire to measure assertive responses. The role-play involved scenarios that were commonly experienced by the psychiatric in-patients who participated in the study, such as 'You're enjoying a favourite television programme when another patient enters the room and bothers you by continually chatting about unimportant things'. The video-recorded responses to these scenarios were blindly rated on four scales for assertion, empathy, anxiety and verbal skills. The questionnaires involved similar situations, with four possible choices of response, including an assertive response. Both measurement approaches were found to have sufficient internal consistency ($\alpha = 0.71–1.00$) and found to be sensitive to social skills treatment effects. The combined approach to the evaluation of interpersonal effectiveness is encouraging, and may allow the identification of social skills deficits and the monitoring of treatment response.

A similar approach to the measurement of interpersonal effectiveness was utilised by Harris & Rice (1984), who examined the social skills and assertiveness behaviours of 13 firesetters and 13 controls matched for age and intelligence. The recorded role-play scenarios involved disputes with a landlord, spouse, family member, hospital staff, an employer and a co-patient. Forensic psychiatric in-patients were rated by an observer for assertiveness on a nine-point scale. Firesetters were found to be less assertive in verbal expressions of anger, disappointment and hurt feelings and tended to be described by others and themselves as more shy and withdrawn. Harris & Rice also found that the arson offenders performed significantly worse than other offenders on the Rathus Assertion Schedule (Rathus, 1973), a self-report questionnaire that measures standing up for personal rights in a public space and initiating and maintaining interactions.

Fire interest

Physical actions that have been found to be temporally close to the incidents of firesetting have tended to be the main focus of functional descriptions of the behaviour; however, some researchers have asked about the offender's emotional reactions before, during and immediately after the firesetting (Harmon *et al*, 1985; Leong & Silva, 1999). Coid *et al* (1999), in their study of self-mutilating prisoners, for example, describe a list of emotions associated with firesetting, some of which may be considered consequential to the act. These included sexual arousal, excitement and symptom relief. One notable account illustrating the fascination firesetting holds for some is the vivid description of the cognitions, emotions and behaviours associated with serial arson provided by Orr (1989*a*,*b*). Interestingly, Orr, who was a professional firefighter with the Glendale (Californian) Fire Department at the time, was subsequently convicted of arson and sentenced to 30 years in prison (Wambaugh, 2003). Wheaton (2001) also provided a relatively comprehensive account of cognitions, emotions and behaviours temporally close to the firesetting act in a case study of her own firesetting. In comparing Orr's and Wheaton's accounts, a common feature is a desire to stay and watch the fire and its aftermath. Both describe feelings of excitement and a fascination with the flames and the trappings of fire (emergency services attending, people watching in awe); over the next several days after the fire the scene is revisited and fantasies about the fire are recreated. Both writers also comment on feelings of disappointment and even anger when the fire is extinguished. Feeling excited at the time of firesetting, and depressed or deflated afterwards, suggests that for serial arsonists there is a strong emotional component to promoting and maintaining the behaviour. The elation experienced at the time of firesetting may be sufficiently positively reinforcing to ensure the behaviour continues.

Consequently, an important feature of the assessment of firesetters is the attempt to elucidate not only those factors likely to explain antisocial behaviour tendencies, but also the elements likely to lead a person with an 'inadequate personality' to use fire as a means of stimulating change in their environment. Several researchers have commented on the association between exposure to fire at an early age (including playing with fire and matches) and subsequent pathological firesetting (Macht & Mack, 1968; MacDonald, 1977; Kolko & Kazdin, 1990; Rice & Harris, 1991; Saunders & Awad, 1991; Hanson *et al*, 1994; Perrin-Wallqvist & Norlander, 2003). An unpublished study by Smith and Bailey (cited by Bailey *et al*, 2001) examined the case notes of 119 adolescent firesetters. They found 21% of cases ($n = 25$) evidenced a history of child fire-play and 11% of individuals ($n = 13$) had been victims of firesetting at some time.

More recently, in an empirical study of 88 Australian incarcerated arsonists Doley (2009) found some important distinctions between serial and one-time arsonists. These included serial arsonists reporting greater psychosocial dysfunction (particularly family dysfunction and educational and occupational maladjustment) and psychiatric disturbance. Doley (2009) found that more arsonists reported playing with fire and obsessing about fire in childhood than did non-arsonists. Further, many more serial arsonists (26%) than one-time arsonists (9%) reported an enduring interest in fire and its trappings from a young age. Finally, while the specific features of the fire offence behaviour did not distinguish serial arsonists in this sample, it appeared that their firesetting had a strong emotive rather than instrumental element, with more reporting setting fires for excitement, supporting the relevance of exploring the emotional component of firesetting as part of a comprehensive assessment.

Gallagher-Duffy et al (2009) developed a modified Stroop task for measuring fire interest. Examinees were shown a series of images on a computer, presented in one of four colours. In response to the stimuli, participants indicated which of the four colours was presented. Among the 49 images, 15 were presented as fire-related stimuli (e.g., campfire, matchbook with smoking matches, fire engine). Based on the interference nature of Stroop tasks, emotionally relevant stimuli should require a longer response time, and decrease accuracy, thereby reflecting an information processing bias. As hypothesised, adolescents referred for firesetting behaviours were less accurate and required more time in responding to fire-related stimuli than were two control groups of adolescents (healthy controls and clinic controls). No significant difference was obtained for the three groups when the stimuli were unrelated to fire. Moreover, the strength of an implicit approach to assess fire interest was reinforced by the finding that self-reported interest in fire and fire-related materials did not significantly differentiate adolescent firesetters from the two control groups.

Assessment of the risk of arson recidivism

Standardised, reliable and valid instruments for appraising risk of continued offending behaviour are often utilised by forensic practitioners. Risk assessment measures for violent offenders and sex offenders that have been cross-validated across samples are available, such as the Violence Risk Appraisal Guide (VRAG; Quinsey et al, 2006) and the Static 99 (Hanson & Thornton, 2000). Risk assessment instruments for arson offenders which have been validated across multiple samples, however, are not currently available. Prospective follow-up studies of recidivism among firesetters are rare. Studies examining arson recidivists have more frequently been retrospective in nature (e.g., Dickens et al, 2009). Quinsey et al (2006) reported follow-up recidivism for 208 adult male arsonists incarcerated in Oak Ridge, a forensic psychiatry facility in Penetanguishene, Ontario.

The men were followed up for an average of 7–8 years. Released firesetters were more likely to commit a non-violent offence (57% of the sample did so) or a sexual or violent offence (31%) than to reoffend by firesetting (16%). While Quinsey et al (2006) were unable to obtain specific details regarding the severity of fires lit by recidivists, they did ascertain that none resulted in human fatality. In this study firesetting recidivism was statistically significantly predicted by childhood firesetting, never having been married, more fires previously set, age at setting first fire and absence of concurrent criminal charge at the time of firesetting (Quinsey et al, 2006). Among the male firesetters, previous convictions for violent offences were associated with an increased risk of violent recidivism, but with a decreased risk of arson recidivism. The inverse association between violence history and firesetting recidivism further highlights the contribution of a lack of personal assertiveness in firesetting risk. Further, arson recidivism was associated with lower levels of intelligence.

Using regression analyses, Quinsey et al (2006) created a risk assessment instrument for arson recidivism consisting of age at the time of first firesetting offence, number of arson offences, presence of firesetting problems in childhood, low IQ, absence of other criminal charges, acting alone in firesetting and a lower rating for aggression. The final firesetting recidivism instrument had a large effect size in predicting future arson offences (receiver operator characteristics area under curve was 0.76, Cohen's $d = 1.1$). Despite the encouraging findings, Quinsey et al cautioned that they were not yet ready to recommend clinical application and identified limited overlap between the significant predictors for arson recidivism, violent recidivism and non-violent recidivism. This finding highlights the importance of using instruments specifically designed for evaluating arson recidivism, as opposed to using generic tools or risk assessment tools for other offending categories.

Studies on arson recidivism and the personality characteristics of arson offenders highlight the importance of considering arson offenders as a distinct category of offender compared with violent offenders. Interpersonally, arson offenders have been described as under-assertive, experiencing difficulties in the expression of anger and socially isolated. Risk factors for repeat firesetting have been differentiated from risk factors for predicting violent behaviour (Quinsey et al, 2006), with a history of violent behaviour associated with lower risk of arson recidivism. This raises concern regarding the potential use of validated instruments designed for predicting violent recidivism among arson offenders, such as the VRAG (Quinsey et al, 2006) and the Historical, Risk, Clinical – 20 (HCR-20; Webster et al, 1995). Only risk assessment procedures which have demonstrated predictive validity with arson offenders should be used. Thus, given Quinsey et al's (2006) caution regarding their tool, this leaves professionals in a difficult situation regarding how they may assess risk.

Arson-specific assessment: into the future

The field of offence-specific assessment for arson is in its infancy relative to that for other types of crime, such as violent and sex offences. There is a range of avenues for future development and in the following discussion we highlight a few of those factors which have not yet been widely explored in arson research but which we consider are pertinent to a comprehensive assessment of firesetters.

Impulsivity

Impulsivity as a personality construct has rarely been investigated in relation to arson offenders. This is surprising, as impulsivity plays a central role in theories of antisocial behaviour (Gottfredson & Hirshi, 1990) and developmental pathways to offending (Moffitt, 1993; Farrington, 1995). The Barratt Impulsiveness Scale (BIS; Patton et al, 1995) is a 30-item self-report measure of impulsivity that is among the most widely used. Research with the BIS indicates acceptable levels of reliability and moderate to high effect sizes in differentiating offender from non-offender samples (Patton et al, 1995; Smith & Waterman, 2006). Importantly, Smith & Waterman's (2006) sample of 123 male and female violent offenders included arsonists. Patton et al (1995) proposed three second-order factors for the interpretation of results: attentional, motor and non-planning. The proposed factor structure, however, has not been replicated in a larger sample of 1103 prisoners (Ireland & Archer, 2008). Consequently, it would be more appropriate to utilise the total BIS score, as opposed to factor scores, for the assessment of arson offenders.

Anger

Anger arousal has been identified as a precursor to firesetting (Kolko & Kazdin, 1991; Stewart, 1993) and as a predictor of arson recidivism among maltreated children (Root et al, 2008). The role of anger in firesetting, however, has not been investigated using well-standardised and validated measures. The Novaco Anger Scale and Provocation Inventory (NAS-PI; Novaco, 2003) and the State–Trait Anger Expression Scale – 2 (STAXI-2; Spielberger, 1999) have been well established in working with offenders generally. Both measure propensity to experience anger, although they differ in the underlying dimensions of anger measured, and there are benefits in using them in combination to evaluate anger-related difficulties. Both the NAS-PI and the STAXI-2 have been validated for use with violent and general offenders (Baker et al, 2008; Mela et al, 2008), although further investigation of their psychometric properties is required for arsonists.

Psychopathy

Psychopathy in relation to firesetting had, until recently, been investigated in only an isolated number of case studies (e.g., Clare *et al*, 1992). Psychopathy reflects a constellation of relatively stable personality characteristics including lack of emotional concern for others, interpersonal deceit, and persistent irresponsible and antisocial behaviour. Labree *et al* (2010) evaluated levels of psychopathy as measured by the Psychopathy Checklist – Revised (PCL-R; Hare, 2003) among 25 arsonists sentenced to a maximum-security hospital in the Netherlands. Derived from file review, the psychopathy scores for arsonists were not found to be statistically significant from those for a comparison sample of 50 non-arsonist offenders. The mean PCL-R score for both groups of offenders (17.4 for arsonists, 18.3 for non-arsonists) is comparable to results reported in the PCL-R manual for scores obtained from file review without conducting an interview (Hare, 2003). Given the substantial amount of research with offender populations using the PCL-R and the centrality of psychopathy in measuring recidivism for various groups of offenders, the construct of psychopathy is likely to have similar relevance for arson offenders.

Cognitive distortions, social perception and empathy

Research with offenders has long evaluated cognitive distortions, antisocial attitudes and justifications for offending behaviour (Sykes & Matza, 1957; Yochelson & Samenow, 1976). Measures of attitudes supporting offending have been found to differentiate violent offenders and sex offenders from non-offenders (Bumby, 1996; Kelty *et al*, 2011). Malamuth *et al* (1995), for example, found that men who scored higher on measures of hostile masculinity as well as impersonal sex were significantly more likely to engage in sexually aggressive acts over a 10-year follow-up than were men who scored lower on hostile masculinity and impersonal sex. Concern, however, has been raised that self-report measures assessing cognitive distortions among offenders may be too easily susceptible to impression management (Arkowitz & Vess, 2003). Research with offenders has advanced towards the use of implicit measures of antisocial cognitions, as these reduce the potential for social desirability bias in responding (Mihailides *et al*, 2004). Research with arson offenders has yet to progress in this area and there is a lack of research and standardised assessment tools for appraising cognitive content supportive of firesetting behaviours.

Blake & Gannon (2010) describe how cognitive distortions influence individuals' social perceptual processes, which then provides the basis for selecting courses of action. Biases and distortions in perceptual processes have been identified in both sex offenders (Malamuth & Brown, 1994) and violent offenders (Holtzworth-Munroe, 1992). As anger, revenge, under-assertion and interpersonal skills deficits have been identified among firesetters, social perceptual processes are likely to be relevant. Attribution of hostile intent refers to the perception of another person's actions as intending harm (physically or psychologically) when the other person's actions may have been accidental or benign (Dodge, 1986). Distortion in information processing has often been identified in individuals with anger-related difficulties (Novaco, 1997; Anderson & Bushman, 2002). As arson offenders have been identified as being under-assertive, they may lack the prerequisite skills to resolve interpersonal conflict appropriately. The selection of courses of action in interpersonal contexts is influenced by both cognitive processes and information processing (Blake & Gannon, 2010). Further development of assessment procedures for arson offenders would benefit from the use of frameworks established with other categories of offenders.

Distortions in social perception and cognitive content may lead to deficits in empathy. Deficits in empathy comprising both cognitive processes (understanding the perspective of others) and affective capacity (emotional reaction in concordance with another's emotional experience) have been hypothesised to contribute to antisocial behaviour. Lower scores on trait measures of empathy have been associated with higher rates of antisocial behaviour (relative to higher levels of trait empathy) (Miller & Eisenberg, 1988; Davis, 1996). Among measures of trait empathy, Davis' (1983) Interpersonal Reactivity Index (IRI) has been widely used. The IRI measures four domains: perspective-taking, fantasy, empathic concern, and personal distress. The role of trait measures of empathy in describing offenders, however, has been disputed. Lindsey et al (2001), for example, found little difference between offenders and non-offenders on perspective-taking, fantasy or empathic concern as measured by the IRI. Significant differences have been found for the personal distress scale, with offenders scoring higher than non-offenders. Elevated personal distress reflects a tendency to become emotionally reactive in intense situations and to become self-oriented in perspective (Lindsey et al, 2001). Further, trait empathy as measured by the IRI has been inversely related to therapists' ratings of adolescent sex offenders' victim empathy (Curwen, 2003). Empathy deficits among offenders may be more specific to empathy for the victim of offending behaviour as opposed to a global deficit in empathy (Tierney & McCabe, 2001).

Some research has examined the role of empathy among convicted arson offenders. For example, Walsh et al (2004) evaluated the prevalence of empathy deficits among 21 male adolescent firesetters in comparison with a control group of 21 adolescent males referred for family counselling. On the Bryant Index of Empathy for Children and Adolescents (Bryant, 1982), both groups had low levels of empathy when compared with the normative sample, although no difference was evident between firesetters and non-firesetters (those referred for counselling). Firesetting behaviour typically occurs when the victim is more distal from the offence, compared with violence and sex offending, where the victim is in the direct vicinity of the perpetrator. Anticipating and understanding the consequences for potential victims of firesetting may therefore require greater abstract reasoning skills and forethought, compared with other types of offence. In conjunction with their low intelligence, understanding the perspective of victims of arson may be difficult for these offenders. Thus, research is needed to investigate procedures for measuring empathy towards victims of arson.

Conclusion

Serial arsonists are distinguished from one-time arsonists primarily, it appears, by degree of disadvantage across antecedent variables such as psychiatric disturbance and family dysfunction and, to a lesser extent, in the nature of their firesetting, with the fire-related acts of serial arsonists being more oriented towards experiencing fire and its trappings (Doley, 2009). This is consistent with the explanation of recidivistic firesetting that proposes arson as a means of effecting desired change in the individual's life circumstances and firesetting being employed by individuals with a deficient skill repertoire. This chapter has provided a guide for the assessment of arsonists and suggested directions for research in this field. Promising new directions include a focus on the social processing and cognitions associated with the firesetting behaviour, as well as the emotions and behaviours temporally close to the fire event.

The assessment of convicted arsonists requires consideration of historical predisposing factors, time-stable individual characteristics, as well as more dynamic characteristics that may precipitate and perpetuate the risk of firesetting. As they would with other offenders, clinicians need to review developmental history, including family history, developmental stages, academic history and performance, and any history of maltreatment. More specific to the approach with firesetters is the need to investigate childhood exposure to fire and fire-related activities. Stable personal characteristics for assessment include mental health disorders, personality disorders and intellectual disability. Due to the potential for assessments to be challenged in legal contexts, forensic practitioners need to utilise validated and standardised measures, as described above. Social skills deficits, especially in relation to limited assertion skills, have been particularly indicated in assessing arsonists. Assessment procedures have included role-play scenarios, as well as valid self-report measures such as the Rathus Assertion Schedule (Rathus, 1973). Comprehensive assessment of prior firesetting behaviours is crucial, including situational circumstances, type of incendiary devices and emotional arousal associated with fire. Recent advances indicate the benefits of utilising indirect, implicit measures of fire interest with firesetters, as these reduce the potential for social desirability bias. Finally, the authors encourage further development in the use of assessment instruments that are widely used with non-arson offenders, including measures of impulsivity, anger, psychopathy, cognitive distortions, social perception and empathy.

In discussing the assessment of adult firesetters, this chapter presents suggestions for 'best practice'. There is an aspirational theme embedded in these recommendations, guided in part by legal and ethical requirements of mental health professionals and informed not just by an understanding of what is accepted about firesetters but also by knowing where the gaps in our current knowledge lie. In many instances, further research is required in order to be able to refine and clarify assessment targets. The focus here has been on adult firesetters in mental health contexts. Further information concerning the assessment of juveniles as well as the assessment of adult arsonists in community-based settings would be relevant to the overall discussion. The limitation of this chapter is one that applies to most texts in this field – the information contained herein describes an ideal but the context of application is dynamic and it can be expected (indeed hoped) that as work continues in this area standards of practice will change and evolve with an advancing scientific base.

References

Alexander, R., Piachaud, J., Odebiyi, L., *et al* (2002) Referrals to a forensic service in the psychiatry of learning disability. *British Journal of Forensic Practice*, **4**, 29–33.

American Psychiatric Association (1952) *Diagnostic and Statistical Manual of Mental Disorders* (1st edn) (DSM-I). APA.

American Psychiatric Association (1968) *Diagnostic and Statistical Manual of Mental Disorders* (2nd edn) (DSM-II). APA.

American Psychiatric Association (1980) *Diagnostic and Statistical Manual of Mental Disorders* (3rd edn) (DSM-III). APA.

American Psychiatric Association (2000) *Diagnostic and Statistical Manual of Mental Disorders* (4th edn, text revision) (DSM-IV-TR). APA.

Anderson, C. A. & Bushman, B. J. (2002) Human aggression. *Annual Review of Psychology*, **53**, 27–51.

Arkowitz, S. & Vess, J. (2003) An evaluation of the Bumby RAPE and MOLEST Scales as measures of cognitive distortions with civilly committed sexual offenders. *Sexual Abuse: Journal of Research and Treatment*, **15**, 237–249.

Bailey, S., Smith, C. & Dolan, M. (2001) The social background and nature of 'children' who perpetrate violent crimes: a UK perspective. *Journal of Community Psychology*, **29**, 305–317.

Baker, M. T., Van Hasselt, V. B. & Sellers, A. H. (2008) Validation of the Novaco Anger Scale in an incarcerated offender population. *Criminal Justice and Behavior*, **35**, 741–754.

Barker, A. (1994) *Arson: A Review of the Psychiatric Literature*. Oxford University Press.

Barnett, W. & Spitzer, M. (1994) Pathological fire-setting 1951–1991: a review. *Medicine, Science and the Law*, **34**, 4–20.

Basco, M. R., Bostic, J. Q., Davies, D., *et al* (2000) Methods to improve diagnostic accuracy in a community mental health setting. *American Journal of Psychiatry*, **157**, 1599–1605.

Blackburn, R. (1993) *The Psychology of Criminal Conduct*. Wiley.

Blake, E. & Gannon, T. (2010) Social perception deficits, cognitive distortions, and empathy deficits in sex offenders: a brief review. *Trauma, Violence and Abuse*, **9**, 34–55.

Bland, J., Mezey, G. & Dolan, B. (1999) Special women, special needs: a descriptive study of female special hospital patients. *Journal of Forensic Psychiatry*, **10**, 34–45.

Bourget, D. & Bradford, J. (1989) Female arsonists: a clinical study. *Bulletin of the American Academy of Psychiatry and Law*, **17**, 293–300.

Bradford, J. (1982) Arson: a clinical study. *Canadian Journal of Psychiatry*, **27**, 188–193.

Bryant, B. (1982) An index of empathy for children and adolescents. *Child Development*, **53**, 413–425.

Bumby, K. M. (1996) Assessing the cognitive distortions of child molesters and rapists: development and validation of the MOLEST and RAPE scales. *Sexual Abuse: A Journal of Research and Treatment*, **8**, 37–54.

Clare, I., Murphy, G., Cox, D., *et al* (1992) Assessment and treatment of firesetting: a single-case investigation using a cognitive–behavioural model. *Criminal Behaviour and Mental Health*, **2**, 253–268.

Coid, J., Kahtan, N., Gault, S., *et al* (1999) Patients with personality disorder admitted to secure forensic psychiatry services. *British Journal of Psychiatry*, **175**, 528–536.

Curwen, T. (2003) The importance of offense characteristics, victimization history, hostility, and social desirability in assessing empathy of male adolescent sex offenders. *Sex Abuse: A Journal of Research and Treatment*, **15**, 347–364.

Davis, M. H. (1983) Measuring individual differences in empathy: Evidence for a multi-dimensional approach. *Journal of Personality and Social Psychology*, **44**, 113–126.

Davis, M. H. (1996) *Empathy: A Social Psychological Approach*. Westview.

DeJong, J., Virkkunen, M. & Linnoila, M. (1992) Factors associated with recidivism in a criminal population. *Journal of Nervous and Mental Disease*, **180**, 543–550.

Dennis, M. L., White, M., Titus, J. C., *et al* (2007) *Global Appraisal of Individual Needs: Administration Guide for the Gain and Related Measures*. Chestnut Health Systems.

Devapriam, J., Raju, L. B., Singh, N., *et al* (2007) Arson: characteristics and predisposing factors in offenders with intellectual disabilities. *British Journal of Forensic Practice*, **9**, 23–27. At http://pierprofessional.metapress.com/content/u24t778607119007 (accessed 21 December 2010).

Dickens, G., Sugarman, P., Edgar, S., *et al* (2009) Recidivism and dangerousness in arsonists. *Journal of Forensic Psychiatry and Psychology*, **20**, 621–639.

Dodge, K. A. (1986) A social information processing model of social competence in children. *Minnesota Symposium on Child Psychology*, **18**, 77–125.

Dolan, M., Millington, J. & Park, I. (2002) Personality and neuropsychological function in violent, sexual and arson offenders. *Medicine, Science and the Law*, **42**, 34–43.

Doley, R. (2003) Pyromania. Fact or fiction? *British Journal of Criminology*, **43**, 797–807.

Doley, R. (2009) *A Snapshot of Serial Arson in Australia*. Lambert Academic Publishing.

Doley, R., Fineman, K., Fritzon, K., *et al* (2011) Risk factors for recidivistic arson in adult arson offenders. *Psychology, Psychiatry and Law*, **18**, 409–423.

Dudeck, M., Kopp, D., Kuwert, P., *et al* (2009) Prevalence of psychiatric disorders in prisoners with a short imprisonment: results from a prison in north Germany. *Psychiatrische Praxis*, **36**, 219–224.

Duncan, A., Sacks, S., Melnick, G., *et al* (2008) Performance of the CJDATS Co-Occurring Disorders Screening Instruments (CODSIs) among minority offenders. *Behavioral Sciences and the Law*, **26**, 351–368.

Enayati, J., Grann, M., Lubbe, S., *et al* (2008) Psychiatric morbidity in arsonists referred for forensic psychiatric assessment in Sweden. *Journal of Forensic Psychiatry and Psychology*, **19**, 139–147.

Farrington, D. P. (1995) The twelfth Jack Tizard memorial lecture. The development of offending behaviour and antisocial behaviour from childhood: key findings from the Cambridge study in delinquent development. *Journal of Child Psychology and Psychiatry*, **360**, 929–964.

Ferster, C. (1965) A functional analysis of depression. *American Psychologist*, **28**, 857–870.

Fineman, K. R. (1995) A model for the qualitative analysis of child and adult fire deviant behavior. *American Journal of Forensic Psychology*, **13**, 31–60.

First, M. B., Spitzer, R. L., Gibbon M., *et al* (1996) *Structured Clinical Interview for DSM-IV Axis I Disorders, Clinician Version (SCID-CV)*. American Psychiatric Press.

First, M. B., Gibbon M., Spitzer R. L., *et al* (1997) *Structured Clinical Interview for DSM-IV Axis II Personality Disorders (SCID-II)*. American Psychiatric Press.

Fridell, M., Hesse, M. & Billsten, J. (2007) Criminal behavior in antisocial substance abusers between five and fifteen years' follow-up. *American Journal of Addictions*, **16**, 10–14.

Fritzon, K., Dolan, M., Doley, R., *et al* (2011) Juvenile fire-setting: a review of treatment programs. *Psychology, Psychiatry and Law*, **18**, 395–408.

Gallagher-Duffy, J., MacKay, S., Duffy, J., *et al* (2009) The Pictorial Fire Stroop: a measure of processing bias for fire-related stimuli. *Journal of Abnormal Child Psychology*, **37**, 1165–1176.

Gannon, T. A. & Pina, A. (2010) Firesetting: psychopathology, theory and treatment. *Aggression and Violent Behavior*, **15**, 224–238.

Geller, J. (1987) Firesetting in the adult psychiatric population. *Hospital and Community Psychiatry*, **38**, 501–506.

Geller, J., Fisher, W. & Bertsch, G. (1992) Who repeats? A follow-up study of State hospital patients' firesetting behavior. *Psychiatric Quarterly*, **63**, 143–157.

Geller, J., McDermeit, M. & Brown, J. M. (1997) Pyromania? What does it mean? *Journal of Forensic Science*, **42**, 1052–1057.

Goren, C., Romanczyk, R. & Harris, S. L. (1977) A functional analysis of echolalic speech: the effects of antecedent and consequent events. *Behaviour Modification*, **1**, 481–499.

Gottfredson, M. R. & Hirshi, T. (1990) *A General Theory of Crime.* Stanford University Press.

Greenspan, S. (1999) What is meant by mental retardation? *International Review of Psychiatry*, **11**, 6–18.

Groth-Marnat, G. (2009) *Handbook of Psychological Assessment* (5th edn). Wiley.

Hanley, G., Iwata, B. & McCord, B. (2003) Functional analysis of problem behavior: a review. *Journal of Applied Behavior Analysis*, **36**, 147–185.

Hanson, M., Mackay-Soroka, S., Staley, S., *et al* (1994) Delinquent firesetters: a comparative study of delinquency and firesetting histories. *Canadian Journal of Psychiatry*, **39**, 230–232.

Hanson, R. K. & Thornton, D. (2000) Improving risk assessments for sex offenders: a comparison of three actuarial scales. *Law and Human Behavior*, **24**, 119–136.

Hare, R. D. (2003) *Hare Psychopathy Checklist – Revised (PCL-R)* (2nd edn). MHS.

Harmon, R., Rosner, R. & Wiederlight, M. (1985) Women and arson: a demographic study. *Journal of Forensic Sciences*, **30**, 467–477.

Harris, G. T. & Rice, M. E. (1984) Mentally disordered firesetters: psychodynamic versus empirical approaches. *International Journal of Law and Psychiatry*, **7**, 19–34.

Heath, G., Hardesty, V., Goldfine, P., *et al* (1985) Diagnosis and childhood firesetting. *Journal of Clinical Psychology*, **41**, 571–575.

Heilbrun, K., Grisso, T. & Goldstein, A. (2009) *Foundations of Forensic Mental Health Assessment.* Oxford University Press.

Hollin, C. (1989) *Psychology and Crime.* Routledge.

Holtzworth-Munroe, A. (1992) Social skills deficits in maritally violent men: interpreting the data using a social information processing model. *Clinical Psychology Review*, **12**, 605–617.

Huff, T. G., Gary, G. P. & Icove, D. J. (1997) *The Myth of Pyromania.* National Center for the Analysis of Violent Crime, FBI Academy.

Hurley, W. & Monahan, T. (1969) Arson: the criminal and the crime. *British Journal of Criminology*, **9**, 4–21.

Inciardi, J. (1970) The adult firesetter: a typology. *Criminology* (August), 145–155.

Ireland, J. L. & Archer, J. (2008) Impulsivity among adult prisoners: a confirmatory factor analysis study of the Barratt Impulsivity Scale. *Personality and Individual Differences*, **45**, 286–292.

Jackson, H. F. (1994) Assessment of fire-setters. In *The Assessment of Criminal Behaviours of Clients in Secure Settings* (eds M. McMurran & J. Hodge), pp. 94–126. Jessica Kingsley.

Jackson, H. F., Glass, C. & Hope, S. (1987a) A functional analysis of recidivist arson. *British Journal of Clinical Psychology*, **26**, 175–185.

Jackson, H. F., Hope, S. & Glass, C. (1987b) Why are arsonists not violent offenders? *International Journal of Offender Therapy and Comparative Criminology*, **31**, 143–151.

Joukamaa, M. & Tuovinen, M. (1983) Finnish arsonists. *Journal of the Forensic Science Society*, **23**, 172–173.

Kelty, S., Hall, G. & Watt, B. (2011) You have to hit some people! Measurement and criminogenic nature of violent sentiments in Australia. *Psychiatry, Psychology and Law*, **18**, 15–32.

Kolko, D. J. & Kazdin, A. E. (1990) Matchplay and firesetting in children: relationship to parent, marital, and family dysfunction. *Journal of Clinical Child Psychology*, **19**, 229–238.

Kolko, D. J. & Kazdin, A. E. (1991) Motives of childhood firesetters: firesetting characteristics and psychological correlates. *Journal of Child Psychology and Psychiatry*, **32**, 535–550.

Kolko, D. J. & Kazdin, A. E. (1992) The emergence and recurrence of child firesetting: a one-year prospective study. *Journal of Abnormal Child Psychology*, **20**, 17–37.

Labree, W., Nijman, H., van Marle, H., *et al* (2010) Backgrounds and characteristics of arsonists. *International Journal of Law and Psychiatry*, **33**, 149–153.

LeJoyeux, M., Arbaretaz, M., McLoughlin, M., *et al* (2002) Impulse control disorders and depression. *Journal of Nervous and Mental Disease*, **190**, 310–314.

Leong, G. (1992) A psychiatric study of persons charged with arson. *Journal of Forensic Sciences*, **37**, 1319–1326.

Leong, G. & Silva, J. (1999) Revisiting arson from an outpatient forensic perspective. *Journal of Forensic Science*, **44**, 558–563.

Lewis, N. O. C. & Yarnell, H. (1951) *Pathological Firesetting (Pyromania)*. Nervous and Mental Disease Monographs no. 82. Coolidge Foundation.

Linaker, O. (2000) Dangerous female psychiatric patients: prevalence and characteristics. *Acta Psychiatrica Scandinavica*, **101**, 67–72.

Lindberg, N., Holi, M., Tani, P., *et al* (2005). Looking for pyromania: characteristics of a consecutive sample of Finnish male criminals with histories of recidivist fire-setting between 1973 and 1993. *BMC Psychiatry*, **5**. (Published online 14 December 2005.)

Lindsay, W. R. (2009) Adaptations and developments in treatment programmes for offenders with developmental disabilities. *Psychiatry, Psychology and Law*, **16**, S18–S35.

Lindsay, W. R. & Macleod, F. (2001) A review of forensic learning-disability research. *British Journal of Forensic Practice*, **3**, 4–10.

Lindsey, R. E., Carlozzi, A. F. & Eells, G. (2001) Differences in the dispositional empathy of juvenile sex offenders, non-sex-offending delinquent juveniles, and nondelinquent juveniles. *Journal of Interpersonal Violence*, **16**, 510–522.

MacDonald, J. (1977) *Bombers and Firesetters*. Charles C. Thomas.

Macht, L. & Mack, J. (1968) The firesetter syndrome. *Psychiatry*, **31**, 277–288.

Malamuth, N. M. & Brown, L. M. (1994) Sexually aggressive men's perceptions of women's communications: testing three explanations. *Journal of Personality and Social Psychology*, **67**, 699–712.

Malamuth, N. M., Linz, D., Heavey, C. L., *et al* (1995) Using the confluence model of sexual aggression to predict men's conflict with women: a 10 year follow-up study. *Journal of Personality and Social Psychology*, **69**, 353–369.

McElroy, S. L., Hudson, J. I., Pope, H., *et al* (1992) The DSM-III-R impulse control disorders not elsewhere classified: clinical characteristics and relationship to other psychiatric disorders. *American Journal of Psychiatry*, **149**, 318–327.

McEwan, T., Doley, R. & Dolan, M. (in press) Bushfires and wildfires: arson risk assessment in the Australian context. In *Arson and Mental Health: Theory, Research and Practice* (eds G. Dickens, P. Sugarman, & T. Gannon). RCPsych Publications.

McKerracher, D., & Dacre, A. (1966) A study of arsonists in a special security hospital. *British Journal of Psychiatry*, **112**, 1151–1154.

Mela, M., Balbuena, L., Duncan, C. R., *et al* (2008) The STAXI as a measure of inmate anger and a predictor of institutional offending. *Journal of Forensic Psychiatry and Psychology*, **19**, 396–406.

Mihailides, S., Devilly, G. J. & Ward, T. (2004) Implicit cognitive distortions and sex offending. *Sexual Abuse: A Journal of Research and Treatment*, **16**, 333–350.

Miller, P. A. & Eisenberg, N. (1988) The relation of empathy to aggressive and externalizing/antisocial behaviour. *Psychological Bulletin*, **103**, 324–344.

Moffitt, T. E. (1993) Adolescence-limited and life-course persistent antisocial behaviour: a developmental taxonomy. *Psychological Review*, **100**, 674–701.

Novaco, R. W. (1997) Remediating anger and aggression with violent offenders. *Legal and Criminological Psychology*, **2**, 77–88.

Novaco, R. W. (2003) *The Novaco Anger Scale and Provocation Inventory: NAS-PI*. Western Psychological Services.

Orr, J. (1989a) Profiles in arson: the revenge firesetter. *American Fire Journal*, 41, 30–32.

Orr, J. (1989b) Profiles in arson: the serial firesetter. *American Fire Journal*, 41, 24–27.

O'Sullivan, G. & Kelleher, M. (1987) A study of firesetters in the south-west of Ireland. *British Journal of Psychiatry*, **151**, 818–823.

Patton, J. H., Stanford, M. S. & Barratt, E. S. (1995) Factor structure of the Barratt Impulsiveness Scale. *Journal of Clinical Psychology*, **51**, 768–774.

Perr, I. (1979) Comments on arson. *Journal of Forensic Sciences*, **24**, 885–889.

Perrin-Wallqvist, R. & Norlander, T. (2003) Firesetting and playing with fire during childhood and adolescence: interview studies of 18-year-old male draftees and 18–19-year-old female pupils. *Legal and Criminological Psychology*, **8**, 151–157.

Pontius, A. (1999) Motiveless firesetting: implicating partial limbic seizure kindling by revived memories of fires in 'limbic psychotic trigger reaction'. *Perceptual and Motor Skills*, **88**, 970–982.

Puri, B., Baxter, R. & Cordess, C. (1995) Characteristics of firesetters: a study and proposed multiaxial psychiatric classification. *British Journal of Psychiatry*, **166**, 393–396.

Quinsey, V. L., Harris, G. T., Rice, M. E., et al (2006) *Violent Offenders: Appraising and Managing Risk* (2nd edn). Washington, DC: American Psychological Association.

Räsänen, P., Hirvenoja, R., Hakko, H., et al (1994) Cognitive functioning ability of arsonists. *Journal of Forensic Psychiatry*, **5**, 615–620.

Raskind, S. (1986) Suicide by burning: emotional needs of the suicidal adolescent on the burn unit. *Issues in Comprehensive Paediatric Nursing*, **9**, 369–382.

Rathus, S. A. (1973) A 30-item schedule for assessing assertive behaviour. *Behavior Therapy*, **4**, 398–406.

Repo, E. (1998) Finnish fire-setting offenders evaluated pretrial. *Psychiatria Fennica*, **29**, 175–189.

Repo, E. & Virkkunen, M. (1997) Outcomes in a sample of Finnish fire-setters. *Journal of Forensic Psychiatry*, **8**, 127–137.

Rice, M. E. & Chaplin, T. C. (1979) Social skills training for hospitalized male arsonists. *Journal of Behavior Research and Experimental Psychiatry*, **10**, 105–108.

Rice, M. E. & Harris, G. T. (1991) Firesetters admitted to a maximum security psychiatric institution. *Journal of Interpersonal Violence*, **6**, 461–475.

Rix, K. J. B. (1994) A psychiatric study of adult arsonists. *Medicine, Science and the Law*, **34**, 21–34.

Rohesnow, D. J. (2008) Substance use disorders. In *A Guide to Assessments That Work* (eds J. Hunsley & E. J. Mash), pp. 319–338. Oxford University Press.

Root, C., MacKay, S., Henderson, J., et al (2008) The link between maltreatment and juvenile firesetting: correlates and underlying mechanisms. *Child Abuse and Neglect*, **32**, 161–176.

Sapsford, R., Banks, C. & Smith, D. (1978) Arsonists in prison. *Medicine, Science and the Law*, **18**, 247–254.

Saunders, E. & Awad, G. (1991) Adolescent female firesetters. *Canadian Journal of Psychiatry*, **36**, 401–404.

Skinner, B. F. (1953) *Science and Human Behavior*. Macmillan.

Slade, P. (1982) Towards a functional analysis of anorexia nervosa and bulimia nervosa. *British Journal of Clinical Psychology*, **21**, 167–179.

Smith, P. & Waterman, M. (2006) Self-reported aggression and impulsivity in forensic and non-forensic populations: the role of gender and experience. *Journal of Family Violence*, **21**, 425–437.

Smith, R. & Churchill, R. (2002) Identification of environmental determinants of behavior disorders through functional analysis of precursor behaviors. *Journal of Applied Behavior Analysis*, **35**, 125–136.

Soltys, S. M. (1992) Pyromania and firesetting behaviors. *Psychiatric Annals*, **22**, 79–83.

Spielberger, C. D. (1999) *STAXI-2: State–Trait Anger Expression Inventory – 2. Professional Manual*. PAR.

Steadman, H. J., Scott, J. E., Osher, F., *et al* (2005) Validation of the Brief Jail Mental Health Screen. *Psychiatric Services*, **56**, 816–822.

Steadman, H. J., Robbins, P. C., Islam, T., *et al* (2007) Revalidating the Brief Jail Mental Health Screen to increase accuracy for women. *Psychiatric Services*, **58**, 1598–1601.

Stewart, L. A. (1993) Profile of female firestarters: implications for treatment. *British Journal of Psychiatry*, **163**, 248–256.

Sykes, G. & Matza, D. (1957) Techniques of neutralisation: a theory of delinquency. *American Sociological Review*, **22**, 664–673.

Tennent, T., McQuaid, A., Loughnane, T., *et al* (1971) Female arsonists. *British Journal of Psychiatry*, **119**, 497–502.

Tierney, D. W. & McCabe, M. P. (2001) An evaluation of self-report measures of cognitive distortions and empathy among Australian sex offenders. *Archives of Sexual Behaviour*, **30**, 495–519.

Ullrich, S., Deasy, D., Smith, J., *et al* (2008) Detecting personality disorders in the prison population of England and Wales: comparing case identification using the SCID-II screen and the SCID-II clinical interview. *Journal of Forensic Psychiatry and Psychology*, **19**, 301–322.

Virkkunen, M., De Jong, J., Bartko, J., *et al* (1989*a*) Relationship of psychobiological variables to recidivism in violent offenders and impulsive fire setters: a follow-up study. *Archives of General Psychiatry*, **46**, 600–603.

Virkkunen, M., De Jong, J. & Linnoila, M. (1989*b*) Psychobiological concomitants of history of suicide attempts among violent offenders and impulsive fire setters. *Archives of General Psychiatry*, **46**, 604–606.

Virkkunen, M., Eggert, M., Rawlings, R., *et al* (1996) A prospective follow-up study of alcoholic violent offenders and fire setters. *Archives of General Psychiatry*, **53**, 523–529.

Volavka, J., Martell, D. & Convit, A. (1992) Psychobiology of the violent offender. *Journal of Forensic Sciences*, **37**, 237–251.

Vreeland, R. & Levin, B. (1980) Psychological aspects of firesetting. In *Fires and Human Behaviour* (ed. D. Canter), pp. 31–46. David Fulton.

Walsh, D., Lambie, I. & Stewart, M. (2004) Sparking up: family, behavioural and empathy factors in adolescent firesetters. *American Journal of Forensic Psychology*, **22**, 5–32.

Wambaugh, J. (2003) Fire lover. *Australian Reader's Digest*, March, 136–151.

Webster, C. D., Eaves, D., Douglas, K. S., *et al* (1995) *The HCR-20 Scheme: The Assessment of Dangerousness and Risk*. University of Toronto.

Wheaton, S. (2001) Memoirs of a compulsive firesetter. *Psychiatric Services*, **52**, 1035–1036.

Yochelson, S. & Samenow, S. E. (1976) *The Criminal Personality. Vol. 1: A Profile for Change*. Aronson.

Zahari, M. M., Bae, W. H., Zainal, N. Z., *et al* (2010) Psychiatric and substance abuse comorbidity among HIV seropositive and HIV seronegative prisoners in Malaysia. *American Journal of Drug and Alcohol Abuse*, **36**, 31–38.

Zoccali, R., Muscatello, M. R. A., Bruno, A., *et al* (2008) Mental disorders and request for psychiatric intervention in an Italian local jail. *International Journal of Law and Psychiatry*, **31**, 447–450.

CHAPTER 11

Bushfire and wildfire arson: arson risk assessment in the Australian context

Troy E. McEwan, Rebekah M. Doley and Mairead Dolan

Deliberately lit vegetation fires have the greatest destructive potential of any intentionally lit blaze. The 'Black Saturday' bushfires of 7 February 2009 in Victoria, Australia, killed 173 people, injured 414 and destroyed 3500 buildings, including two entire towns (Teague *et al*, 2010). Even before the fires had abated, police and firefighters revealed that several had been deliberately lit (Silvester, 2009). The subsequent Royal Commission attributed four of the large fires to arson. These four fires caused 52 deaths and burnt approximately 2000 km² of land, an area slightly larger than that of Greater London (Teague *et al*, 2010). The community was united in its outrage that anyone would intentionally set a bushfire, particularly on a day with the most severe fire danger rating in over 20 years. The question of why anyone would set such fires is, unfortunately, not easy to answer, as there has been little investigation of those who deliberately light bushfires, especially in Australia. The lack of research in this area is somewhat surprising, given that events like Black Saturday are not uncommon in Australia and other fire-prone regions. The Australian Institute of Criminology estimates that 25 000–30 000 bushfires are deliberately lit in Australia each year (Bryant, 2008). Disaster-level bushfires (those resulting in more than $10 million in damage) cost the Australian economy an annual average of $77 million, even before the associated costs of police and courts and the intangible human and social costs wrought by large fires are considered (Department of Infrastructure, Transport, Regional Development and Local Government, 2001). Estimates from the USA suggest that between 20% and 25% of wildfires are deliberately lit, with rates dependent on location (Federal Emergency Management Agency, 1994; Hall, 1998). Even in the UK, where vegetation fires rarely result in the type of widespread destruction seen elsewhere, it is thought that some 20% of fires in open countryside are the result of arson (Lewis, 1999).

In areas such as south-eastern Australia, where bushfire is a seasonal hazard responsible for significant property loss, there is little tolerance for deliberate firesetting. Public pressure on law-enforcement agencies and government to prevent bushfire arson is becoming increasingly intense. The criminal justice system and media frequently seek the expertise of mental health professionals to explain what seems inexplicable, yet, without a solid base of research in the field, experts can speak only in generalities about these offenders. Few bushfire arsonists are identified and even fewer are apprehended and sent to prison or hospital. We know most about those offenders who have contact with criminal justice or mental health systems and it is highly likely that these individuals are not representative of the arson offending population generally. The low police apprehension rate for fire-related offences also means little can be said about the typical offending patterns of arsonists (e.g., consistency in their offences), the likelihood of recidivism or the assessment of risk. Assessment procedures currently in place tend to be general ones used for other types of offender, as is the limited treatment available to firesetters. With the paucity of evidence informing practice, there can be little confidence in assessment procedures or that psychological interventions are effective in reducing the risk of arsonists (including bushfire arsonists) reoffending. The purpose of this chapter is to provide readers with an understanding of what *is* currently known about bushfire arson. We first provide some background to bushfires generally and the role of environmental features in bushfire arson, then discuss what is known about people who deliberately light bushfires, approaches to psychological assessment and treatment options for bushfire arsonists. Ultimately, we aim for greater understanding of the risks and treatment priorities associated with this unique group of firesetters.

Bushfires and the context in which they occur

A bushfire (or wildfire, as they are usually known in the USA) is any fire that burns unchecked in an outdoor area (Commonwealth Scientific and Industrial Research Organisation, 2002). They are typically classified by the dominant type of vegetation in the area – most often scrub, forests or grassland. Bushfires are closely linked to particular world regions, notably the western USA and Canada, the Mediterranean basin (including countries such as Greece and Spain), parts of central and southern Africa, and south-eastern Australia. Examples in this chapter are largely drawn from south-eastern Australia, partly because it is where the authors live, but also because its particular environment makes this the most fire-prone region in the world (Pyne, 1995).

Geographic and environmental context

Any examination of bushfire arson must include discussion of the environment in which it occurs. Fires are endemic to the Australian environment and pre-date European colonisation. Prior to European settlement, fire was routinely used by indigenous Australians to manage the land and controlled burning took place with regularity. With the arrival of Europeans in the late 18th century, the frequency, size and impact of bushfires underwent dramatic change. From the mid-19th century, as indigenous Australians were pushed out of their lands, Europeans massively restructured Australian fire regimes and removed the tradition of almost constant and minor controlled burns (Pyne, 1991). At the same time there was an increase in the population living in and around forested areas and conflagrations became more common, even after controlled burns were reintroduced in the mid-20th century. From the mid-19th century the history of south-eastern Australia has been marked by disastrous blazes, beginning with the 'Black Thursday' fires of 1851 and continuing ever since (see Table 11.1). Major fire events are rarely restricted to the catastrophic day that earns their moniker. Large bushfires typically burn in rugged country for many weeks or even months, coating hundreds of kilometres of surrounding land with smoke and ash. Australia is fortunate to enjoy many inner-city parks and reserves in urbanised areas and these too are subject to the attentions of bushfire arsonists.

In all cases of arson, the damage wrought by the fire may far outweigh the original intentions of the firesetter. The disjunction between intent and

Table 11.1 Major bushfires in south-eastern Australia since European settlement

Year	Region	Fire name	Area burned (km²)	Fatalities
1851	Victoria	Black Thursday	50 000	15
1898	Victoria	Red Tuesday	2 600	12
1905/09	Victoria			12
1926	Victoria	Black Sunday	4 000	60
1938/39	NSW[1]		730	13
1939	Victoria	Black Friday	20 000	71
1943/44	Victoria		10 160	51
1951/52	NSW[1]		40 000	11
1952	Victoria		10 500	10
1962	Victoria – Melbourne		454 homes	32
1967	Tasmania – Hobart	Black Tuesday	2 650	62
1968/69	NSW[1]		20 000	14
1969	Victoria		2 500	23
1983	Victoria & South Australia	Ash Wednesday	4 180	75
2002/03	NSW[1]		14 640	2
2003	Victoria		13 000	1
2003	ACT[2] – Canberra	Canberra Firestorm	160	4
			500 homes	
2006	South Australia		14 500	9
2009	Victoria	Black Saturday	4 350	173

[1] New South Wales.
[2] Australian Capital Territory.

Source: GeoScience Australia (2010); Department of Sustainability and Environment (2010), Teague *et al* (2010).

effect is exacerbated in cases of bushfire arson, where weather and geography play defining roles in the behaviour of the fire, more so perhaps than is the case with urban or structural fires. Significant bushfires are most likely to occur in the context of severe drought, low atmospheric humidity, high daytime temperatures and strong winds (Muller, 2009). For instance, on Black Saturday the temperature was 46.4°C (115°F), the relative humidity was less than 6%, the wind speed sometimes went over 100 km/h and there had been 12 years of drought and record low rainfall in the winter and spring of 2008 (Teague *et al*, 2010). It is these environmental factors more than the specific actions of individual arsonists that made the fires on that day so particularly devastating. Despite a widely held view that bushfire arsonists are more active on days of severe fire danger (where the above conditions are present), the evidence indicates that this is not the case (Mees, 1991; Hennessy *et al*, 2005).

It does seem, however, that deliberately lit vegetation fires tend to be larger than accidental or natural fires occurring in similar weather conditions. There is evidence to suggest that some bushfire arsonists target areas and times that are more likely to result in large fires. A review of fire location in forested areas around Melbourne showed that fires were predominantly lit in areas that would promote rapid fire growth; for example, the slope of the land was in the direction of the prevailing wind and the gradient tended to be more extreme (vegetation fires travel more rapidly uphill) (Willis, 2004). Thus, while bushfire arsonists do not necessarily target days of severe fire danger, at least some light fires with the intention of guaranteeing ignition and spread. The interaction between environment and behaviour is of relevance to clinicians, as it has implications for the design and content of psychological interventions and relapse prevention models of offender treatment (discussed further under 'Assessment and treatment', below).

Beyond weather and topographical characteristics, a number of geographic and demographic characteristics have been associated with deliberately lit vegetation fires. Such fires seem more likely to occur in and around major urban centres than in rural areas. In New South Wales, deliberately lit bushfires are more common within 10 km of the Sydney city fringe than in the rest of the state (Muller, 2009). While the 'urban–rural fringe' is commonly cited the area at greatest risk of deliberately lit bushfires, it may be that these figures are an artefact of the greater visibility of fire in these areas. In the second author's interviews with incarcerated bushfire arsonists, many reported lighting and extinguishing numerous undetected fires in remote locations, which attracted little attention. Where they do occur in close proximity to residential areas, deliberately set vegetation fires have been found to be most likely in regions marked by low socio-economic status and high rates of poverty (Prestemon & Butry, 2005). In the area around Sydney, suburbs with a high proportion of children aged between 5 years and 15 years, larger numbers of people who left school early with no educational qualifications, lower average income, higher rates of unemployment and higher rates of rental accommodation were more likely to experience deliberately lit fires (Nicolopoulos, 1997). The link between social deprivation and general firesetting has been shown in other studies, notably in a UK Home Office report into firesetting behaviour, where arson was 31 times more likely in areas of low socioeconomic status (Home Office, 1999).

Public perceptions of bushfire arson

It is worth noting that not all or even the majority of bushfires are started by arsonists. The reality is that, with or without arson, the forests of south-eastern Australia and regions with similar environments will regularly burn, and reducing bushfire arson will prevent only a proportion of these fires. Yet the frequency with which large unchecked fires occur in south-eastern Australia and the amount of damage they cause provides a very particular social context for the actions of bushfire arsonists. In 2001 the Australian Model Criminal Code Officers Committee recommended the creation of a specific bushfire offence, since enshrined in the Australian Model Criminal Code (Model Criminal Law Officers Committee, 2009). The proposed offence prohibits intentional, reckless or negligent conduct that causes or risks bushfire ignition. Legislation was subsequently adopted in the various state and territory jurisdictions across southern Australia, although to date it has been relatively rarely used, as identifying and prosecuting bushfire arson remain difficult (Muller, 2009). The reasoning behind the introduction of the bushfire offence was captured by the New South Wales Attorney-General, who noted that the legislation was not introduced to overcome a perceived gap in the existing arson law, but rather 'to seek to emphasise society's abhorrence and condemnation of the deliberate lighting of bushfires by making specific provisions against it' (*NSW Legislative Assembly Hansard*, 12 April 2002). The Attorney-General's statement hints at the contempt with which bushfire arson is viewed in Australia.

Individuals who set bushfires in Australia are targets of public outrage and vilification. For example, in the days following Black Saturday the Australian Prime Minister described the arson as acts of 'mass murder' and stated that the perpetrators should 'rot in jail' (Malkin, 2009). Direct comparisons were drawn between arsonists and paedophiles as the most despised individuals in society (O'Leary, 2009). More disturbing were the threats to kill a man accused of setting a fatal bushfire that were posted on social networking sites. Despite a court order suppressing his identity, photographs of the accused were taken from his Facebook profile and distributed widely on the internet in the days following his arrest, accompanied by threats to his ex-girlfriend and family (Milovanovic, 2009). It has since been alleged that he was attacked by other prisoners while held on remand (Lowe, 2010).

The emotional fallout from bushfires extends well beyond the immediate aftermath of the fires themselves. In October 2009 the Victorian State opposition leader called for those imprisoned for arson to be subject to 'extended supervision orders' similar to those applied to repeat child sex offenders (Johnston, 2009). In a similar vein it has been suggested that arsonists' names should be recorded on registries to aid police investigation and prevent recidivism, as is done in some US jurisdictions (Dunn, 2009; McClelland & O'Conner, 2010). As Griffiths (2009) notes, in Australia, 'arsonists, it seems, are actually "terrorists". The fires, we tell one another, are "a threat to national security".' Just as mental health clinicians are increasingly being asked to provide opinions about the 'dangerousness' of structural arsonists (Barnett *et al*, 1999), courts in bushfire-prone regions ask forensic psychiatrists and psychologists for recommendations about risk and treatment of bushfire arsonists. Given the vitriol directed towards these offenders, clinicians working with bushfire arsonists must be able to make dispassionate recommendations based on evidence about the likelihood of recidivism and response to treatment. Unfortunately, their ability to do so is limited, as research on bushfire arsonists is scarce.

Characteristics of bushfire arsonists

Challenges in drawing on wider arson research

While arson is acknowledged in many urbanised nations, empirical research in the field originated in the USA and UK and the focus of this work was on urban rather than rurally based arson. Whether the findings are generalisable to those who set bushfires is unknown. Some authors have suggested that bushfire arsonists may be a distinct group, with different motivations and behaviours from structural arsonists (Teague *et al*, 2010). Shea (2002) suggested that the primary difference between bushfire and other forms of arson is the lack of purely instrumental reasons for fire-setting among the former group. This claim is unsubstantiated and other authors propose that a significant proportion of vegetation fires may be set for instrumental reasons, such as land clearance or even as an (illegal) attempt to prevent larger and more dangerous fires (Willis, 2004).

The reasons why individuals set vegetation fires are poorly understood. Willis (2004) tentatively outlined potential motivations for bushfire arson in his review for the Australian Institute of Criminology (see Table 11.2); however, he acknowledged that this was based on a combination of information from fire services and police, and a large amount of supposition. The broad motivational categories of Willis's typology are similar to those proposed for other forms of arson and encompass revenge, vandalism, excitement and a range of other commonly proposed motives, such as profit and crime concealment; Willis also included mental illness and a cry for

Table 11.2 Willis's bushfire motivational classification system

Category	Subtypes
Bushfires lit to create excitement or relieve boredom	Vandalism: by individuals or groups Stimulation: the firesetter seeks the excitement and stimulation of seeing the fire crews, and possibly the media, arrive Activity: fires are lit by firefighters or others in order to generate activity and relieve the boredom or tension arising from waiting for a naturally occurring fire to break out
Bushfires lit for recognition or attention	Heroism: fires are lit to create the possibility that the firesetter will gain positive recognition and rewards Self-esteem/impress others: fires are lit in response to feelings of inadequacy, or to gain a feeling of power and control, and to demonstrate these qualities to others Pleading: fires are lit as a 'cry for help'
Bushfires lit for a specific purpose or gain	Anger: fire is lit to secure revenge or as an expression of anger or protest Pragmatic: fires are lit for purposes such as land clearing Material: fires are lit for material gain, such as by firefighters seeking overtime or other payments Altruistic: the fire is lit to achieve an aim the firesetter believes will benefit others
Bushfires lit without motive	Psychiatric: fires are lit in response to psychological or psychiatric impulses directly derived from mental illness Children: fires are lit as a form of play or experimentation but without any form of malicious intent or belief that the fire will spread
Bushfires lit with mixed motives	Multiple: fires are lit on the basis of several of the above motives arising at one time Incidental: bushfires result from the spread of a fire that was lit with malicious intent but without an expectation of a bushfire occurring

Source: Willis (2004). Reproduced with the permission of the Australian Institute of Criminology

help as categories. Unfortunately, in echoing the motivations proposed for other forms of arson, Willis's system also suffers from many of the identified shortcomings of other classification systems (Doley, 2003). For example, Gannon & Pina (2010) noted that classifying any arson as 'motiveless' may be a semantic contradiction, given that children or those who suffer from a major mental illness are likely to have some motive for setting the fire, even if it is not discernible or logical to others. These authors also question the utility of generating multiple typological categories that overlap and are not validated, particularly when even the more sophisticated categorisations of motive imply that arson is driven by a single motivating force, which is unlikely given the complexity of the behaviour and the situations in which it occurs. As with any typological classification, categorising bushfire arsonists is useful to clinicians only if the categories provide information that can guide the direction of assessment or indicate the need for specific management or treatment options. At present, motivational classification systems such as that proposed by Willis are not sufficiently validated, and their contribution to the understanding of firesetting is questionable. Even if further research does show that a motivational typology can assist the assessment of risk and the identification of management strategies, understanding an offender's motivation alone will be insufficient to guide clinical practice in any particular case of bushfire arson (Gannon & Pina, 2010).

It is probable that there are multiple direct and indirect reasons for bushfire arson, as there appear to be for other forms of firesetting behaviour (Jackson et al, 1987a; Jackson, 1994). Gannon & Pina (2010) provide a thorough review of the evidence for factors thought to contribute to firesetting behaviour generally. These include early maladjustment, deficits in assertiveness and communication, low self-esteem, high impulsivity, specific types of psychopathology (personality disorder and schizophrenia particularly), other offending and substance misuse. In the absence of any studies of psychopathology or criminogenic factors among vegetation firesetters, it is unclear whether this group has unique risk factors for recidivism or particular types of criminogenic need.

Studies of bushfire arsonists

Only two studies have examined bushfire arsonists as a specific group. Muller (2008) examined the court records of 1232 individuals appearing in court in New South Wales on charges of arson in the 5 years to September 2006, of whom 133 (11%) were charged with bushfire arson. The majority of the sample was male: 88% of general arsonists and 94% of bushfire arsonists. Comparison of the two groups showed that while their mean age was similar (26 years), the distribution of age differed markedly, with bushfire arsonists 1.5 times more likely be aged under 18 (95% CI = 1.04 to 2.28). The majority of juvenile bushfire arsonists were aged between 15 and 17 years. In Muller's study 56% of all arson offenders and 37% of bushfire arson offenders had a previous recorded conviction. Prior convictions for arson were relatively rare (3% of the general arson group and 4% of the bushfire arson group). Two bushfire arson offenders had previous convictions for bushfire arson at the time of their court appearance. Echoing findings in broader samples of arson offenders (Rice & Harris, 1996; Soothill et al, 2004) a variety of prior criminal convictions were present. The most common prior conviction was for a personal offence (homicide, sexual assault, assault, robbery, other acts intended to cause injury, and dangerous or negligent acts endangering persons), present in 40% of arsonists and 29% of bushfire arsonists. Prior drug offences, which may provide some information about substance misuse, were present for 17% of arsonists and 7% of bushfire arsonists. The nature of the court data meant that information on mental disorder was unavailable.

Doley (2009) conducted the only clinically based empirical research into Australian arsonists to date. In a national study she analysed police files recording a total of 187 offenders and 226 of their arson or fire-related offences across two Australian policing jurisdictions (Victoria and Queensland) and interviewed 88 incarcerated offenders across three Australian states (South Australia, Queensland and Victoria). A range of personal, psychological, social and environmental characteristics were examined, in addition to criminal history and firesetting behaviour. Within this sample was a subgroup of nine arsonists interviewed while in prison who described 20 bushfire offences they were responsible for, as well as information about a further ten offenders convicted of lighting another 20 bushfires that was gleaned from the review of police files. In a preliminary analysis, in comparison with other arsonists in this sample, bushfire arsonists were older, with an average age of 25–27 years, and, despite reporting an extensive and long-standing firesetting history, very few had criminal records for fire-related offences, although many had records for property offences (mainly stealing or receiving stolen goods). Further analysis of the data is pending, although the small sample size limits the generalisability of the findings and further research focused on the subgroup of bushfire arson offenders is warranted.

Others have theorised about the characteristics of bushfire arsonists but with little evidence to support their claims. Shea (2002) notes the potential role of mental illness, but draws attention to the fact that identifying direct links between the symptoms of illness and firesetting is often difficult, and those with a major mental illness may well light bushfires for reasons entirely unrelated to their symptoms. He also notes the disinhibiting effects of drugs and alcohol, and the potential role of impulsivity and failure to examine consequences associated with a variety of mental disorders. Campbell (2009) describes a range of psychological characteristics attributable to bushfire arsonists, arguing that they are phenomenologically different to urban arsonists. He posits roles for 'sociopathy', narcissism and pyromania, and makes claims as to the psychological mechanisms that underlie bushfire arson (e.g., 'inexpressible resentment', p. 31; poor internal locus of control, sensation-seeking). While he cites case studies of interviews with bushfire arsonists, the evidence base for his claims is unclear and his conclusions have not been empirically tested.

Firefighter arson

The issue of firefighter arson is addressed in Chapter 8 but because it is a central point for consideration in any discussion of bushfire arson it is also briefly discussed here. In bushfire-prone regions the issue of fires set by firefighters has drawn significant public attention, perhaps due more to the perceived breach of trust than to the actual number of incidents. Although the incidence of firefighter arson is relatively rare in comparison with the total number of currently serving firefighters, the impact on community faith and fire service morale is disproportionately great. For example, a New South Wales police bushfire arson taskforce investigated 1600 suspicious bushfires between 2001 and 2004 and charged 50 individuals, 11 of whom were volunteer firefighters (Willis, 2004).

Firefighter arsonists are rarely studied and knowledge of their existence and behaviour owes more to anecdotal evidence held within fire services and law-enforcement agencies than to scientific research (for examples see Stambaugh & Styron, 2003). This may be due in part to the fact that these individuals are frequently not inclined to admit their guilt after detection. Further, offenders are not categorised by occupation; therefore it is difficult to gather information through official records unless the circumstances of a particular offender are known personally to the researcher, such as through a pre-trial assessment order or treatment programme. The few studies that have examined firefighter arsonists have been based in the USA and have not conducted comparisons with other offenders, making it difficult to draw conclusions about the defining characteristics of this group. The second author conducted interviews with a number of senior fire officers and convicted firefighter arsonists to identify common characteristics of firefighter arsonists from New Zealand ($n = 17$) and Australia ($n = 14$). Most of those studied were volunteer male firefighters, with an age range of 18–42 years. The number of fires set varied from 2 to 55; however, this is likely to be an underestimate, given that these figures represent fires with which the individual was charged and exclude any which were undetected or for which there was insufficient evidence for charges to be laid. With few exceptions, each individual was responsible for more than 12 fires.

It has been acknowledged that, as a group, volunteers may be at greater risk of setting fires than career firefighters, due to more rigorous screening processes for the latter group (Victoria Police, 2009). This is of some concern, given the ratio of volunteer to career firefighters in fire-prone regions. In the USA, approximately 75% of the 30000 fire services are volunteer based, while in Australia there are approximately 220000 volunteer firefighters across eight state and territory rural fire services (130 volunteers to every career firefighter) (McLennan & Birch, 2005). Accordingly, the US National Volunteer Fire Council (NVFC) commissioned an investigation of firefighter arson in 1994, in the wake of an apparent increase in cases across the USA. A national survey of fire services was undertaken to measure the size of the problem, achieving an 85% response rate. It found that most fire services did not keep records of firefighter arson. Moreover, respondents indicated that while education and screening of volunteer firefighters was important, few jurisdictions had firm policies in this area and many states had no programmes to raise awareness of firefighter arson within their training (Newton, 1994). This situation has since improved somewhat and a number of US state fire services now have procedures in place both to screen potential recruits and to educate existing members about the dangers of firefighter arson (Stambaugh & Styron, 2003).

The only published study of firefighter arsonists (not all of whom set bushfires) was undertaken by the US Federal Bureau of Investigation (FBI) in 1993 (Huff, 1994). The National Center for the Analysis of Violent Crime (NCAVC) polled fire investigators attending training workshops and identified 25 cases of firefighter arson. These cases involved 182 fires across seven US states and a Canadian province, which were attributed to 66 offenders in total (16 cases involved lone offenders). Interviews with the investigators formed the basis of data collection. All offenders in this sample were male. Among lone offenders the average age was 23, with all but two aged between 18 and 30. Where groups of firefighters set fires together, the average age was 19 (range 16–35). There was greater evidence of planning among group offenders, who frequently drove and brought incendiary devices or accelerants to the ignition location. There were differences in the backgrounds of lone versus group offenders, with lone offenders more likely to have a criminal record and broader social, employment and academic problems. In the investigators' opinion, the majority of firefighter arsonists in this sample were motivated by a need for excitement (89% of group offenders and 56% of lone offenders), followed by profit (as volunteers, they were paid overtime and received continued employment if the fire season continued). A revenge motive was noted in a minority of cases.

Subsequent to the NCAVC study, two 'profiles' of firefighter arsonists were published, one developed by the FBI's Behavioural Analysis Unit, the other by the South Carolina Forestry Commission (Stambaugh & Styron, 2003). Both identified 'typical' characteristics of firefighter arsonists, such as being young, male and White and having a background of early maladjustment and interpersonal problems. The utility of these profiles is questionable, given that these characteristics are typical of the vast majority of offenders. The only firefighter-specific variable appears to be a fascination with fire and fire services. These profiles have not been empirically tested and their predictive validity is unknown.

Assessment and treatment

It is clear from the above review that there is insufficient evidence to draw firm conclusions about best practice in the assessment or treatment of those who deliberately light bushfires. However, given the publicity surrounding bushfire arson in those jurisdictions where it occurs, it is unlikely that courts will be dissuaded from asking for expert opinion in these cases, nor will the lack of an adequate evidence base to support expert assessment prevent bushfire arson offenders from being referred for forensic psychological or psychiatric review and treatment. How then should clinicians proceed? In the absence of evidence suggesting a markedly different approach for bushfire arson, we recommend that clinicians adopt an approach similar to that advocated by Gannon & Pina (2010) for the assessment of other forms of arson.

Gannon & Pina (2010) provide a comprehensive review of risk factors for recidivistic arson and conclude that clinicians involved in firesetting risk prediction can proceed in one of two ways. First, if the offender appears to have been intentionally using firesetting to cause physical or psychological harm to others, an existing generic violence risk assessment tool such as the HCR-20 may be useful in providing a structure for assessing risk of future violence using firesetting. Alternatively, where the risk is that of firesetting *per se*, that is, in the absence of violent intent, Gannon & Pina recommend using Fineman's (1995) framework to assess an individual's risk of recidivism. Fineman advocates collecting information from multiple sources on a range of individual behavioural and historical character-istics, including psychopathology, interpersonal interactions, history of fire-related behaviour, characteristics of the index firesetting, cognitive distortions regarding the firesetting, emotional arousal associated with the firesetting, substance misuse, and triggers and reinforcers of firesetting behaviour. As Gannon & Pina note, this framework for data collection is consistent with research on structural arsonists which indicates that 'paramount predictors for recidivist firesetting tended to be fire-specific variables' (p. 233) and interest in or excitement associated with fire may be particularly important.

We suggest that in addition to the detailed individual assessment of fire-related risk factors recommended by Fineman (1995), risk assessment of those who set bushfires might be aided by the use of a structured risk assessment tool for general non-violent recidivism, such as the Level of Service/Case Management Inventory (LS/CMI; Andrews *et al*, 2004). While there are few studies specifically examining risk factors for firesetting recidivism, examinations of arsonists' offence histories shows that fire-setting is typically only one of a range of offending and antisocial behaviours and that firesetters appear more similar to property offenders than to violent offenders (see Gannon & Pina, 2010, for review). Dickens *et al* (2009) reported that recidivistic structural firesetters commonly had developmental histories of violence or substance misuse, early age at first criminal offence, relationship problems and more previous convictions for property offences, but were not more likely than one-time firesetters to have convictions for violent or sexual offences. Using a structured tool to guide judgements about the general risk of recidivism will likely provide clinicians with useful information about the scope of the firesetter's broader criminogenic needs, which may contribute to increased risk of firesetting, as well as ensuring comprehensive attention to potential responsivity factors. The results of the structured risk assessment can then be considered in conjunction with specific fire-related variables such as those outlined by Fineman, and the combination used to make judgements about an individual's propensity for recidivistic firesetting.

In addition to incorporating existing structured tools into risk assessment of bushfire arsonists, we also recommend adopting a formulation approach when communicating the results of a clinical assessment. Formulation is an approach to conceptualising problems with a view to specifying interventions (Lewis & Doyle, 2010). When formulating, clinicians apply a systematic method to organise information and make hypotheses about possible causal mechanisms underlying a problem. Their hypotheses are based on a theoretical model explaining the problem. For example, a formulation of a depressive episode that makes use of the cognitive–behavioural model will emphasise the role of the individual's appraisals and evaluations of situations in understanding their depressed mood. A common framework for organising a formulation is the 'four Ps', which orients the clinician to consider factors that *predispose* the individual to the problem, *precipitate* particular occurrences of the problem, *perpetuate* the problem once it has begun, and *protect* the individual against the problem or reduce its impact (Weerasekera, 1996, 2009). In the forensic field, formulation approaches have been used to explain the nature, origin and maintenance of risky behaviour (e.g., violence; Lewis & Doyle, 2010). The formulation provides the link between the atheoretical risk assessment and risk judgement about the likelihood of a behaviour (e.g., low, moderate, high) and the development of plans to manage those judged to be at high risk. A theoretically oriented formulation explains (hypothesises) how and why risk factors and other individual characteristics interact to produce offending behaviour for a particular individual in a particular situation.

A formulation of firesetting behaviour based on the four Ps would examine the origins, development and maintenance of the firesetting and hypothesise which risk factors are most relevant to precipitating and maintaining firesetting for that individual. These then become the primary targets for intervention and the accuracy of the formulation is tested by the efficacy of treatment. This approach is consistent with that advocated by Jackson *et al* (1987*a,b*), who examined firesetting behaviour within a functional analysis and social learning framework. In our view, both the risk assessment and theory-based formulation are essential components of the clinical assessment. A formal risk assessment directs attention towards high-risk offenders (ensuring those at highest risk are provided with more intensive treatment), while the formulation provides hypotheses about the links between various criminogenic needs and responsivity factors and the firesetting behaviour, which can then be incorporated into the treatment plan.

As discussed by Gannon & Pina (2010), treatment for firesetting, including bushfire arson, would be likely to involve a combination of interventions targeting needs associated with general offending (e.g., assertiveness and social skills training, problem-solving, emotional regulation), as well as fire-specific interventions examining the specific cognitive and emotional precipitants of firesetting behaviours, attitudes towards firesetting, and factors that reinforce firesetting for that individual. These fire-specific interventions would include the development of an explanatory analysis of offending (offence chain) for the individual's particular firesetting behaviour, and a specific relapse prevention plan addressing idiographic factors related to increased risk of firesetting. For bushfire arsonists, it may be necessary to place particular attention on environmental conditions when developing offence chains and constructing relapse prevention plans. Bushfire arson may be more dependent on the offender's location than other forms of arson, and this presents opportunities to limit the client's ability to set fires on days when their offending behaviour is likely to be most damaging. For example, a relapse prevention plan for a bushfire arsonist might explicitly cover the offender's emotional state and behaviours on days of high fire danger, and help them to recognise 'seemingly irrelevant' decisions that could place them in high-risk situations and locations associated with lighting bushfires.

Until further research is conducted examining specific risk factors for recidivistic firesetting, and comparing structural and vegetation firesetters, the foundation for the evidence-based assessment and treatment of bushfire and other arson offenders remains of concern. Structuring assessment of firesetters using existing risk assessment tools such as the HCR-20 and LS/CMI, supplemented with Fineman's (1995) guidelines and functional analysis of the firesetting behaviour as advocated by Jackson *et al* (1987a,b), appears to be a reasonable stop-gap measure until tools specific to firesetting are developed. Given the underdeveloped nature of research in this area, it is essential that clinicians are able to provide fully reasoned and justified explanations for their conclusions. Communicating results using a systematic formulation makes the assessment transparent and accountable, and provides a flexible means of showing change in risk state over time.

Future research

The lack of investigation of bushfire arson to date means that there are numerous avenues for future research in this area. There is a clear need to better describe bushfire arsonists as a specific group and determine whether they are representative of the wider arsonist population or have different offending profiles, risk factors and treatment needs. Given the difficulties of collecting information on bushfire arson, pooling data on vegetation arsonists may be a useful avenue for developing larger data-sets and producing more robust findings. For practitioners in bushfire-prone regions, it is essential to know whether findings from other locations can be generalised to their offender populations. Even in non-bushfire-prone environments, the literature could benefit from differentiating structural and vegetation firesetters in data collection and analysis, to begin to establish whether the results from one group can be applied to the other.

If it can be shown that bushfire and other arsonists come from the same underlying population, classifying arsonists according to motive or type of offence target may be less useful than considering them as a homogeneous group on a continuum of risk, with judgements of high risk made considering both likelihood of offending and potential for harm, based on the intensity, magnitude, targets and frequency of potential blazes. In this model, bushfire arson could arguably be considered to be one of the highest-risk firesetting behaviours, as bushfires are so heavily influenced by the environments in which they occur and there are many elements outside the control of the offender that affect the size and scope of the fire. As such, even those bushfire arson offenders who are judged to have low to moderate likelihood of reoffending may be targets for treatment, owing to their potential to cause significant harm should they reoffend.

To be able to make accurate judgements about risk, we need vastly to improve our understanding of risk factors for adult and juvenile recidivistic firesetting. Currently the literature tells us more about why an individual might light a fire than about what differentiates a one-time firesetter from a serial arsonist, or what causes some to cease firesetting, while others continue. Routine collection and comparison of data from single versus multiple firesetters may reveal information about static and dynamic risk factors for recidivistic firesetting. Understanding more about the processes involved in choosing fire, but also about factors that maintain (and escalate) firesetting behaviour, can also help identify the treatment needs of high-risk offenders and facilitate the development of targeted offence-specific treatments and community-based intervention programmes. While recognising that detection and imprisonment rates for arson and bushfire arson are low, and that identified offenders may not represent the wider arsonist population, a better understanding of those arsonists who are in custody or under supervision can only aid in the development of appropriate in-custody assessment and rehabilitative interventions. Current treatment services for arson offenders are piecemeal and often not validated (Palmer *et al*, 2007). In some locations, including Australia, there are no specific treatments offered to incarcerated arsonists. Community-based interventions, recognised in other areas of offender treatment to have greater effect than interventions delivered in custodial settings (Andrews & Bonta, 2006), appear virtually non-existent (the authors are aware of community-based psychological services for arsonists in Victoria and Western Australia, although there are no available data about treatment efficacy). Given the lack of validated treatment programmes and outcome data for incarcerated firesetters, there are legitimate questions about whether current criminal justice approaches will actually have any rehabilitative effect for arson offenders, or reduce their risk of reoffending.

Conclusion

The greatest need for scientific research into bushfire arson is in areas where the phenomenon is most damaging. Unfortunately, those regions most able to produce such research, Australia, Canada and the USA, have paid little systematic attention to the issue. In Australia there is no national system that consistently records information about arson or bushfire arson across states and territories, and while interest in the technicalities of deliberate ignition is consistent, interest in the psychology of arson appears to wax and wane with public opinion. When the devastation caused by deliberately lit fires is immediate, as in the aftermath of Black Saturday, there is strong public sentiment that 'something must be done' to stop such offences. This interest and associated funding for research wanes as bushfires recede in public memory. To develop evidence-based clinical approaches to bushfire arsonists, consistent and coordinated research is required to uncover the characteristics of bushfire arson. Greater cooperation between courts, mental health, fire, law-enforcement and corrections services will be essential both to facilitate research and to enable the successful implementation and evaluation of assessment and intervention protocols. Somewhat tongue in cheek but with an underlying plea (and with apologies to John F. Kennedy's famous speech), we ask you to consider not what the arson literature can do for you, but rather what you and your agency can do to contribute to this sorely under-researched yet vitally important aspect of our community and practice.

Acknowledgements

The authors are members of the Australian Bushfire Arson Prevention Initiative, which receives support from Monash University and the Royal Automobile Club of Victoria (RACV).

References

Andrews, D. A. & Bonta, J. (2006) *The Psychology of Criminal Conduct* (4th edn). Anderson Publishing.

Andrews, D. A., Bonta, J. & Wormwith, S. (2004) *The Level of Service/Case Management Inventory (LS/CMI)*. Multi-Health Systems.

Barnett, W., Richter, P. & Renneberg, B. (1999) Repeated arson: data from criminal records. *Forensic Science International*, **101**, 49–54.

Bryant, C. (2008) *Deliberately Lit Vegetation Fires in Australia*. Trends and Issues in Criminal Justice no. 350. Australian Institute of Criminology.

Campbell, A. (2009) Bushfire arsonists: who are they and why do they do it? *Psychotherapy in Australia*, **15**, 30–36.

Commonwealth Scientific and Industrial Research Organisation (CSIRO) (2002) *Bushfires – Type, Measurement and Fuel*. CSIRO. At http://www.csiro.au/resources/BushfireTypes.html (accessed 17 December 2010).

Department of Infrastructure, Transport, Regional Development and Local Government (2001) *Economic Costs of Natural Disasters in Australia*. Report 103. Australian Government Department of Infrastructure and Transport. At http://www.bitre.gov.au/info. aspx?ResourceId=199&NodeId=22 (accessed 17 December 2010).

Department of Sustainability and Environment (2010) *Bushfire History – Major Bushfires in Victoria*. Department of Sustainability and Environment. At http://www.dse.vic. gov.au/DSE/nrenfoe.nsf/childdocs/-D79E4FB0C437E1B6CA256DA60008B9EF?open (accessed 17 December 2010).

Dickens, G., Sugarman, P., Edgar, S., *et al* (2009) Recidivism and dangerousness in arsonists. *Journal of Forensic Psychiatry and Psychology*, **20**, 621–639.

Doley, R. (2003) Making sense of arson through classification. *Psychiatry, Psychology and Law*, **10**, 346–352.

Doley, R. (2009) *A Snapshot of Serial Arson in Australia*. Lambert Academic Publishing.

Dunn, M. (2009) Baillieu backs call for register of arsonists. *The Age*, 14 February.

Federal Emergency Management Agency (1994) *Southern Californian Firestorms: Hazard Mitigation Survey Team Report*. United States Fire Administration.

Fineman, K. R. (1995) A model for the qualitative analysis of child and adult fire deviant behavior. *American Journal of Forensic Psychology*, **13**, 31–60.

Gannon, T. A. & Pina, A. (2010) Firesetting: psychopathology, theory and treatment. *Aggression and Violent Behavior*, **15**, 224–238.

Geoscience Australia (2010) *Major Historic Bushfires*. Geoscience Australia. At http://www. ga.gov.au/hazards/bushfire/historic.jsp (accessed 17 December 2010).

Griffiths, T. (2009) 'An unnatural disaster'? Remembering and forgetting bushfire. *History Australia*, **6**, 35.1–35.7.

Hall, J. R. (1998) The truth about arson. *National Fire Protection Association Journal*, November/December, 59–67.

Hennessy, K., Lucas, C., Nicholls, N., *et al* (2005) *Climate Change Impacts on Fire – Weather in South-East Australia*. CSIRO.

Home Office (1999) *Safer Communities: Towards Effective Arson Control. The Report of the Arson Scoping Study*. Home Office.

Huff, T. (1994) *Fire-Setting Fire Fighters: Arsonists in the Fire Department – Identification and Prevention*. National Volunteer Fire Council. At http://www.nvfc.org/news/hn_ firefighter_arson.html (accessed 17 December 2010).

Jackson, H. F. (1994) Assessment of fire-setters. In *The Assessment of Criminal Behaviours in Secure Settings* (eds M. McMurran & J. Hodge), pp. 94–126. Jessica Kingsley.

Jackson, H. F., Glass, C. & Hope, S. (1987*a*) A functional analysis of recidivistic arson. *British Journal of Clinical Psychology*, **26**, 175–185.

Jackson, H. F., Hope, S. & Glass, C. (1987*b*) Why are arsonists not violent offenders? *International Journal of Offender Therapy and Comparative Criminology*, **31**, 143–151.

Johnston, M. (2009) Opposition leader Ted Baillieu announces plans to place arsonists on extended supervision orders. *The Herald–Sun*, 12 October.

Lewis, A. (1999) *The Prevention and Control of Arson*. Fire Protection Association.

Lewis, G. & Doyle, M. (2010) Risk formulation: what are we doing and why? *International Journal of Forensic Mental Health*, **8**, 286–292.

Lowe, A. (2010) Churchill arson accused 'attacked in custody'. *The Age*, 31 May.

Malkin, B. (2009) Australian bushfires: death toll rises to 130 as Kevin Rudd calls arson 'mass murder'. *The Telegraph*, 9 February.

McClelland, R. & O'Conner, B. (2010) National Bushfire Arson Forum joint media release. Attorney-General's Department. At http://www.ag.gov.au/www/ministers/ mcclelland.nsf/Page/MediaReleases_2010_SecondQuarter_3May2010-2010National BushfireArsonForum (accessed 17 December 2010).

McLennan, J. & Birch, A. (2005) A potential crisis in wildfire emergency response capability? Australia's volunteer firefighters. *Environmental Hazards*, **6**, 101–107.

Mees, R. (1991) Is arson associated with severe fire weather in southern California? *International Journal of Wildland Fire*, **1**, 97–100.

Milovanovic, S. (2009) Online hate mail threat to arson case. *The Age*, 17 February.

Model Criminal Law Officers Committee (2009) *Model Criminal Code*. Standing Committee of Attorneys-General.

Muller, D. A. (2008) *Offending and Reoffending Patterns of Arsonists and Bushfire Arsonists in New South Wales*. Australian Institute of Criminology.

Muller, D. A. (2009) *Using Crime Prevention to Reduce Deliberate Bushfires in Australia*. Australian Institute of Criminology.

Newton, K. (1994) *National Volunteer Fire Council Meets with FBI on Firefighter Arson*. National Volunteer Fire Council. At http://www.nvfc.org/news/hn_firefighter_arson. html (accessed 17 December 2010).

Nicolopoulos, N. (1997) *Socio-economic Characteristics of Communities and Fires*. NSW Fire Brigades.

O'Leary, T. (2009) Ultimately, arsonists need our help. *The Age*, 11 February.

Palmer, E. J., Caulfield, L. S. & Hollin, C. R. (2007) Interventions with arsonists and young fire setters: a survey of the national picture in England and Wales. *Legal and Criminological Psychology*, **12**, 101–116.

Prestemon, J. P. & Butry, D. T. (2005) Time to burn: modeling wildfire arson as an autoregressive crime function. *American Journal of Agricultural Economics*, **87**, 756–770.

Pyne, S. J. (1991) *Burning Bush. A Fire History of Australia*. Henry Holt & Co.

Pyne, S. J. (1995) *World Fire. The Culture of Fire on Earth*. Henry Holt & Co.

Rice, M. E. & Harris, G. T. (1996) Predicting the recidivism of mentally disordered firesetters. *Journal of Interpersonal Violence*, **11**, 364–375.

Shea, P. (2002) The lighting of fires in a bushland setting. *Judicial Officers' Bulletin*, **14**, 1–4.

Silvester, J. (2009) Police taskforce to hunt arsonists, fears bushfire toll may double. *The Age*, 9 February.

Soothill, K., Ackerley, E. & Francis, B. (2004) The criminal careers of arsonists. *Medicine, Science and the Law*, **44**, 27–40.

Stambaugh, H. & Styron, H. (2003) *Special Report: Firefighter Arson*. Department of Homeland Security, US Fire Administration.

Teague, B., McLeod, R. & Pascoe, S. (2010) *Victorian Bushfires. Royal Commission Final Report*. Parliament of Victoria. At http://www.royalcommission.vic.gov.au (accessed 17 December 2010).

Victoria Police (2009) *Arson Investigation and Offender Management*. Victoria Police.

Weerasekera, P. (1996) *Multiperspective Case Formulation: A Step Towards Treatment Integration*. Krieger.

Weerasekera, P. (2009) A formulation of the case of Antoinette: a multiperspective approach. In *Clinical Case Formulation: Varieties of Approaches* (ed. P. Sturmey), pp. 145–156. Wiley-Blackwell.

Willis, M. (2004) *Bushfire Arson: A Review of the Literature*. Australian Institute of Criminology.

CHAPTER 12

Arson: treatment and interventions

Clive R. Hollin

In England and Wales, the act of arson is included in the Criminal Damage Act 1971 as a crime in which a fire is deliberately set with the intention of destroying or damaging property. The act of arson may also endanger life. In Scotland the legal term for the act of deliberately setting a fire is *fire-raising*. The generic term *firesetter* is often used in the context of children below the age of criminal responsibility who deliberately set fires (e.g., Fineman, 1980). The issue of terminology is complicated with offenders who have a mental disorder: first, these offenders may not fall under the rubric of criminal law, so technically they are not arsonists (although convicted arsonists may be transferred from prison to mental health facilities); second, there are international variations in law, so that terminology varies; third, there are variations in the use of terms across the literature. For simplicity the term 'arson' is used here in a generic sense to refer to deliberately setting fires, an act that brings about significant harm to people and property at a considerable financial cost (Palmer *et al*, 2010).

Fire: basic figures

The government statistics for England and Wales, published by the Office of the Deputy Prime Minister (Arson Control Forum, 2003), show that since the early 1990s there have been more than 3500 incidents of arson, causing 32 000 injuries and 1200 deaths. On average, arson brought about 55 injuries and two deaths a week, most of which occurred when the fire was in a dwelling. In 2006 there were 68 deaths attributed to arson in a place of residence (Department for Communities and Local Government, 2008). There may also be large financial costs associated with arson. For example, when a fire destroys a public building, such as a school or a hospital, the costs of rebuilding and replacing equipment are substantial. A fire in a factory may destroy equipment and stock, again with heavy costs. Indeed, many businesses close permanently after a fire, adding job losses to the costs.

Firesetting populations

The empirical literature on those who set fires, which directly informs evidence-based practice, falls into the three groupings of juveniles, adults and psychiatric populations.

Juveniles

Juvenile firesetters are most likely to be male; they often display a variety of problem behaviours, including violence, cruelty to animals, and drug and alcohol misuse. They have typically been fascinated with fire from a very early age, playing with matches and setting off fire alarms (Kolko *et al*, 2006). They often have poor interpersonal skills, are impulsive and have high levels of anger and poor assertion and problem-solving skills (Chen *et al*, 2003). Firesetting is also associated with several childhood psychiatric and behavioural problems, including antisocial behaviour, anxiety, conduct disorder, hyperactivity and substance misuse (Martin *et al*, 2004; Dadds & Fraser, 2006). Juvenile firesetters are likely to have disturbed family lives – their early experience marked by low levels of parental control and high levels of punitive and abusive treatment (Root *et al*, 2008) – together with a disrupted education (Hollin *et al*, 2002).

Adults

As reviewed by Prins (1994, 1995), there is a body of research, focused on adult populations, concerned with motivations for arson. These motivations can be grouped into six broad types:

1   *concealing a crime* by using fire to destroy any incriminating evidence at the scene of a crime
2   *economic*, where the fire may be followed by a fraudulent insurance claim, for financial profit or to eliminate debt or to close a failing business (arson may also be an effective means by which to eliminate a business rival)
3   *excitement*, when the individual finds the sight and sound of fire, together with the arrival of the firefighters and the general chaos, a source of thrills and a sense of power (the scale of the arson attacks may escalate as the arsonist becomes tired of setting nuisance fires and seeks greater excitement with larger fires in homes and industrial buildings)
4   *politically motivated* fires, which are set in the name of a political, social, or even religious cause
5   *revenge*, exacted through the damage and fear caused by fire, especially against a particular person, a group of people, an institution such as a school, or society in general

6   *vandalism*, often associated with juvenile firesetters, who set fires for
     fun, with peer group pressure an obvious factor, typically targeting
     schools, empty buildings or woodland.

In their report to the Office of the Deputy Prime Minister, Canter & Almond
(2002) noted that arson is mainly committed either for financial gain or to
cover up evidence of another crime. Canter & Almond identified three types
of arsonist who set fires for financial profit: (1) 'professional' arsonists, who
are paid to set fires; (2) business or property owners who aim to profit from
a fraudulent insurance claim; and (3) business owners who are attempting
to cover their losses. Such 'arson for profit' is likely to be efficiently planned,
with the fire ignited at several points in the building to achieve maximum
destruction, and the use of accelerants (Flanagan & Fisher, 2008). When
the motivation for arson is to cover up a crime, a fire may be used to add
confusion regarding what was stolen in a burglary, or with murder a fire
may be used to destroy evidence and obscure the victim's identity (Davies
& Mouzos, 2007).

Psychiatric populations

Prins (1995) notes that there is a high incidence of psychiatric court
reports in cases of arson, suggesting that the likelihood is increased that
mental disorder will be identified for this offence. The disposition for the
arsonist with a mental disorder is typically detention in a secure hospital.
Statistics for Finland (Repo *et al*, 1997), Sweden (Fazel & Grann, 2002)
and the UK (Coid *et al*, 2001) suggest that about 10% of those admitted to
forensic psychiatric services have committed arson. Psychiatrists' concerns
about the dangers posed by firesetters are greatest when the fire was set
to occupied buildings with the intention to endanger life (Sugarman &
Dickens, 2009).

Several types of mental disorder are frequently observed in arsonists.
Rice & Harris (1991) reviewed the clinical files of 243 male arsonists (98
were apprehended for setting a single fire and 145 were repeat firesetters)
in a Canadian maximum-security psychiatric facility. Personality disorder
was the most common diagnosis, evident in over half the sample, followed
by schizophrenia in about a third. The repeat arsonists were younger, with
more disturbed histories, including other types of criminal behaviour. When
the arsonists were compared with a control group from the same facility but
without a history of firesetting, the arsonists were younger, more often had
a lifetime history of an unusual interest in fire, were more likely to have
been involved in violence, and were more likely to have spent time in an
institution.

Jayaraman & Frazer (2006) examined the pre-trial psychiatric reports of
34 arsonists: there were high levels of mental disorder and frequent use of
alcohol and drugs before and during the offence. A Finnish study of over 400
arsonists referred for pre-trial psychiatric assessment (Lindberg *et al*, 2005)

found high levels of personality disorder. Lindberg *et al* also reported that comorbid alcohol misuse and dependency was a particular feature of their sample, and a significant number of fires were set when the individual was in a condition of acute alcohol intoxication.

Enayati *et al* (2008) reviewed the diagnostic information on 214 arsonists (59 women and 155 men) referred for in-patient psychiatric assessment in Sweden. The most frequently observed diagnoses for both male and female arsonists were substance use disorders, personality disorders and psychosis (typically schizophrenia). Schizophrenia is often associated with arson (Ritchie & Huff, 1999), perhaps particularly so with women (Jamieson *et al*, 2000). A Swedish study reported by Anwar *et al* (2011) examined the incidence of schizophrenia among 1340 men and 349 women convicted for arson. When compared with a control group from the general population, those with schizophrenia showed a significantly increased risk of being convicted for arson. Anwar *et al* noted that the likelihood of being diagnosed with schizophrenia was 20 times greater for the arsonists than for the controls. In keeping with the trend reported in the literature, Anwar *et al* found a higher rate of schizophrenia among the female arsonists.

Arson is also prevalent among people with an intellectual disability (Murphy & Clare, 1996). Dickens *et al* (2008) looked at the relationship between low IQ and arson in a sample of 202 men and women referred for psychiatric assessment. They reported that 88 of the sample had an IQ of 85 or below: these low-IQ arsonists set more fires than individuals with a higher IQ, although often to items such as waste rather than buildings. Dickens *et al* suggest that this higher rate of firesetting may reflect the enduring complications this population experiences in coping with social and other difficulties in life.

Rice & Harris (1996) used their 1991 data-set to generate a typology of arsonists with a mental disorder and identified four types:

1 the largest group they called *psychotics*, characterised by a high frequency of schizophrenia and alcohol problems
2 *unassertives* were the next largest grouping, consisting of men charac- terised by ordinary family and employment backgrounds, with little or no contact with the criminal justice system, who had set fires in a state of anger or to gain revenge
3 *multi-firesetters* were the youngest, with the most disturbed back- grounds and a diverse pattern of setting fires
4 *criminals* had the most extensive criminal history, including violence, and were the most likely to commit other offences, including arson, after release.

At an 8-year follow-up after discharge there was, across the whole sample, a low rate of recidivism for arson (16%). The strongest predictors of recidivistic firesetting were associated with the intensity of the individual's firesetting history. The younger firesetters of lower intelligence without a history of violent behaviour but *with* a high incidence of firesetting had the highest risk of further firesetting.

Dickens *et al* (2009) examined predictors of recidivism in 167 male and female adult arsonists referred to psychiatric services in England. When compared with those who had set a single fire, the multiple arsonists were younger and had histories characterised by disrupted education and family life as well as by higher levels of contact with the criminal justice system. Diagnoses of personality disorder and intellectual disability were more frequent among the multiple firesetters.

There is one psychiatric diagnosis, *pyromania*, that is explicitly concerned with fire.

Pyromania

The psychiatric condition of *pyromania* is described by DSM-IV-TR (American Psychiatric Association, 2000) as a morbid fascination with setting fires as a source of pleasure and tension release (see Box 12.1).

Lindberg *et al* (2005) applied the DSM-IV-TR criteria to the 90 repeat arsonists within their larger sample of 401 arsonists. Of these 90 arsonists they excluded 56 individuals with any diagnosis of psychosis, intellectual disability, organic brain syndrome or antisocial personality disorder. Twelve of the remaining 34 arsonists fulfilled the diagnostic criteria for pyromania. Of these 12 a further nine were excluded because of acute alcohol intoxication when committing the arson (as specified by DSM-IV-TR), leaving three pyromaniacs, or less than 1% of the original sample of 401, and just over 3% of the repeat arsonists. Similarly, Rice & Harris (1991) reported that only one of 243 male arsonists in their sample fulfilled the diagnostic criteria for pyromania. It is reasonable to conclude that genuine pyromania is a rare phenomenon.

Box 12.1 DSM-IV-TR diagnostic criteria for pyromania

- Deliberate and purposeful firesetting on more than one occasion.
- Tension or affective arousal before the act.
- Fascination with, interest in, curiosity about, or attraction to fire and its situational contexts (e.g., paraphernalia, uses, consequences).
- Pleasure, gratification, or relief when setting fires, or when witnessing or participating in their aftermath.
- The firesetting is not done for monetary gain, as an expression of sociopolitical ideology, to conceal criminal activity, to express anger or vengeance, to improve one's living circumstances, in response to a delusion or hallucination, or as a result of impaired judgement (e.g., in dementia, intellectual disability, substance intoxication).
- The firesetting is not better accounted for by conduct disorder, a manic episode, or antisocial personality disorder.

Reproduced with permission from the American Psychiatric Association (2000)

Prevention

As indicated above, arson is perpetrated for a diverse range of motives by a broad cross-section of the population. The consequences of arson are severe in terms of both human and financial costs. There is therefore much to be gained from the successful implementation of preventive measures that reduce the incidence of arson. There are three approaches which have been used to prevent firesetting: situational crime prevention; education; and treatment.

Situational approaches

Situational approaches to crime prevention are based on the proposition that a crime takes place when an individual and a target coincide to provide a low-risk opportunity (Clarke, 1983). The application of this reasoning to arson suggests that it may be effective to control the environment to limit opportunities to set fires, to increase the risk of detection and to raise the legal penalties for the offence.

Situational crime prevention strategies to reduce arson may involve a risk assessment to identify and inform control of specific vulnerabilities or fire hazards. Typical 'hot spots' include abandoned vehicles, piles of flammable waste and weaknesses in property security that an arsonist could exploit. The measures to eliminate or control risk may include removing flammable liquids and clearing away refuse and abandoned vehicles. Security measures, particularly for commercial sites, may involve controlled access to the site, maintenance of perimeter fencing and the use of CCTV, fire detectors and smoke alarms.

An example of the implementation of situational measures to reduce arson can be found in the initiative successfully implemented by Northumbria Police and Tyne and Wear Fire Service in 1998. A regional arson task force was established to reduce the high levels of arson in the west of the city of Newcastle. These environmental initiatives included the removal of waste from public spaces, boarding-up empty properties and removing abandoned vehicles from streets and parks. Educational and diversionary schemes were also established as part of the scheme.

The national Arson Control Forum (ACF) – a government-led body that aims to reduce arson by encouraging partnership working between the government, fire services, local authorities, the police and insurance companies – now promotes initiatives such as the one in Newcastle. The ACF's New Projects Initiative has been successful in helping to establish a number of local partnerships which, assisted through the award of grants and provision of expert advice, have successfully implemented several local arson-prevention schemes (Home Office, 2006a,b).

The deterrent consequences for arson are contingent upon the severity of the offence: arson can range from minor acts of 'simple arson', to 'reckless arson', where there is no concern whether lives were put at risk, and 'arson with intent', where the aim is to endanger life. The sentences for arson range accordingly from an antisocial behaviour order (ASBO), through various community sentences, to a custodial sentence, including life imprisonment if lives are threatened or lost.

Educational approaches

The basis of educational interventions is that arson can be reduced by providing potential firesetters with information about the dangers of fire and their acquisition of fire safety skills. Educational programmes are often delivered by fire and rescue service personnel. It may be advisable for the young person's family to be actively involved in the programme (Pinsonneault, 2002).

An educational approach to prevention has proved to be popular in work with young people, both as a general strategy with, say, school populations and as an intervention targeted at known juvenile firesetters. The weight of the evidence for educational (and treatment) approaches is with juvenile populations (Kolko, 2001a, 2002).

The American Federal Emergency Management Agency (1994) evaluated the effect of a juvenile firesetting educational programme. Eleven months after completion of the programme the recidivism rate for arson was 1.25%. An evaluation of the effect of attending an educational fire safety workshop also reported a low rate (2.1%) of recidivism for arson (Faranda *et al*, 2001). There are several other positive evaluations of educational programmes (e.g., Franklin *et al*, 2002; Cole *et al*, 2004), including evaluations with child psychiatric populations (e.g., DeSalvatore & Hornstein, 1991), and two UK programmes are described in more detail below. This evaluative research faces practical problems, such as establishing matched control groups, and the extant studies also have short follow-up periods and rely on official convictions, which may or may not accurately reflect actual behaviour.

The FACE programme

Canter & Almond (2002) describe the Fire Awareness Child Education (FACE) programme, initially implemented by the Merseyside fire and rescue service (Broadhurst, 1991). FACE is an educational programme for children and adolescents and has been adopted by number of UK fire and rescue services. FACE was later adapted in partnership with Liverpool's Youth Justice Department as the FACE UP programme for arsonists aged 10–17 years. The FACE programme has been adopted as a 'crime reduction toolkit' for arson by the Home Office (Home Office, n.d.). As such, FACE provides a good example of an educational programme.

The target group for FACE is children aged from 2 to 18 years with a history of playing with fire, or using fire with criminal intent, or making hoax telephone calls, or setting off fire alarms. The programme is delivered to the child and immediate family and participation is voluntary. The main aim of FACE is to change the child's understanding of the risks of fire while also giving the parents or guardians guidance on fire safety.

The programme consists of a home visit by a trained person, a 'fire friend', during which the child and family are guided through a discussion of the dangers of fire, using prompts such as pictures and film clips. The child and siblings are given 'projects', such as colouring books and quizzes, designed to enhance their awareness of fire safety. The opportunity is taken to review the presence of smoke alarms in the home, the parents' monitoring of matches and lighters in the home, and the family's fire escape plan.

Once the child has completed the projects and their fire play has stopped there is a visit to a fire station: they are also told that their fire friend will keep in touch with their parents to ensure all is well. If the family's difficulties are seen to extend beyond the child's interest in fire, then a referral to other agencies may be made. This aspect of FACE relies upon a functioning local multi-agency network, including agencies as diverse as local authority children's services departments, educational welfare, fire and rescue services, juvenile justice, mental health, police and Sure Start. It is likely that collaborative efforts between community agencies contribute appreciably to efforts to reduce arson (Kolko, 2001a; Lambie *et al*, 2002).

The Muckley programme

Canter & Almond (2002) also note the programme developed by Andrew Muckley for juvenile firesetters. This manualised programme, based on a combination of education and counselling, is delivered by trained professional staff. The programme begins with an assessment of the child's firesetting, which determines the level of intervention and the need for referral to other agencies. The child's parents may receive fire safety advice in addition to the work with the child. Canter & Almond estimated that around one-third of fire and rescue services in England and Wales have programmes based on Muckley's approach.

Therapeutic approaches

The mainstream psychological theories have formulated explanations of fire-setting which have informed therapeutic practice. Freud (1932) suggested an interplay between fire and sexual desire and other psychodynamically orientated accounts of arson have drawn on instinctual drives, such as aggression and anxiety, to explain firesetting (Kaufman *et al*, 1961; Macht & Mack, 1968).

Jackson *et al* (1987) outlined a behavioural conceptualisation of arson with a focus on the reinforcing consequences of setting fires. They suggested that the consequences of firesetting can be positively reinforcing, as seen with the social rewards when arson is committed with peers, or the reward of watching people's reactions to the fire and the appearance of the fire services. Alternatively, the consequences of setting fires may be negatively reinforcing: that is, the fire provides a means by which the individual can avoid, say, the difficulties of debt, insolvency or the many demands of school.

Social learning theory suggests that models play an important role in the acquisition of behaviour and there may be models that make fire appear attractive. An American study reported by Curri *et al* (2003) pointed out the paradox that on the one hand children are taught that fire is dangerous and has to be treated with caution, but on the other hand there are images directed at children on toy packaging that depict fire as fun and exciting. Curri *et al* examined the packaging on toys for images of flames; they found that video-games and toy cars and trucks most frequently used pictures of fire. Almost all the fire imagery was targeted at males. Curri *et al* suggested that young boys are being shown through advertising that fire is fun and that such advertisements contribute to the higher incidence of fire play and fire-related injuries in boys.

Another American study, by Greenhalgh & Palmieri (2003), considered media accounts – categorised as comics, advertisements, written articles or television shows – that portrayed behaviour that would risk burn injuries. In keeping with social learning theory, Greenhalgh & Palmieri argued that media portrayals of fire as fun and of little real consequence can influence the behaviour of children, particularly boys, as many of the advertisements using fire were aimed at them.

While educational approaches are reasonably widely used, particularly with children, several commentators have made the point that, despite the theoretical formulations and the growing empirical base, therapeutic practice is not well developed for adult arsonists (Gannon & Pina, 2010), including mentally disordered populations (Swaffer *et al*, 2001). This lack of interventions for adult arsonists was highlighted in a national survey, funded by the Office of the Deputy Prime Minister, conducted in England and Wales in 2005 (Palmer *et al*, 2005, 2007). The organisations that participated in the survey included fire and rescue services, probation services, youth offending services, forensic mental health units (including Special Hospitals and other Secure Forensic Services), the Home Office Mental Health Unit, the Offending Behaviour Programmes Unit of the Prison Service, the Research Development and Statistics Directorate of the Home Office and the National Association for the Care and Resettlement of Offenders (NACRO). Some forensic mental health units provided interventions, but no specialist provision for arsonists was available in the Prison Service or probation services. A specialist intervention for arsonists, along with an associated needs analysis, has begun development in the south-east of England by Gannon and colleagues and was due to be piloted and evaluated in 2011/12 across a number of adult male prisons. The development of this programme is still at a relatively early stage and the content of the programme and the results of the evaluation will become available over the next few years.

Finally, the Arson Control Forum (2006) has reported that 33 of the 47 fire services in England and Wales had intervention schemes for young firesetters. The majority of these interventions were, as might be anticipated given the target population, aimed at early prevention of firesetting behaviours.

While the literature is limited, there are nonetheless examples of therapeutic work with arsonists.

Behavioural practice

Interventions based on behavioural theory and practice, primarily directed at young firesetters, have used a range of techniques, including aversion therapy, over-correction and satiation procedures (e.g., Kolko, 1983; Wolff, 1984; Hardesty & Gayton, 2000).

In an example of such a procedure, Daniel (1987) described an intervention with a young male offender serving a 2-year custodial sentence for arson. The young offender had a long history of firesetting, including starting a blaze in his own home. In the penal institution it was observed that he habitually carried matches, although he did not smoke. The intervention was based on stimulus satiation, a technique where the individual can, under controlled conditions, engage in the problematic behaviour. In this instance the procedure was that matches could be struck, but only one match at a time, which had to be held with arm extended and allowed to burn out before being placed in a metal bin before the next match was struck. The young man could spend as much of each weekly 50-minute session striking matches as he wished. At the fourth session all 50 minutes were spent striking matches. This continued for the next two sessions, then the time spent began to decline so that by session 11 the young man refused to strike any more matches, complaining that it was 'boring' and that he was beginning to burn his fingers (which was not the case in the earlier sessions). His refusal to continue with the sessions coincided with him no longer carrying matches. Daniel reported that 6 months after discharge from prison the young man had no further convictions related to arson.

Psychosocial interventions

Psychosocial interventions have been used with arsonists; these typically address several of the psychological and social factors associated with arson. As with educational approaches, psychosocial interventions have mainly been used with young firesetters.

This type of intervention typically includes a range of techniques drawn, for example, from anger control training, behavioural family therapy and contingency management (e.g., Cole *et al*, 1983; Kolko & Ammerman, 1988; Cox-Jones *et al*, 1990; Adler *et al*, 1994). With respect to contingency management, the studies on the effects of advertising discussed above serve as reminders of the potency of modelling. It is incumbent upon those living and working with arsonists, whether in the home or in a residential setting, consistently to model appropriate behaviour with respect to fire.

Hollin & Epps (1996) present a case study, with an adolescent arsonist, in which cognitive–behavioural methods were used, such as anger control and problem-solving, alongside a fire safety and awareness educational programme. The young man also participated in sexual abuse counselling and offence counselling as part of a comprehensive treatment package. The intervention started in secure residential accommodation, then continued in open conditions, with the addition of life-skills training and family work. At a 1-year follow-up there were no recorded instances of firesetting and the young man had entered full-time education.

Schwartzman *et al* (1998) describe a psychosocial programme called Community Alternatives To Commitment Hazards (CATCH). The CATCH programme, developed by the Department of Youth Services in Oregon, is for juveniles aged 13–17 years who have been adjudicated for arson. The 16-session CATCH programme aims to help young firesetters to understand their firesetting behaviour through the use of anger management, assertiveness training, confrontation of thinking errors, coping skills training, empathy development and identification of feelings. CATCH is delivered in a group setting by a fire service professional and a youth counsellor. The child's parents are involved to help develop their parenting skills and for them to understand and reinforce the skills their children are acquiring. In a process with overtones of restorative justice, the young people are required to identify and interview the victims of their fire. A report on the interviews, presented to the court and youth services, is written by the young people to show that they understand the effect of the fire on their victims. Schwartzman *et al* reported that the evaluation of CATCH showed that at 1-year follow-up 93% of those participating had not committed another act of arson. Further, 67% of those involved had no further criminal behaviour at all.

Adler *et al* (1994) conducted a randomised study with 138 young firesetters: half received a home visit from fire and rescue service staff for educational input on fire safety; the other half participated in a multi-component programme consisting of visits from fire and rescue service staff, the provision of educational material on fire safety, behavioural satiation and parent training in dealing appropriately with firesetting behaviours. A 1-year follow-up showed that the frequency and severity of firesetting had fallen by similar degrees in both conditions.

Kolko (2001*b*) compared the effects of three types of intervention in a study where 46 young male firesetters, aged 5–13 years, were randomly assigned to one of three conditions: (1) fire safety education (FSE), which comprised fire safety skills training and discussion of motives for firesetting with firefighters; (2) cognitive–behavioural treatment (CBT), consisting of training in self-control, problem-solving, coping skills and prosocial behaviours; (3) a brief home visit by a firefighter (HVF) to simulate routine fire service practice. There were significant positive changes for all three conditions, as assessed by self-report and parent report of firesetting and match play at the end of treatment and at 1-year follow-up. Across conditions,

CBT and FSE showed better outcomes than HVF; CBT particularly led to a decrease in fire interest, while FSE enhanced fire safety skills.

The effectiveness of an intervention is likely to be moderated by child and family factors such as degree of exposure to fire materials, modelling of appropriate behaviours and family dysfunction (Kolko et al, 2006). In order to ensure a good response to an intervention, such factors should be allowed for when treatment is matched to the needs and characteristics of the firesetters and their families.

Interventions with psychiatric populations

Palmer et al (2007) noted that there were a small number of interventions, delivered on a group-work basis, in forensic mental health services. These programmes were targeted at young males with intellectual disabilities and at adults in high security.

Taylor et al (2004) presented case studies of four male firesetters with developmental disabilities who took part in a group-based intervention. The 31-session intervention focused on a range of targets, including coping skills, self-esteem, increasing the understanding of the risks posed by fire and the development of personalised relapse prevention plans. Taylor et al reported that the four patients all completed the programme but that their scores on fire-specific measures did not change markedly.

The same programme was used with six female arsonists with intellectual disabilities (Taylor, et al, 2006). As with the males, the female patients all completed the intervention. The scores on the fire-related measures improved after the programme and at 2-year follow-up none of the women had set another fire.

Swaffer et al (2001) describe a 62-session structured programme for arsonists with a mental disorder living in conditions of high security. Following Jackson et al, the programme had four modules, delivered in the following sequence as described by Swaffer et al (p. 469):

(1) Dangers of fire – assessing and developing insight (12 sessions); (2) Skills development – coping without firesetting (24 sessions); (3) Insight and awareness – assessing and developing (12 sessions); (4) Practical strategies to help break offence cycles (14 sessions).

The programme used a broad range of assessments, ranging from the Fire Interest Rating Scale (Murphy & Clare, 1996) to the Novaco Anger Scale (Novaco, 1994). Swaffer et al use a case study to illustrate the positive application and outcome of the programme with a female patient. A longer-term outcome study of this programme has not yet been published.

Conclusion

While research has revealed a considerable amount of information about both arson and arsonists, it appears that practice and its evaluation rather lag behind the data – a point which is particularly pertinent for mentally disordered populations. The majority of interventions take an educational approach and are aimed at young firesetters. The evaluations of these educational programmes indicate some promising outcomes but are limited by weak methodologies and short follow-up. Furthermore, most of the empirical evidence is from North America, which raises the issue of the degree to which the findings will generalise to countries with different legal systems and cultural standards.

The lack of provision in the criminal justice system for arson, an offence with such well-documented harmful consequences, is particularly notable given the investment and sustained progress in the treatment of other groups of serious offenders (Mann & Fernandez, 2006; Polaschek, 2006).

The treatment of arsonists in mental health services is not well advanced, which, at face value, is a curious state of affairs. Substantial numbers of patients who have set fires are admitted to secure mental health facilities. It is also the case that some of these patients will commit more acts of arson after they are discharged. The evidence base on the predictors of repeat instances of firesetting, while not extensive, gives some indication of how treatment may be configured. In particular, the work of Rice & Harris points to subgroups of arsonists with mental disorders: it may be that these subgroupings offer a basis from which to develop treatments suited to particular types of arsonist.

It may be, of course, that therapeutic work with the primary mental health diagnosis alongside attention to comorbid diagnoses, as with alcohol use, is in itself sufficient to prevent arson. The specific issue raised by this point is that there is, particularly in the UK, a weak evidence base with respect to understanding the association between arson and mental disorder. The consequence of this lack of knowledge is a paucity of evidence-based treatment and attendant outcome studies and clinical trials.

When considered in relation to research and practice with other serious offences committed by adults, it is difficult to resist the conclusion that arson has been neglected. A national research programme to develop our understanding of arson and our ability to intervene effectively with arsonists is overdue.

References

Adler, R. G., Nunn, R. J., Lebnan, V. M., *et al* (1994) Secondary prevention of childhood firesetting. *Journal of the American Academy of Child and Adolescent Psychiatry*, **33**, 1194–1202.

American Psychiatric Association (2000) *Diagnostic and Statistical Manual of Mental Disorders* (4th edn, text revision) (DSM-IV-TR). APA.

Anwar, S., Långström, N., Grann, M., *et al* (2011) Is arson the crime most strongly associated with psychosis? A national case–control study of arson risk in schizophrenia and other psychoses. *Schizophrenia Bulletin*, **37**, 580–586 .

Arson Control Forum (2003) *Annual Report*. Office of the Deputy Prime Minster.

Arson Control Forum (2006) *Youth Training and Diversion Schemes*. Arson Control Forum Research Bulletin no. 8. Office of the Deputy Prime Minister.

Broadhurst, S. (1991) Fighting arson. *The Magistrate*, **55**, 104–105.

Canter, D. & Almond, L. (2002) *The Burning Issue: Research and Strategies for Reducing Arson*. Office of the Deputy Prime Minster.

Chen, Y., Arria, A. M. & Anthony, J. C. (2003) Firesetting in adolescence and being aggressive, shy, and rejected by peers: new epidemiologic evidence from a national sample survey. *Journal of the American Academy of Psychiatry and Law*, **31**, 44–52.

Clarke, R. V. (1983) Situational crime prevention: its theoretical basis and practical scope. *Crime and Justice: A Review of Research*, **4**, 225–256.

Coid J., Kahtan, N., Gault, S., *et al* (2001) Medium secure forensic psychiatry services: comparison of seven English health regions. *British Journal of Psychiatry*, **178**, 55–61.

Cole, R. E., Laurenitis, L. R., McAndrews, M. M., *et al* (1983) *Final Report of 1983 Fire-Related Youth Project*. New York State Office of Fire Prevention and Control.

Cole, R. E., Crandall, R. & Kourofsky, C. (2004) We can teach young children fire safety. *Young Children*, **59**, 14–18.

Cox-Jones, C., Lubetsky, M., Fultz, S. A., *et al* (1990) Inpatient treatment of a young recidivist firesetter. *Journal of the American Academy of Child Psychiatry*, **29**, 936–941.

Curri, T. B., Palmieri, T. L., Aoki, T. H., *et al* (2003) Playing with fire: images of fire on toy packaging. *Journal of Burn Care and Rehabilitation*, 24, 163–165.

Dadds, M. R. & Fraser, J. A. (2006) Fire interest, fire setting and psychopathology in Australian children: a normative study. *Australian and New Zealand Journal of Psychiatry*, **40**, 581–586.

Daniel, C. J. (1987) A stimulus satiation treatment programme with a young male firesetter. In *Applying Psychology to Imprisonment: Theory and Practice* (eds B. J. McGurk, D. M. Thornton & M. Williams), pp. 239–246. HMSO.

Davies, M. & Mouzos, J. (2007) *Fatal Fires: Fire-Associated Homicide in Australia, 1990–2005*. Trends and Issues in Crime and Criminal Justice no. 340. Australian Institute of Criminology.

Department for Communities and Local Government (2008) *Fire Statistics, United Kingdom 2006*. Department for Communities and Local Government.

DeSalvatore, G. & Hornstein, R. (1991) Juvenile firesetting: assessment and treatment in psychiatric hospitalisation and residential placement. *Child and Youth Care Forum*, **20**, 103–114.

Dickens, G., Sugarman, P., Ahmad, F., *et al* (2008) Characteristics of low IQ arsonists at psychiatric assessment. *Medicine, Science and the Law*, **48**, 217–220.

Dickens, G., Sugarman, P., Ahmed, F., *et al* (2009) Gender differences amongst adult arsonists at psychiatric assessment. *Medicine, Science and the Law*, **47**, 233–238.

Enayati, J., Grann, M., Lubbe, S., *et al* (2008) Psychiatric morbidity in arsonists referred for forensic psychiatric assessment in Sweden. *Journal of Forensic Psychiatry and Psychology*, **19**, 139–147.

Faranda, D. M., Katsikas, S. L. & Lim, N. (2001) Communities working together: an evaluation of the intervention program for juvenile firesetters and arsonists in Broward County, Florida. *American Journal of Forensic Psychology*, **19**, 37–62.

Fazel, S. & Grann, M. (2002) Older criminals: a descriptive study of psychiatrically examined offenders in Sweden. *International Journal of Geriatric Psychiatry*, **17**, 907–913.

Federal Emergency Management Agency (1994) *The National Firesetter/Arson Control and Prevention Program*. US Fire Administration.

Fineman, K. R. (1980) Firesetting in childhood and adolescence. *Psychiatric Clinics of North America*, **3**, 483–499.

Flanagan R. J. & Fisher, D. S. (2008) Volatile substance abuse and crime: data from UK press cuttings 1996–2007. *Medicine, Science and the Law*, **48**, 295–306.

Franklin, G. A., Pucci, P. S., Arbabi, S., *et al* (2002) Decreased juvenile arson and firesetting recidivism after implementation of a multidisciplinary prevention program. *Journal of Trauma, Injury, Infection and Critical Care*, **53**, 260–266.

Freud, S. (1932) The acquisition of power over fire. *International Journal of Psychoanalysis*, **13**, 405–410.

Gannon, T. A. & Pina, A. (2010) Firesetting: pathology, theory and treatment. *Aggression and Violent Behavior*, **15**, 224–238.

Greenhalgh, D. G. & Palmieri, T. L. (2003) The media glorifying burns: a hindrance to burn prevention. *Journal of Burn Care and Research*, **24**, 159–162.

Hardesty, V. A. & Gayton, W. F. (2000) The problem of children and fire: an historical perspective. In *Handbook on Firesetting in Children and Youth* (ed. D. J. Kolko), pp. 1–13. Academic Press.

Hollin, C. R. & Epps, K. J. (1996) Adolescent firesetters. In *Clinical Approaches to Working with Young Offenders* (eds C. R. Hollin & K. Howells), pp. 197–207. Wiley.

Hollin, C. R., Epps, K. & Swaffer, T. (2002) Adolescent firesetters: findings from an analysis of 47 cases. *Pakistan Journal of Psychological Research*, **17**, 1–16.

Home Office (2006a) *Tackling Arson: Home Office Guide*. Home Office.

Home Office (2006b) *Arson Control Forum: Annual Report 2006*. At http://www.communities.gov.uk/documents/fire/pdf/154145.pdf (accessed 8 November 2011).

Home Office (n.d.) Crime reduction toolkits. At http://tna.europarchive.org/20100413151441/crimereduction.homeoffice.gov.uk/toolkits/ (accessed 8 November 2011).

Jackson, H., Glass, C. & Hope, S. (1987) A functional analysis of recidivistic arson. *British Journal of Clinical Psychology*, **26**, 175–185.

Jamieson, E., Butwell, M, Taylor, P., *et al* (2000) Trends in special (high-security) hospitals. 1: Referrals and admissions. *British Journal of Psychiatry*, **176**, 253–259.

Jayaraman, A. & Frazer, J. (2006) Arson: a growing inferno. *Medicine, Science and the Law*, **46**, 295–300.

Kaufman, I., Heims, L. & Reiser, D. E. (1961) Are-evaluation of the psychodynamics of firesetting. *American Journal of Orthopsychiatry*, **31**, 123–136.

Kolko, D. J. (1983) Multicomponent parental treatment of firesetting in a six year old boy. *Journal of Behavior and Experimental Psychology*, **14**, 349–354.

Kolko, D. J. (2001a) Firesetters. In *Handbook of Offender Assessment and Treatment* (ed. C. R. Hollin), pp. 391–414. Wiley.

Kolko, D. J. (2001b) Efficacy of cognitive–behavioral treatment and fire safety education for children who set fires: initial and follow-up outcomes. *Journal of Child Psychology and Psychiatry*, **42**, 359–369.

Kolko, D. J. (ed.) (2002) *Handbook on Firesetting in Children and Youth*. Academic Press.

Kolko, D. J. & Ammerman, R. T. (1988) Firesetting. In *Child Behavior Therapy Casebook* (eds M. Hersen & C. G. Last), pp. 243–262. Plenum Press.

Kolko, D. J., Herschell, A. D. & Scharf, D. M. (2006) Education and treatment for boys who set fires: specificity, moderators, and predictors of recidivism. *Journal of Emotional and Behavioral Disorders*, 14, 227–239.

Lambie, I., McCardle, S. & Coleman, R. (2002) Where there's smoke there's fire: firesetting behaviour in children and adolescents. *New Zealand Journal of Psychology*, **31**, 73–76.

Lindberg, N., Holi, M. M., Tani, P., *et al* (2005) Looking for pyromania: characteristics of a consecutive sample of Finnish male criminals with histories of recidivist firesetting between 1973 and 1993. *BMC Psychiatry*, **5**, 47. At http://www.biomedcentral.com/1471-244X/5/47 (accessed 21 December 2010).

Macht, L. B. & Mack, J. E. (1968) The firesetter syndrome. *Psychiatry*, **31**, 277–288.

Mann, R. E. & Fernandez, Y. M. (2006) Sex offender programmes: concept, theory, and practice. In *Offending Behaviour Programmes: Development, Application, and Controversies* (eds C. R. Hollin & E. J. Palmer), pp. 155–177. Wiley.

Martin, G., Bergen, H. A., Richardson, A. S., *et al* (2004) Correlates of firesetting in a community sample of young adolescents. *Australian and New Zealand Journal of Psychiatry*, **38**, 148–154.

Murphy, G. H. & Clare, I. C. H. (1996) Analysis of motivation in people with mild learning disabilities (mental handicap) who set fires. *Psychology, Crime and Law*, **2**, 153–164.

Novaco, R. W. (1994) Anger as a risk factor for violence among the mentally disordered. In *Violence and Mental Disorder: Developments in Risk Assessment* (eds J. Monahan & H. J. Steadman), pp. 21–59. University of Chicago Press.

Palmer, E. J., Caulfield, L. S. & Hollin, C. R. (2005) *Evaluation of Interventions with Arsonists and Young Firesetters*. Office of the Deputy Prime Minister.

Palmer, E. J., Caulfield, L. S. & Hollin, C. R. (2007) Interventions with arsonists and young firesetters: a survey of the national picture in England and Wales. *Legal and Criminological Psychology*, **12**, 101–116.

Palmer, E. J., Hollin, C. R., Hatcher, R. M., *et al* (2010) Arson. In *Handbook on Crime* (eds F. Brookman, M. Maguire, H. Pierpoint & T. Bennett), pp. 380–392. Willan Publishing.

Pinsonneault, I. L. (2002) Fire safety education and skills training. In *Handbook on Firesetting in Children and Youth* (ed. D. J. Kolko), pp. 219–260. Academic Press.

Polaschek, D. L. L. (2006) Violent offender programmes: concept, theory, and practice. In *Offending Behaviour Programmes: Development, Application, and Controversies* (eds C. R. Hollin & E. J. Palmer), pp. 114–154. Wiley.

Prins, H. (1994) *Fire-Raising: Its Motivation and Management*. Routledge.

Prins, H. (1995) Adult fire-raising: law and psychology. *Psychology, Crime, and Law*, **1**, 271–281.

Repo, E., Virkkunen, M., Rawlings, M., *et al* (1997) Criminal and psychiatric histories of Finnish arsonists. *Acta Psychiatrica Scandinavica*, **95**, 318–323.

Rice, M. E. & Harris, G. T. (1991) Firesetters admitted to a maximum security psychiatric institution: offenders and offenses. *Journal of Interpersonal Violence*, **6**, 641–675.

Rice, M. E. & Harris, G. T. (1996) Predicting the recidivism of mentally disordered offenders. *Journal of Interpersonal Violence*, **11**, 364–375.

Ritchie, E. C. & Huff, T. G. (1999) Psychiatric aspects of arsonists. *Journal of Forensic Science*, **44**, 733–740.

Root, C., MacKay, S., Henderson, J., *et al* (2008) The link between maltreatment and juvenile firesetting: correlates and underlying mechanisms. *Child Abuse and Neglect*, **32**, 161–176.

Schwartzman, P., Stambaugh, H. & Kimball, J. (1998) *Arson and Juveniles: Responding to the Violence*. US Fire Administration Technical Report Series USFA-TR-095. US Fire Administration.

Sugarman, P. & Dickens, G. (2009) Dangerousness in firesetters: a survey of psychiatrists' views. *Psychiatric Bulletin*, **33**, 99–101.

Swaffer, T., Haggertt, M. & Oxley, T. (2001) Mentally disordered firesetters: a structured intervention programme. *Clinical Psychology and Psychotherapy*, **8**, 468–475.

Taylor, J. L., Thorne, I. & Slavkin, M. L. (2004) Treatment of fire-setting behaviour. In *Offenders with Developmental Disabilities* (eds W. R. Lindsay, J. L. Taylor & P. Sturmey), pp. 221–240. Wiley.

Taylor, J. L., Robertson, A., Thorne, I., *et al* (2006) Responses of female fire-setters with mild and borderline intellectual disabilities to a group intervention. *Journal of Applied Research in Intellectual Disabilities*, **19**, 179–190.

Wolff, R. (1984) Satiation in the treatment of inappropriate firesetting. *Journal of Behavioral Therapy and Experimental Psychiatry*, **15**, 337–340.

CHAPTER 13

Arson and mental health: case reports from psychiatric practice

Tim Rogers

Most crimes of arson are committed by a small number of prolific offenders, many of whom are under 18 and who commit other offences also. The majority of these individuals do not experience mental illness. Research does, however, place arson in the same category as homicide in respect of the magnitude of the increase in risk of such offending that mental illness confers (Anwar et al, 2011). This increase is much higher than those reported for other violent crimes. Intellectual disability in particular also greatly increases a person's risk of committing arson. Mental health professionals therefore frequently encounter arsonists of both a dangerous and a recidivist nature. The courts often seek specialist advice when sentencing arsonists.

In formulating risk management plans it is frequently necessary to put in place approaches to rehabilitation and recovery that address the criminogenic needs which pertain to firesetting. The literature distinguishes two broad groups of such interventions, namely educational approaches (seeking to inform individuals about the risks of fire) and psychosocial approaches (with the aim of modulating some aspect of precipitant or behaviour) (Palmer *et al*, 2005).

This chapter presents two anonymised case studies to illustrate the ways in which offences of arson can arise in psychiatric patients. Their multidisciplinary treatment and management are described in detail. All personal details, dates, locations and other information that might identify the individuals in question have been either omitted or made fictitious to ensure no breach of confidentiality.

Case 1. Psychosis driving arson

Mr S is the son of two African professionals. His parents have, however, never lived together. Mr S was raised by his mother and had only sporadic contact with his father. There is a family history of serious mental illness, although not in first-degree relatives. There is no known family history of criminal behaviour.

Mr S was born by normal delivery and attained normal developmental milestones. From the age of 6 months he attended day nursery while his mother worked. His mother describes him as a respectful child who was not initially aggressive in character. From an early age he found it difficult to concentrate in class and became a disruptive pupil, however. He played truant and fought on a number of occasions, often being suspended. He received special support at times during his education and performed most successfully in small classes. There was a brief, unsuccessful referral to a child and family guidance clinic but his behaviour continued to be disruptive while he was in secondary education. Mr S's memories of his mother appeared to be dominated by descriptions of adverse interactions such as 'just getting beat when I done wrong'. It was his belief that she had habitually used excess force in disciplining him. He alleged that she had stamped upon him and used her hands to smack or hit him too often. Asked whether she would comfort him when distressed he responded, 'I know she didn't cuddle me – I have a good memory'. He recalled that he had not sought solace in his mother when upset as a child, instead being 'more likely to go on the run'.

Mr S is known to have used cannabis since around the age of 11 years. He left school at 16, without formal qualifications. Difficulties in the education system coincided with his increasing offending behaviour around this time; he received convictions for theft, assault with intent to resist arrest, supplying cannabis and eventually robbery, which led to his brief incarceration at a young offender institution. Mr S developed a pattern of regular crack cocaine use from this point, reportedly spending hundreds of pounds each week during his heaviest periods of intake. This was funded largely through acquisitive offending. Although crack cocaine was his drug of choice, he also experimented with ecstasy and amphetamines (without using these more regularly). There appears to have been no significant history of alcohol misuse. Mr S did not resume education until his early 20s, when he took a carpentry course. Employment did not materialise from this and Mr S found it difficult to sustain work or other vocational activities, complaining of boredom or 'too much travel'. Mr S had no significant history of physical ill health such as asthma, diabetes, epilepsy or hypertension. He had no history of head injuries aside from plating of his jawbone after a fracture at the age of 20 years.

Mr S is exclusively heterosexual in orientation. He has had a number of sexual encounters but no more significant or long-term intimate relationships. He has no children. An allegation of rape was made against him at the age of 20 years that resulted in his arrest and remand in custody. He received the injury above while in prison, from an attack at the hands of his co-defendant, who wished to coerce him into accepting all responsibility for the allegation. Mr S was found not guilty at trial.

Around this time, Mr S was observed by others to show evidence of gradual change in character. He would lose his temper and become angry more quickly. He lived with his mother in a troubled inner-city neighbour-hood and unfortunately was witness to a killing in the local area. He made the necessary initial reports to the police but, fearing reprisals, was unhappy about cooperating further as a prosecution witness. Tremendous pressure was applied upon him in order that he do so. He experienced further stress in the context of unemployment, low income and the absence of a structure or role in his life. He began to spend days in bed, to exhibit signs of low mood and to be verbally aggressive at times. This escalated into his refusal to leave the house. In conversation with others he would voice fears that strangers were looking and laughing at him. Over a period of months his mental state deteriorated further, to the extent that those close to him described the onset of 'ranting and raving gibberish and nonsense' and of 'an obsession with the oppression of Black people'. Mr S suddenly developed religious beliefs and began to talk about his possession of 'spiritual powers'. With the encouragement of his mother, he agreed to attend his local mental health unit for out-patient appointments. Around this time it was reported that he had destroyed a number of possessions in his bedroom.

It was initially difficult to engage Mr S in treatment. He agreed to take the antidepressant amitriptyline but no other treatment, as he felt that his difficulties consisted of depression and poor sleep only. He was offered monitoring and follow-up and soon presented to services again. His complaint was once more of depression but also of 'feeling unsure who he was'. He was verbally aggressive on one occasion and threatened to shoot a member of staff. Around this time he agreed to a period of voluntary in-patient hospital care. Under observation he complained of racing thoughts, difficulty with sleep and further uncertainty about his own identity. He appeared guarded, suspicious and when interviewed he became verbally aggressive, threatening 'you lot will go to hell, you psychologists playing your mind games!' Urine drug screening revealed no illicit substances at this stage. A number of aggressive incidents occurred, including an unprovoked assault upon a fellow patient and the making of threats to kill his consultant and to shoot another staff member. He was persuaded to commence olanzapine antipsychotic medication. After 5 days of adherence to this treatment plan and no further adverse incidents, it was agreed by the clinical team that he could spend some time outside in the grounds of the hospital. He did not return to the unit.

It later emerged that the following sequence of events had ensued. Mr S travelled to a local petrol station, where he purchased a plastic petrol can, fuel and a carbonated beverage in a bottle. A short time later his mother, who was at home in an upstairs room, heard the sound of breaking glass from downstairs. She called the police. A neighbour, who had also heard the sound, witnessed Mr S placing an item into a rubbish bin. This was later discovered to be the plastic petrol can. Flames were soon evident at the downstairs window. Curtains had been ignited and were blowing in and out of the broken pane.

Mr S was seen to run off down the street by the observing neighbour, who, fortuitously, had access to an extinguisher and put out the fire. Crime-scene examination revealed that a brick had been thrown through the window. It lay together with an empty beverage bottle. This was charred and smelled strongly of petrol. As police were dealing with the incident they were contacted by hospital staff, who informed them that Mr S had returned there and had spoken about setting a fire at his mother's address. Police officers attended the ward and asked Mr S if he knew why they had come to speak with him. He replied 'Yeah, it's because I set fire to my mother's place'. He was arrested. He assaulted, spat upon and dismissed his solicitor during their consultation. A decision was made by police not to interview him after he continued to appear highly disturbed. Mr S was charged with <u>arson being</u> reckless as to whether life was endangered.

Following his arrest Mr S was remanded in custody and immediately located in the prison hospital wing. He began to discuss the incident in more detail and gave an account consistent with the known facts. He reported the intention of burning down his mother's home and was able to convey his motives for doing so. He would typically reply 'It's the war, the White man has to pay for what he did, enslaved us, murdered our babies, raped our ancestors and made them suck their dicks'. He believed that his family had been in league with the oppression of other Black people, despite their own African origins. He believed that they had also been 'playing psychological games' and had framed him such that he had been charged with rape. He believed that this persecution at the hands of his own family had enabled him to discover his true identity and mission in life ('they helped me discover who I was and what my mission is'). He had taken the stage name of a New York 'hip-hop' lyricist but believed he was a prophet and leader of all Black people, with a unique mission to lead them 'to America, and then to Africa to line them up for war'. Mr S believed that he had set a fire in his mother's home as a necessary part of his war against White men. There was evidence of disordered thinking. He was also experiencing constant auditory hallucinations in the form of voices talking in both the second and third person. He was hearing derogatory comments, echoes of his own thoughts and a running commentary about all his actions.

Mr S refused to accept that any of these experiences might relate to mental illness, but nonetheless appeared to be accepting of the olanzapine antipsychotic treatment offered to him in custody. He threatened that he might behave in a similarly dangerous way in future, as the issues which concerned him had not been resolved. He often appeared perplexed and agitated when asked to describe events leading to the alleged arson. He tended to produce rambling accounts, difficult to follow, of his actions, saying things like 'my family are refusing me, I have to be with God, a rape has been done and starvation has been done, arson needed to be done'. Mr S told clinicians that he would have committed the offence sooner had he not had to wait several days in order to obtain the money necessary to purchase petrol. He admitted to having broken a window in his mother's house on a previous occasion. It appeared that he had refrained from setting a fire then because he had noticed men in a nearby car, whom he assumed were plain-clothed police officers. The fact that he had not been arrested on this occasion had prompted him to conclude 'They wanted me to do it, it's my destiny'. He spoke of having interpreted innocuous-sounding comments from a mental health worker prior to the fire as giving him a coded message to commit arson. Mr S expressed surprise at his arrest, believing that he had been acting with the approval of the police. He explained his belief that it remained his role to repeat the experiences of the oppression of the tribes of Africa by carrying out certain actions. Furthermore, he believed that burning down his mother's home would have prevented his enemies from knowing about his own home location. Mr S's adherence to first olanzapine and then risperidone treatment (at therapeutic doses) appeared to allay the behavioural manifestations of his illness but not significantly to affect his perceptions and thought content.

It was concluded that Mr S was likely to be suffering from paranoid schizophrenia, given his presentation with an approximately 6-month history of behavioural change characterised by increasing irritability, the experience of a number of abnormal perceptions, including auditory hallucinations, thought echo, thought interference, disordered thought form and a complex paranoid delusional system. He was eventually transferred for urgent treatment under section 48 of the Mental Health Act 1983 to a medium-security hospital.

At his subsequent sentencing the court accepted that, in believing he had been a prophet with a unique mission to avenge the suffering of Black people in history, Mr S had been labouring under such a defect of reason, from disease of the mind, as not to know what he was doing was wrong. In meeting the strict 'M'Naughten' test, Mr S was subsequently found not guilty by reason of insanity. He was made the subject of a hospital order restricting discharge without limit of time under the Criminal Procedure (Insanity and Unfitness to Plead) Act 1991.

At the outset of his sentence, physical examination and a comprehensive array of blood tests (including HIV and auto-antibody screening) on admission revealed nothing of concern. Electrocardiography revealed sinus tachycardia but was otherwise normal. Magnetic resonance brain images revealed no space-occupying lesions, demyelinating or other pathological abnormalities. Waking electroencephalography recordings were unremarkable. At this point Mr S appeared less chaotic and disorganised compared with his time in custody, but he remained conspicuously deluded, despite apparent adherence to oral risperidone. Auditory and other hallucinations remained but had become less intensely experienced. Mr S's symptoms included a feeling of 'detachment' from himself. He said that he did not believe that he was part of himself. He wished to know who he was, so that he could 'get back to himself'. He added that when he looked in the mirror, he saw a stranger. He described the sensation of insects crawling under his skin. Therapeutic trials of treatment with oral quetiapine, injectible zuclopenthixol decanoate and flupenthixol decanoate were all undertaken as alternatives to risperidone, which had proven only partially effective. Amitriptyline was replaced with paroxetine, at therapeutic doses also.

On the ward Mr S needed encouragement to attend occupational therapy groups. He was observed to be quiet and at times restless. Initially he needed encouragement to speak and would rather keep to himself, but some months after admission to hospital he had become more active and spontaneous in his communications. Mr S, however, continued to make complaints of detachment, a sensation so pervasive that he described feeling that it was 'impossible to not focus on these or to get away from them'. He described 'a nightmare situation' that caused him to feel depressed in mood and unable to see any real future. Approaching 1 year after admission, he had improved to a certain extent but continued occasionally to describe seeing 'demon shadows' across the wall in front of him or on the floor, in the form of 'pairs of human eyes'. He was by now far less preoccupied with feelings of depersonalisation. He denied any of the more florid psychotic symptoms that he had experienced around the time of his index offence.

He often experienced fleeting suicidal thoughts but made no actual attempts at suicide or self-harm. He tended to articulate his concerns in a blunted and emotionally detached way. There was evidence of poverty of thought and a lack of spontaneity in his thinking.

Psychometric testing with Mr S had revealed evidence of a deterioration in cognitive functioning such that his intellectual level (borderline range) was slightly lower than expected given his educational and occupational history. Mr S performed poorly on tasks assessing working memory and information processing, indicating that his immediate retention and encoding of verbal and visual information and his ability to learn following repeated trials were rather poor. It appeared that negative symptoms of schizophrenia were having some adverse effects on aspects of his cognitive functioning. It was suggested that Mr S's cognitive functioning be retested in all areas once improvements in his mental state were observed. It was further recommended that it was important to limit the amount and complexity of information given to him at any one time and to repeat information as necessary.

Mr S gained significant weight while detained in hospital, despite exercising in the gym fairly regularly. He was found to be mildly hypertensive. He complained of impotence as a further side-effect of antipsychotic medication, which remained under review as a therapeutic and tolerable longer-term prescription was sought. Sildenafil (Viagra) was prescribed but with limited benefit.

Further efforts were made to engage Mr S in psychological interventions, including insight-oriented treatments and relapse-prevention planning. Initial sessions focused on the ongoing feelings of detachment. Mr S adopted a negative attitude to the possibility that this symptom might change and it was felt that too rigid a focus on it might be counterproductive. Subsequently Mr S was able to identify early symptoms of his mental illness and outline these in a relapse-management plan. By this stage, when speaking about the index offence he would express some ideas about having been unwell at the time of the arson. He was, however, much less willing to discuss other aspects of his character and episodes of previous offending. With time, the therapeutic alliance he had developed with the psychologist began to diminish and he became less engaged in their sessions. He spoke about 'feeling fed up' and came to believe that he had spent sufficient time in hospital. A timeline review was used to try to explore other aspects of his life. Mr S described events in purely factual terms and saw no need for further discussion. It was concluded that further work was indicated regarding insight into both his illness and his offence but that this work would be reviewed after Mr S had had a break from psychological treatment. Mr S admitted to using cannabis early in the course of his admission. This was an intermittent problem, particularly at times of stress or loss. He participated in occupational therapy, including use of the gym, horticulture, music therapy and a mental health awareness group but needed much encouragement and prompting, particularly for morning sessions. Mr S was granted a progressively increasing programme of leave away from the ward. There were no incidents of violence but his body language was often intrusive and he would frequently engage in horseplay with other patients. Around this time it appeared that Mr S had been involved in encouraging other patients to abscond from the ward. It was the perception of nursing staff that he engaged in bullying also. These behaviours ceased after he was counselled about them. Mr S had a further period of contact with the clinical psychology department. During this period he undertook further work regarding his understanding of both his illness and his offence. Mr S was able to speak more openly about the areas of his history which he had previously found difficult to discuss. He developed good insight into his mental illness and the need for long-term medication, demonstrating an awareness of the impact of illicit stimulants upon his mental state and offending. He felt less certain about whether or not cannabis use would be likely to have an adverse impact on his mental state. He was able to speak with relative ease about the arson at his mother's home. Although he had come to believe that it was related to his mental state at the time, and although he was able to demonstrate empathy when reflecting upon how his mother might have felt, the context of the fire still appeared to be confusing for him.

Mr S continued to utilise day leave from the hospital without incident and presented no other management problems around this time, approaching 2 years after admission. He moved to reside in a part of the hospital set up as independent flatlets, where he adjusted well to his responsibilities and increased independence. He came to be regarded as a conscientious and courteous house-mate and he took a lead role among residents there. He attended a therapeutic drug and alcohol group each week, demonstrating commitment to attendance and contribution. Of concern remained his reluctance to accept that cannabis had had an equally serious role as illicit stimulants in his mental deterioration. When the point was raised he appeared to become slightly defensive. It was therefore felt that he might require some support with his decision to abstain from cannabis once in the community. There remained no significant evidence of psychotic symptoms around this time. Such was Mr S's progress in treatment that his supervising clinicians decided, some 2 years after first admission, to move towards planning his eventual discharge.

Around this time Mr S suffered a sudden and dramatic relapse in illness. No aspect of his care had been altered. It appeared that this had been precipitated by the experience of intense stress, both about the implications of discharge and the need for increased self-reliance and about the prospect of reconciling his relationship with and managing his feelings towards his mother. It came to light that Mr S's outward appearance of stability concealed the true extent of psychotic symptoms, which he had been able to disguise from clinicians. It proved possible to plan once more for Mr S's discharge only after the introduction of clozapine medication and also the completion of systemic family therapy involving his mother.

Discussion

Most of those who develop schizophrenia are not violent, are not liable to set fires and do not otherwise pose a significant danger to others. Mr S is therefore unusual. He perpetrated a murderous attack upon his mother, although the court sentence recognised that he bore no guilt in law. It is of interest to examine what differentiates Mr S from other people with a major mental disorder who do not offend. Most obvious are the indicators of early maladjustment. He gave a history of harsh and inconsistent parenting. His mother had to raise him as a single parent and attachment difficulties developed between them. He developed a variety of features of childhood conduct disorder, found in many studies to be associated with later offending on the part of people who are mentally ill (Dunedin Multidisciplinary Health and Development Research Unit, 2010). The misuse of illicit substances was probably responsible both for precipitating the onset of illness in him and for maintaining it and increasing its symptomatic floridity. The features of his illness comprised some 'threat/control override symptoms'. These are experiences of a person feeling that others are trying to harm them and that their minds are being influenced by others. Some studies have reported correlations between these symptoms and violence (Link & Stueve, 1994).

The evidence of purposive firesetting inherent in Mr S's use of fuel as an accelerant is a likely indicator of his potential dangerousness in comparison with other arsonists (Dickens *et al*, 2009). Both Mr S and his mother suffered in the course of the events described above. His later relapse is testament to this, seemingly brought about by stress at the prospect of his returning to live in the community and arising from ongoing family difficulties. While the need to treat his psychotic symptoms is plain, the case of Mr S serves as a good illustration of the need for a multidisciplinary approach to safe rehabilitation and recovery that addresses the other aspects of an offender's life. It also emphasises the importance of caring for victims. Following significant input and therapeutic work, Mr S's mother has felt able to begin to take a part in his care once more. She now meets him outside hospital unaccompanied. She has, however, never allowed him to return to her home.

Case 2. Complex firesetting

Mr A is a White European man, now in his mid-30s. He was born and raised in a remote, rural setting. He is the fourth of seven full siblings. He has two younger half-siblings from his mother's subsequent relationship. His mother was a homemaker, a 'happy and relaxed' woman who 'never stopped talking'. His father was a labourer, said to have been violent towards the family in the context of persistent alcohol misuse. Mr A's older brother developed a similar pattern of problem drinking, aside from which he reports no other family history of substance misuse, psychiatric illness, learning difficulty or criminality.

Mr A's birth was uncomplicated. At the age of 3 years, he suffered the loss of his older sister, who was said to have died after choking on chewing gum while asleep. He reportedly achieved developmental milestones appropriately but was nonetheless considered to be a 'slow learner' while at primary school. There are descriptions of hyperactivity in him as a child, which precipitated frequent beatings with a stick or 'slaps about the head' at the hands of his father. As a child, Mr A attended a single-sex primary school, from where he began to truant around the age of 8. He came into repeated contact with local police while engaging in shoplifting and other antisocial behaviours, which included a number of incidents involving fire. In this context he was transferred to a special school to attend as a day pupil. He disliked lessons, failed to complete homework and was regularly placed 'on report' by teachers for talking, eating or otherwise being disruptive in class. His truanting continued. There was some history of cruelty to animals in that on one occasion he 'swung a goat around by its ears'.

Mr A self-harmed on a number of occasions while still a child. He attributes this to the physical abuse he suffered at the hands of his father. He recalls that his mother used to berate him for 'always doing stupid things and looking for attention'. He states that cutting, like firesetting, made him feel better and 'got rid of anger and stress'. His most dramatic act of self-injury involved a laceration to his neck, inflicted at the age of 12 after drinking cider to excess. 'It sends me loopy and more aggressive.'

From the age of 11 Mr A developed further conduct problems. He was arrested for acquisitive offences and began sniffing glue and gas. At the age of 12 he started using alcohol regularly and experimented with cannabis soon after. Around this time his parents separated and he had no further contact with his father, who moved abroad. He was expelled from his school at the age of 14 in the context of further firesetting. He went on to attend a number of different schools due to his ongoing difficult behaviour and formally left education before the age of 16. Mr A spent a number of short periods in a young offender institution after being convicted of offences such as burglary and assault with intent to commit robbery. He absconded on occasion from non-secure institutions. He once attempted suicide by hanging while in custody but was cut down by officers who discovered him, before neurological damage could ensue.

Mr A enrolled upon a youth training scheme and learnt some skills in upholstery. He attended this intermittently for around 2 years but continued to set fires while not at work, on one occasion receiving a community service order after setting light to an unoccupied building. He was able to obtain some paid work in unskilled trades, held various short-term jobs as a cleaner but found no further employment beyond his early 20s. During his late teenage years his illicit drug use escalated to include infrequent use of ecstasy, cocaine powder and amphetamines but he said that he had not become a regular user of such substances because 'they really weren't that great'. He further stated that he did not use opiates, for fear of dangerous overdose.

Mr A is heterosexual in orientation and has had around 20 relationships, most lasting no more than a few months. He has no children.

In early adulthood Mr A moved from a rural to an urban environment, where he lived for a few weeks with a family member before moving into a hostel placement. When this arrangement ended after a few months, he slept rough on the streets, consuming illicit drugs and misusing alcohol with other rough sleepers. He was eventually able to return to hostel dwellings before being allocated a small home of his own by the local authority. He lived there for around a year but, in the context of relationship breakdown, set fire to this also. He had done this with the intention of ending his life, as he had felt depressed and abandoned. He was intoxicated with alcohol at the time. He escaped unhurt but caused severe structural damage to the building and received a conviction for arson.

For the first time (and as a result) he was detained in a non-secure local hospital under section 37 of the Mental Health Act 1983. He was believed to suffer from depression together with dissocial personality disorder and a mild intellectual disability. While in hospital, he went on to set a number of further fires in the grounds, resulting in further convictions and his transfer to conditions of secure care. An order restricting his discharge under section 41 of the Act was added, with the result that he undertook specialist programmes aimed at reducing his risk of arson and future problem drug and alcohol use. This appeared to have taken effect after around 2 years, when he had lived safely for a period in conditions of less secure care, and his conditional discharge to the community was being planned. The practical issues of release, such as funding, accommodation and aftercare, precipitated some delay. In the context of frustration he consumed a large amount of alcohol and set fire to his room. This resulted in his return to conditions of greater security. Mr A has a history of absconding and typically drinks alcohol to intoxication when this occurs. Drinking has also precipitated acts of self-harm and attempted suicide while in hospital.

Throughout Mr A's various hospital admissions he has engaged in psychological therapies aimed at understanding and addressing his fire-related offending. He has full recollection of such events and is able to discuss them. Mr A has always stated that he began setting fires around the age of 4. It is suspected that this was shortly after the loss of his older sister (then aged 5). He stated that he lit his first fire while in his bedroom 'playing' as his mother prepared supper downstairs.

He recalls a fascination with matches that began before this. Although his parents hid them in high cupboards he had managed to obtain a packet. He managed to ignite a blanket in his room and enjoys the recollection of his mother mistakenly believing that she had burnt the supper. Mr A was severely punished for this and as a result set no further fires in the family home, instead doing so elsewhere, in unoccupied areas or in cars he knew to have been abandoned. As he neared the end of primary education he had set fires in 'lots of hay barns'. He is prone to boasting about the ease with which he evaded discovery by hiding the accelerants he had begun to use. His offending increased in breadth as he began setting fire to cars belonging to strangers, if doors or windows had been left open or if he was able to break into them. He recalled that acts of arson had often been planned, to the extent that he would 'stake out' an area for its potential targets and the ease of his escape. He continued to secrete petrol, white spirit and matches where his parents were unable to find them. At his most prolific, he claimed to have set four to five fires each day while truanting from primary school, mostly acting alone.

Mr A has been able to discuss why he thought he had set these fires as a younger child. He speaks about 'being angry and fed up generally', stating 'it was my way of dealing with things'. With further exploration he has been able to describe a direct alteration in mood after setting light to something – 'the anger went'. Mr A reports having set many more fires while his father remained at home, before such behaviours diminished in frequency during mid-adolescence. Mr A recalls disliking school intensely, developing few friendships with male peers and being the victim of bullying. He believes that his parents dressed him in 'hippy clothes, flower power', which led to him being singled out. His recollection is that his older siblings did not protect him, despite having been taller and not therefore victims in the same way. He recalls confrontations with his father: 'I was the only one to give out to my old man. He made me angry. I wanted to get him back and that made him angry too.' Mr A describes a constant desire for vengeance as a child: 'I didn't want to hurt others, so I set fires instead'.

In sessions with clinicians Mr A has variously reported setting between 100 and 200 fires in total. The most significant of these relates to a chemical factory that he claims to have burnt to the ground after drinking heavily, resulting in £25 million worth of damage. He has no conviction for any such offence. Mr A speaks of bearing witness to serious fires for which he has not been responsible but 'really enjoying them' nonetheless. In discussion he will compare and contrast well known fires, ordering them in terms of the degree to which they capture his imagination.

During more recent periods of hospitalisation, Mr A demonstrated periods of excellent progress, engaging in occupational therapy, group-based alcohol and firesetting interventions, demonstrating problem-solving skills and undertaking self-catering. He demonstrated his ability to express anger in appropriate ways, including verbally. Abnormalities in mood were consistently absent, with no known attempts to set fires or obtain alcohol. Phrases such as 'model patient' were used by staff. From time to time, however, there remained minor breaches of rules and procedures, such as lighters being found in his possession or his not using leave within the terms agreed. He would rationalise such instances, saying for example that he had kept the lighter so he could show he 'should be trusted by staff' and prove he was not a fire risk. Such instances precipitated feelings of frustration, boredom and complaints that he had been 'in the system' for too long, following which he would abscond from leave altogether, use alcohol and experience depressive cognitions.

Following one such period of leave Mr A was returned to the unit by local police. After an extended period of stability he had been granted permission to use unescorted community leave by the Ministry of Justice. The first time that he took such leave, he did not return to the unit for some days. It emerged subsequently that he had set a number of fires, including in a wheelie bin in a local park and in several rooms of an empty house that was being renovated nearby. He spoke in a dismissive way about the punitive sanctions that might be applied to him. He stated his belief that there could 'be no cure' for his firesetting, describing himself as 'untreatable', although this label had not been put to him by his clinicians. He was again able to discuss and recount the circumstances of the fires in remarkable detail. Of note on this occasion was his recollection that, given the long period he had achieved without setting a fire, he had been overwhelmed by the urge to 'treat' himself to a further spate of arson. He continues to be detained in hospital.

Discussion

Mr A has had repeated assessments of his cognitive functioning during his various hospital stays. Estimates of his full-scale IQ have varied between 65 and 74, placing him around the threshold for a diagnosis of mild intellectual disability. In terms of function, deficits in some of the skills that contribute to the overall level of intelligence, such as language and social abilities, are at times evident. At other times he displays significant resourcefulness, the ability to deceive others and to apply careful thought to firesetting in particular. He has been able to develop a limited history of employment and to participate in in-patient programmes of occupational therapy with appropriate support. While not insignificant, the elements of cognitive impairment in him are not the primary driver of risk or functional impairment.

It appears that Mr A suffered significant childhood victimisation and that he, more than his siblings, developed a disturbed attachment with a violent father. Problem drinking was established in other members of his family. At a very young age he suffered the loss of his closest sibling, an event that, with the benefit of hindsight, seems to have been the precipitant for the onset of a serious childhood conduct disorder. This comprised acts of aggression, cruelty to animals, firesetting, stealing, repeated truancy from school, marked disobedience and difficulties in his relationships with other children (particularly males).

As an adult, his personality has been characterised by a tendency to act impulsively and without consideration of the consequences; his mood is often unpredictable, with a tendency towards self-destructive behaviour, including suicide gestures and attempts. He has developed a number of short-lived, intense and unstable intimate relationships. He has variously demonstrated his disregard for social obligations and callous unconcern for the feelings or safety of others. His offending behaviour has not been readily modifiable by adverse experience, including punishment. He has a tendency to place the blame for this with others, in particular his father. There exist in him elements of both emotionally unstable and dissocial personality disorders. On a number of occasions it appears that the fluctuations in mood he experiences have persisted, such that depressive illness has developed. A clear risk of suicide remains in the longer term.

Problem drinking is also a significant concern. Negative emotions, boredom, rejection, relationship difficulty and also feelings of excitement are all triggers for his alcohol misuse. During one period of individual cognitive–behavioural therapy, the links between these situations, feelings, behaviour and coping strategies were elucidated. A vicious cycle of alcohol use and firesetting was defined in which alcohol initially alleviates such difficulties but it becomes quickly apparent to Mr A that the 'problem hasn't been solved'. Mr A was able to identify a long-standing, well-established but maladaptive coping strategy for the subsequent feelings of loss of control: resorting to starting a fire.

It is clear, however, that this is not the only mechanism by which arson arises in him. Of concern is the description of a build-up of tension and the desire to set a fire. Acts of arson can be accompanied by intense excitement and enjoyment, and indeed he has come to view them as 'a treat'. He sustains a persistent preoccupation with subjects related to fire and burning, evidenced by the ordering in his own mind of famous or high-profile fires according to the appeal they hold for him. His many acts of, or attempts at, setting fire to property or other objects have frequently been without obvious motive. These features are among those that describe pyromania within the terms of DSM-IV-TR (see Box 12.1, page 228).

The precipitants for, intention behind and culprits behind deliberate fires are notoriously difficult to establish. Although Mr A consistently describes intentional moderation of his targets for firesetting in order to reduce the likelihood of harm to human life, the presence of some features of pyromania, the evidence of multi-point firesetting and the use (and secretion of) accelerants are indicative of high levels of dangerousness. He has derived benefit from the many different approaches to arson risk reduction that he has participated in but this therapeutic effect has been both incomplete and not sufficiently sustained to facilitate his conditional discharge into the community.

References

Anwar, S., Långström, N., Grann, M., *et al* (2011) Is arson the crime most strongly associated with psychosis? A national case–control study of arson risk in schizophrenia and other psychoses. *Schizophrenia Bulletin*, **37**, 580–586 .

Dickens, G., Sugarman, P., Ahmad, F., *et al* (2009) Recidivism and dangerousness in arsonists. *Journal of Forensic Psychiatry and Psychology*, **20**, 621–639.

Dunedin Multidisciplinary Health and Development Research Unit (2010) *Welcome to the Dunedin Multidisciplinary Health and Development Research Unit*. DMHDRU. At http://dunedinstudy.otago.ac.nz (accessed 17 December 2010).

Link, B. & Stueve, A. (1994) Psychotic symptoms and the violent/illegal behavior of mental patients compared to community controls. In *Violence and Mental Disorder* (eds J. Monahan & H. Steadman), pp. 137–159. University of Chicago Press.

Palmer, E. J., Caulfield, L. S. & Hollin, C. R. (2005) Evaluation of Interventions with Arsonists and Young Firesetters. Office of the Deputy Prime Minister.

CHAPTER 14

Fire risk and fire safety in psychiatric care

Allan Grice

Any fire within a hospital has the potential to create a far more challenging situation for local managers and care staff than one which occurs in premises where all persons are fit and able bodied. Where occupants are diagnosed with mental disorder, and may be especially vulnerable, the seriousness can be compounded to a significant degree. This chapter identifies why fires, including deliberately set fires, are a problem for providers of mental health services. The history of fires in psychiatric premises in the UK is briefly reviewed, and the increased risks associated with people resident in psychiatric units are explained. Recent, major changes in UK fire safety legislation are described and the implications for psychiatric practitioners and managers are identified. Practical steps to employ when conducting a fire risk assessment are described and the legal responsibilities of care providers under the new legislation are detailed. It is vitally important that staff receive appropriate training to ensure the safety of persons from fire, and that a fire safety culture is developed and maintained.

Fires in UK psychiatric premises: a brief history

Over the last 100 plus years a number of major fires involving loss of life have occurred in UK psychiatric premises. One of the worst was at the Colney Hatch Lunatic Asylum in north London in 1903, when 51 persons perished and all five wards were burned down (see Rollin, 2003). In 1988, at the same location, but then known as Friern Barnet Hospital, two fatalities resulted from a fire in a ward. In 1968, at Shelton Hospital in Shropshire, a major blaze killed 21 patients and injured 14 others when what was believed to be a cigarette end discarded by a patient in a locked secure ward ignited combustibles. A subsequent inquiry (*Hansard*, 1968) revealed that the night staff at Shelton had not received training in fire evacuation procedures for over 20 years. This incident also graphically illustrated the importance of promptly alerting the emergency services: the inquiry found that a 10-minute delay had occurred before a nurse who had first noticed smoke called the fire brigade. In hospital settings many patients may be unable to make their escape unaided, and therefore a sufficient staff:patient ratio can be crucial in the prevention of death and injury. The Shelton fire inquiry further highlighted this when the investigation reported that the ward was understaffed on the night of the fire. Just one year later, in 1969, four patients lost their lives in a blaze at Carlton Hayes Hospital in Leicestershire, and 30 patients died in a fire at Coldharbour Hospital in Dorset in 1972. Seven patients resident on a psychogeriatric ward at Warlingham Park Hospital in Surrey died in a fire in October 1981.

More recently, within Greater London in 2008 there were five major fires in National Health Service hospitals, one of which was in a medium-security psychiatric unit at Chase Farm Hospital. In May 2010 a fire occurred at Stockton Hall hospital in York and over 100 occupants had to be evacuated but thankfully no injuries occurred. All of these incidents illustrate the importance of proactive fire emergency planning in order to prevent deaths and serious injuries.

Fire and increased risk in psychiatric populations

During 2007 a total of 489 fires involving 30 non-fatal casualties at psychiatric hospitals in the UK were attended by fire and rescue services (FRS) (Department for Communities and Local Government, 2009). This number has fallen since, which is clearly a welcome development. The number of fires attended in psychiatric hospitals – about one in three fires in hospitals attended in 2007 – is, however, disproportionately large when compared with the proportion of hospital beds that are accounted for by mental health services – less than one in five hospital beds in England in 2007 (Department of Health, 2010). Fires are therefore more likely to be attended by FRS in psychiatric premises than in other hospital premises.

There appears to be a heightened risk of firesetting in psychiatric in-patient populations. In a study of 279 adult in-patients resident in a psychiatric hospital in the USA, researchers found evidence of fire-related risk behaviour during adulthood in the medical case notes of 27% of the population and 18% had actually engaged in deliberate firesetting (Geller *et al*, 1992). Other identified fire risks included non-deliberate but nevertheless risky behaviours such as careless smoking, falsely setting off fire alarms and falsely reporting fires to the fire department. In the community, 15% of victims in a sample derived from 535 UK fatal fire reports were judged to have mental impairment, according to the Department for Communities and Local Government (2006a). The Department concluded that 'alongside the immediate causes of a fire (e.g., carelessly discarded cigarettes), alcohol, mobility, and mental illness are the biggest single influences on whether a fire starts and/or whether it has fatal consequences'.

UK fire safety legislation: Fire Safety Order 2005

Pre-2006 legislation

UK fire safety legislation exists so that an enforcing fire authority (a statutory body comprising a committee of local councillors and advised by the chief fire officer, who is responsible for FRS policy and service delivery) can exert legal control to ensure that persons are not needlessly placed in danger from fire and its deadly products of heat, smoke and toxic gases. Until 1997, when the Fire Precautions (Workplace) Regulations (FPWPR) came into force, the FRS were responsible for delivering a prescriptive regime of fire safety enforcement and advice. Between 1997 and 2006, when the Regulatory Reform (Fire Safety) Order 2005 (Statutory Instrument no. 1541, known more simply as the Fire Safety Order) came into effect, the FRS were responsible for enforcing a mix of prescriptive and self-complying fire safety legislation.

The prescriptive regime had served well for over 30 years and was grounded in the application of fire safety law by specialist fire service staff, whose decisions were informed by first-hand experience of the effects of fire on persons and property. Under this prescriptive regime the local authority fire safety inspectors set the minimum levels of fire safety provision which they assessed as being necessary within the premises in question. The prescriptive regime drew on multiple pieces of legislation, the main one being the Fire Precautions Act 1971. Other enabling legislation, arising in the wake of fires involving loss of life in the ensuing period, followed the 1971 Act and was designed to ensure that occupants would be able to make good their safe escape in the event of fire. Owners of designated premises were required to apply to the fire authority for a fire certificate, which was issued only when the prescribed minimum provisions had been installed. Interestingly, hospitals were not identified as designated premises under the Act except where they had within their boundaries an office, shop or factory in which the criteria for fire certification were met, in which case a certificate could be issued but only in respect of that office, shop or factory.

Although some fatal fires did occur after the introduction of these regulations, the diligence of the UK fire services prescriptive regime, and regular on-site inspections to monitor compliance and enforce the fire safety laws, vastly improved the fire safety record of most of those premises to which they applied. Indeed, such was the scale of this success that central government came to the conclusion that there might not be a continuing need for such prescriptive legislation.

Background to the introduction of Fire Safety Order 2005

The thinking described above was bolstered by European Union Directives (89/391/EEC and 89/654/EEC) which required member states to legislate in respect of workplace safety. The central tenet of these Directives was a shift from fire service prescription to a regime in which the burden of responsibility rests on business employers, because any hazards within their premises arise from their own activities, processes and operations. To avoid any doubt, a 'hazard' is something which has the potential to cause harm, and 'risk' is the mathematical probability of the harm from any hazard arising and causing injury to persons. As mentioned, the FPWPR came into force in 1997 and up until 2006 an unsatisfactory overlap of fire safety legislation existed by virtue of the fact that some categories of premise were subject to the requirements of both the 1971 Act and the 1997 FPWPR. Even though a survey by the Chief and Assistant Chief Fire Officers Association (Office of the Deputy Prime Minister, 2002, p. 91) revealed that, several years after their introduction, only 58% of premises had still to self-comply with the FPWPR (which threw doubt on the entrusting of fire safety to a self-determining regime), further public consultation led to the application of regulatory reform legislation, and those effective fire service prescribed laws of the previous 40 or so years were repealed.

About 100 separate pieces of fire safety legislation were brought under the umbrella of the Regulatory Reform (Fire Safety) Order 2005. The Fire Safety Order captures within its net virtually all non-domestic premises, including hospitals and care premises, and came into force in October 2006. Although the local fire authority is still statutorily obliged to enforce the requirements of the legislation, and to provide certain fire safety advice if requested, the unconditional responsibility for adequate standards of premise occupant safety resides with a nominated 'responsible person', who is usually the employer, and is usually not an expert in fire matters. This person, along with certain 'other persons', is required to self-comply with this legislation and to ensure that adequate levels of fire safety exist for all occupants of premises at all material times, so that no person (in a hospital, patients, staff or visitors) are ever placed at risk of death or serious injury from fire (article 5(3) of the Order).

Underlying principles of the Order

At the heart of the Fire Safety Order are three key principles:

1   the carrying out of a *suitable and sufficient* fire risk assessment (FRA)
2   the imposition of legal burdens of responsibility and accountability on a nominated *responsible person*
3   The recording of *significant findings* in premises where five or more persons are present, where any licence is in force or where the FRS have served an 'alterations notice' under the Order.

The concept of a making the employer responsible for self-determining the degree of safety provision required is not new in the UK. Since the Health and Safety at Work Act 1974 and its subsequent legislative progressions and developments, workplace safety legislation has followed this route of employer self-compliance, which gives employers a clear duty to have in place reasonably practicable safety provisions. It also places responsibilities upon individual employees in respect of their own safety, and that of others who might be affected by their acts or omissions.

Such fire safety provisions are essential when they are in premises used for treatment and care, and particularly where sleeping accommodation is provided. The UK fire service has, in the main, applied a 'high risk' category to premises in which persons sleep because it is during the sleeping hours, when persons are oblivious to their surroundings, that they are more vulnerable to the hazards of fire. These hazards are further compounded where psychiatric patients are accommodated.

Fire risk assessment: prevention first

The 2005 Fire Safety Order is not without its critics but perhaps one of its strongest suits is that the prevention of fire is integral, whereas the old regime focused on ensuring that occupants could escape after a fire had started. Central to this preventive process is the FRA. Those charged with assessing the degree of fire risk arising from an actual or perceived hazard must weigh up a range of factors when making their evaluation. The Order requires the FRA to be 'suitable and sufficient' and, should any doubt exist as to the rigour to be employed, then, relative to the hazards existing, it is prudent to use a critical approach, especially in sleeping-risk psychiatric premises.

The decisions made during the fire hazard identification and FRA process by individuals holding a responsibility for implementing the legal requirements of the Order will be informed by their own experiences and knowledge relevant to fire dynamics and thus will be better assisted if they have solid practical experience of the dynamics of fire and smoke. Any serious shortfall in experience, or unsound technical knowledge, could have life-threatening repercussions should fire occur. For example, the less experienced assessor may observe a hazard such as combustible materials within a seemingly fire-resisting room fitted with self-closing fire doors and conclude that the risk to persons is reduced should a fire start, because of the fire-resisting doors. However, if the assessor failed to notice that the room contained a shaft which was part of an air circulation installation, and was not fitted with fire detectors or fire dampers, this could allow smoke and heat from a fire to travel to other locations, with serious consequences (Grice, 2008).

Article 18 of the Order 2005 requires the 'responsible person' to nominate competent persons to assist them in the discharge of their preventive and protective duties. 'Competence' is currently defined in relation to the Order as a person who has 'sufficient training and experience or knowledge and other qualities to enable him properly to assist in undertaking the preventive and protective measures'. Ideally, that competence should reside *within* the organisation because an employee will be more familiar with the physical layout of the premises, and the locations within the premises where the greatest risks exist, than an external advisor (Grice, 2008, p. 172).

Content of fire risk assessment

Central government has produced guidance documents to assist those carrying the burdens of responsibility, including a guide specifically relevant to hospital premises (Department for Communities and Local Government, 2006*b*). The advice within the appropriate guides, along with that to be found in other publications, should be followed closely. Box 14.1 displays

---

Box 14.1 Content of a 'suitable and sufficient' fire risk assessment

- The number and location of 'high risk' and 'vulnerable' patients and the adequacy of staff:patient ratios for assisting these in safe evacuation
- The numbers and location of 'lower risk' patients and the adequacy of staff:patient ratios for assisting these in safe evacuation
- The provision of properly positioned fire exits and fire-protected escape routes which accord with national guidance, including hospital fire safety codes, in terms of exit dimensions and the distances to be travelled to reach a place of safety
- The number and type of staircases and whether they are protected or unprotected
- The evacuation strategies in force, that is, whether horizontal or vertical (i.e., an escape route all on one horizontal level or via a staircase), or a mixture. Whether the evacuation is to a place of ultimate or relative safety and whether it will be a full or partial evacuation, using a staged exiting procedure relative to the severity and size of the fire. A place of relative safety is, for example, to the security of a set of fire doors which holds back fire and smoke. A place of ultimate safety is outside the affected building and in a position out of danger from fire products
- The existence of competently trained fire marshals and fire wardens wearing readily identifiable surcoats, able to ensure safe evacuation to suitably illuminated and secure assembly and refuge points
- A sound staff training programme in fire awareness and fire emergency routines and which includes every employee and which is refreshed often
- A consideration to educate patients and hostel residents of fire dangers
- Secure and prominently indicated 'Fire Evacuation Assembly Points'
- Adequate patient supervision to ensure that no one re-enters the premises, with a particular regard to the most vulnerable patients
- Provision of fire-detection and warning systems suitable for patients and which take into account any hearing or sight impairment
- A clear understanding by all staff of the emergency evacuation routines and an unambiguous understanding of any fire alarm signals to be used
- Early and ongoing liaison with the fire service in respect of fire and rescue
- Early and ongoing liaison with any authority other than the fire service that holds responsibilities in respect of fire safety

---

considerations for inclusion in a 'suitable and sufficient' FRA within a psychiatric care premise. This list is not exhaustive. Box 14.2 displays considerations for a critical fire hazard and risk assessment of all parts of the premises.

Collective and individual safety

The 2005 Fire Safety Order places greater weight on the collective safety of persons than on that of individuals alone, and within our increasingly litigious society, where we are constantly reminded about our 'duty of care', an organisation needs to be able to withstand the most rigorous external

---

Box 14.2 Considerations for a critical fire hazard and risk assessment of all parts of the premises

- Every floor level, every room, cupboard, roof space, false ceiling, hatch and shaft at each level
- Location and type of combustible/ flammable materials discovered
- Location and type of heating boilers, waste incinerators and associated ducting
- Location of refuse and pathogenic waste disposal areas, and arson-secured refuse containers and chutes
- Heating, ventilation and air-conditioning systems and ducting, and whether fitted with fire detection/fire damping features
- Location of isolating switches and valves to electricity, gas and medical gases
- Location of medical gas cylinder compounds
- Approved locations where smoking is permitted
- Evidence of surreptitious smoking in wards, day rooms and bathroom areas
- Location of bedding and mattress stores and their security against arson
- Evidence of poor housekeeping such as combustible refuse or furniture on escape routes
- Defective closing devices on fire and smoke doors
- Fire and smoke doors warped and not fully closing or seals defective
- Obstructions next to fire doors held open on fire-detector-linked magnets
- Failures to close fire and smoke doors during sleeping hours
- Policies for permitting patients to circulate in corridors unsupervised
- Evidence of tampering with fire and smoke detectors
- Evidence of tampering with fire-fighting equipment
- Clear marking of fire-fighting equipment
- Clear records of regular testing of fire detection and alarm systems
- Clear records of regular testing of emergency escape lighting
- Provision of sufficient numbers of fire exit signs visible in all light conditions
- All fire exits unobstructed internally and externally
- Clear policies about opening of secure fire exits in 'high risk' patient areas (i.e., secure or locked wards)
- Premise's fire safety policies to accord with current fire safety guidance issued by central government and by appropriate primary care trusts
- The presence of a comprehensive emergency plan known to all parties and which is subjected to regular review and testing

---

scrutiny should a serious fire occur. This means that, within psychiatric care premises, the potential for disruptive false fire alarms as a result of patients actuating wall-mounted call points needs to be taken fully into account.

Consideration could be given to replacing call points with the appropriate type of ceiling smoke or heat detector, to securing call points with covers which only nominated unit staff can access as part of a pre-planned emergency routine, or other initiatives which will ensure early warning of fire but which cannot be easily actuated by patients. Any failure to implement such initiatives could result in frequent false alarms. Not only does this cause major disruption created by evacuations, not only does it unnecessarily agitate patients, but it can create a 'cry wolf' mentality, with all the dangers of a dilution of the urgency of the response should a genuine emergency occur.

However, any decision to modify arrangements for detecting fire and for sounding an alarm should never be taken lightly, especially within psychiatric healthcare premises, and especially in premises in which persons sleep. Where doubts as to the safety of premise occupants exists as a consequence of measures to limit the potential for false alarms, there must be liaison with the FRS, even though unconditional responsibility under the Fire Safety Order rests with the responsible person(s). The principles which underpin healthcare premise fire safety codes need to be taken fully into account by all caught by the definition within article 5(3).

Responsibilities of psychiatric care staff and managers

Article 5(3) of the Fire Safety Order 2005 defines those members of staff and other persons on whose shoulders the Order imposes a burden of responsibility. All those responsible within the psychiatric care premise must make themselves thoroughly familiar with the life-protecting principles which lie at the heart of this dynamic legislation. For this new law is indeed dynamic and the old, non-retrospective nature of the UK fire safety law regime, in which a legitimate but inadequate standard could be frozen in time, has now gone. The 2005 Order (article 9) requires any FRA to be under constant review so as to ensure that at all material times the levels of preventive and protective provisions to ensure no person is placed at risk of death or serious injury are reasonable and practicable. Such a dynamic concept best ensures that any new scenario arising is subjected to the hazard and risk assessment process.

At the time of writing there is a need for some judicial elucidation in respect of some of the definitions and terminology used within the 2005 Fire Safety Order. While only the courts can interpret what the law was intended to mean, we can state that the 'other persons' mentioned in the Order may well be managers and supervisors, who, when on duty, have to ensure that the general fire safety provisions of the Order are being complied with (article 5(3); see also Grice, 2008). By way of example, one of the requirements of the Order is to ensure that fire exit routes are unobstructed.

If a nursing sister observed obstructions along the exit route from her ward and failed to have these removed, she might be liable if her omission placed any person at risk of death or serious injury. It is also likely that external contractors may be one of these 'other persons'. Given that the Order places such unconditional burdens of responsibility on the nominated 'responsible person', as well as on others, it is essential that all within the psychiatric care premise managerial arena are clear as to what the Order requires, and the following are key elements of this legislation.

All employees have a legal responsibility under the Fire Safety Order. Without this clarity there is the very real possibility that shortfalls might exist within the fire safety provisions for the premises, which could endanger occupants. Each person has an individual legal responsibility for the safety of themselves and others, and this applies from chief executive level down to the most junior member of staff (article 23).

Fire does not have to occur for an offence to have been committed. It cannot be overemphasised that all within the managerial hierarchy who are caught within the net of the Order need to be aware that a fire does not have to occur for offences to have been committed. The 'responsible person' or those 'other persons' mentioned can be liable by placing any person at risk of death or serious injury *even if no fire occurs.*

Limits of responsibility of the fire authority

Although the local fire service is statutorily obliged to enforce the requirements of the 2005 Fire Safety Order, and to provide free advice in respect of fire safety, it cannot carry out the FRA, which is the unconditional responsibility of the 'responsible person'. Even where an external fire safety consultant is instructed, the 'responsible person' cannot use as a defence if charged with committing an offence under the Order, any failing on the part of such a consultant (article 32.2–11(b)). In addition, should the fire authority charge a 'responsible person' with a failure to make adequate fire preventive and protective provisions, it is for the 'responsible person' to prove to the court why it was not reasonable or practicable to make those provisions. Traditionally, up until the introduction of the 2005 Order, it was for the enforcing fire authority to prove that an offence had been committed.

Recording of significant findings

Where five or more persons are employed, or where the fire authority has served an alterations notice, or where any licence is in force, a record of the 'significant findings' of the FRA must be made. To avoid any misunderstanding, an alterations notice is a notice served upon the responsible person of a premise when the enforcing authority are of the opinion that the premise or its contents, services, fittings, construction or usage, are such that a serious risk to persons exists. The notice requires the responsible person to notify the enforcing authority before any changes are made in respect of those parameters which could significantly increase the risk to relevant persons, which means persons within, or within the immediate vicinity of the premises. A licence in force is any licence which is required and is in force on the premise, for example, licence to store petroleum, hazardous substances, to serve alcohol, etc. There is no definition within the Fire Safety Order 2005 of what constitutes a 'significant finding', and this is a second area needing judicial clarification. In practice, however, 'significant finding' is likely to mean something which is of significance to the overall process of implementation of 'general fire precautions' (see article 4 for a definition of 'general fire precautions'). By way of example, some or all of the hazards discovered and assessed in terms of the degree of risk during the FRA would be 'significant findings'. Where the premises contain provisions which are vital to the fire safety of occupants, such as an automatic fire detection and warning system, fire and smoke doors which automatically shut should fire and smoke be detected, then these would be 'significant findings' to be recorded also during the FRA process, especially if the removal or dilution of these could place occupants at risk of death or serious injury.

Importance of staff training

The Fire Safety Order 2005 includes a requirement that all employees (including those at the highest managerial levels) receive suitable and adequate training at periodic intervals. The Home Office FRA guidance manual sets out the sort of topics to be included within employee fire safety training (Department for Communities and Local Government, 2006b). However, the actual wording within the Order does not, in the opinion of some, sufficiently emphasise that training can be crucial to the achievement of requisite standards of person safety. Specifically, the requirement that training 'be repeated periodically where appropriate' (article 21.2(b)) is a loose term and an organisation could carry out staff training every 5 years and claim to be undertaking training 'periodically'. Historically, within the UK fire service, it has been the policy to advise responsible persons within such premises that twice a year is the absolute minimum. However, the practical experience of FRS operational officers when attending fires in premises housing many people such as hospitals indicates that what is imparted at fire safety staff training sessions can soon be forgotten. Accordingly, and especially where there is high staff turnover, one session every 3 months is a better option, and all new employees must receive appropriate fire and safety induction on the first day. Additionally, the issuing of pocket-size *aide-mémoire* cards to trainees, who should be advised always to have these on their person, can play an important part in ensuring sound fire safety knowledge exists. Fire safety training must also relate to the findings of the FRA.

General fire safety training is of little use unless the person delivering it is able clearly to communicate the importance of key factors. This author has found that a role-play scenario, underpinned by explanations and video imagery about what it is actually like to be in a building filling with heat and smoke, is probably a more effective training tool than lectures alone. However, the Fire Safety Order makes it clear that fire safety training is to be carried out in work time. In a busy hospital, time is critical and it is not always possible to be able to engage in time-consuming participatory role-play. On balance, this author has concluded that four short but emphatic training sessions a year (i.e., every 3 months), augmented by pocket prompt cards, better ensure that effective emergency actions are carried out than only one or two longer training sessions per year. By the end of a training session, staff should, as a minimum, be aware of how fires can start, how they can spread, how they can be prevented and basic firefighting operations, and have an understanding that fire evacuation drills are conducted to audit the overall effectiveness of training given (Grice, 2008).

Importance of vigilance via frequent monitoring

In a psychiatric premise it is vital to augment hazard identification with a clear awareness that deliberately ignited fires may occur, and to ensure that appropriate vigilance is kept via frequent physical patrols. Psychiatric premises require that those carrying out the FRA must employ a critical and rigorous approach at all stages. No stone should be left unturned in the identification of fire hazards, including the potential arsonist.

Importance of regular fire evacuation drills

Senior management must ensure that fire drills are carried out regularly in order to ensure that, when the alarm sounds, evacuation routines, calling the fire service and emergency firefighting operations are enacted without fail. In psychiatric hospitals, where the risk is potentially high, it will not be overkill to have fire drills at least four times a year, but their planning and implementation must take into account the category and vulnerability of patients and there must be a clear written policy communicated to all employees in respect of the existence and rationale behind them.

The behaviour of people in fire emergencies

One of the most important things for all those holding fire safety responsibilities to recognise is the psychology of people's behaviour in respect of hearing a fire alarm, or of noticing fire and smoke. Some academic research has been carried out on this (Canter, 1980) and this author has witnessed at first hand how human reaction to fire can be blunted almost as if those seeing flame and smoke do not really believe what they are observing.

During the early stages of the 1979 Manchester Woolworths fire, it was reported that some customers eating in the store's restaurant were reluctant to evacuate even when heavy smoke was evident because they wanted to finish their meals! The fire resulted in ten fatalities. Such experience and academic study findings of personal behaviour in fire emergencies is one of the factors behind the appointment of fire marshals and fire wardens to ensure safety in the event of an emergency evacuation.

Liaison with fire and rescue services

An important element of training is liaison with the FRS ahead of any emergency. Indeed, the 2005 Fire Safety Order makes this a legal requirement of the 'responsible person' (article 13(3)). The Fire and Rescue Services Act 2004 places a duty on the local fire authority to visit premises to obtain information which will assist in their fire and rescue operations. It is important for the premise fire safety manager to realise that such visits will not normally be concerned with an audit of fire safety regulations but rather with those features of the premises which will help FRS to carry out their fire and rescue tasks effectively. Fire crews will note the layout of the premises and any special hazards. They will note where internal hydrants or other water supplies are located. They will need to know how many persons occupy the premises and their locations, including those in secure units. The position of assembly points to which occupants rendezvous on evacuating must be known, as well as the challenges faced by nursing and medical staff in managing patients during a serious fire and ensuring the premises are vacated with no one re-entering (Grice, 2008).

The importance of a fire and safety culture

It is imperative that a fire safety culture is developed and maintained. It is only by way of effective and regular inputs via face-to-face staff training, positive but easily understood written policy statements, and emergency plans (which are legal health and safety requirements), plus ongoing audit of all elements of the fire preventive and fire protective processes, that an organisation will be best protected, as a result of every member of staff being inculcated with the safety culture and preventive ethos.

Fire and its deadly by-products of toxic smoke and gases can often need a more intensive regime and culture than other health and safety situations. The whole business of hazards to persons has resulted in what many would argue is a neurotic and irrational focus on personal safety, to the extent that one can hardly make a cup of coffee in one's office without going through a risk assessment process! Although such critical approaches might be grounded in good intentions, the experienced and intelligent assessor of risk knows that it is all too easy to engage in over-provision, which can border on the ludicrous. However, the process of hazard assessment and risk evaluation when dealing with fire can be a good deal more involved than other areas of personal safety. Within hospital and care premises where the psychiatric patient is accommodated, FRAs have to cover the whole list of elements set out above, and this requires not only adequate time but also a high level of technical and practical competence on the part of those on whose shoulders the burdens for self-compliance with the Fire Safety Order are imposed.

Balance between life quality of patients and overt safety measures

Within a hospital and care premise the quality of the daily life of patients has also to be considered. If safety provisions become too impractical to implement, or lead to individual or collective discomfort, people may resort to their own measures superficially to improve their situation at the expense of potentially jeopardising fire safety provisions. By way of example, during very hot weather occupants may resort to propping or wedging open fire doors in order to get cooling air into the building. Those charged with fire risk and general safety assessments must be able to prioritise intelligently which aspects of safety need to be addressed first. In this case, the potential effect of negating the fire-resisting properties of the doors far outweighs immediate considerations of comfort, and alternative solutions (i.e., air conditioners) should be sought. The prioritisation and selection of the most safety-critical tasks must be made to best ensure that all responsibilities under the Order are being fully complied with. The skill in this prioritisation lies in those carrying out an FRA having enough experience and knowledge to know what is under-provision and what is over-provision in terms of fire preventive and protective mechanisms. Where fire safety is carried out by a dedicated in-house safety manager, there must be a foolproof system in place in which, during his or her absence, a fully competent reserve manager is available at all material times.

Information handover procedure

In organisations where safety responsibilities are shared, say because of a shift system, it is vital that, at the change-over of duties, all information relevant to fire and general safety is fully and clearly handed over, with a dedicated handover log system used which can withstand external scrutiny should an emergency occur. The Fire Safety Order places a legal duty on responsible persons to cooperate and coordinate with each other (article 22).

Sound handover procedures have been an integral part of the world-renowned effectiveness of the UK FRS for decades. For the detailed reasons set out within this chapter, these handover measures assume even greater criticality. For example, if defects were reported in respect of any of the fire safety protective provisions during the day shift, say a fault on the automatic fire detection system, this information must be handed over to the night shift so that all are aware of the situation and of any interim safety procedures.

Relationship between FRS emergency attendance and the fire safety of occupants

Although a prompt response by the FRS has never been a reason for an organisation to shirk its fire safety responsibilities, it has been the case, especially within the larger urban areas, that a rapid response of fire pumps could offset imperfect fire safety provisions. However, since 2004 the UK fire services have had to produce what are called 'integrated risk management plans' as an element in the most effective and efficient allocation of finite resources. One outcome of these risk-based plans has been a reduction in the speed and weight of fire appliances attending reports of fire. Hospital staff who hold responsibilities under the Order need to liaise with the FRS to establish how long, in normal circumstances, it will take for the first crews to arrive on scene. They will need to bear in mind that if an emergency has happened elsewhere, then fire appliances may have to come from a greater distance, during which time a fire may spread. It will be a naïve manager who fails to appreciate that a slower or reduced attendance has a bearing on the need for all fire safety systems to be of the highest level, especially in hospital and care premises. It would also be a naïve employer and manager who failed to appreciate that any central government decisions to impose significant financial cuts, for whatever reason, could have consequences for staffing and resource levels for both the FRS and the health services, and thus impact on fire safety. The above pointers are of importance in any premise in which people sleep, and the larger the complex and the greater the number of occupants, then the greater will be the burden on those holding fire safety responsibilities. Within psychiatric hospitals and other care and treatment centres these burdens will be increased, especially where high-risk or vulnerable persons are present, some of whom may have a history of firesetting.

Enforcement of the Fire Safety Order 2005

The responsible fire authority is statutorily obliged to enforce the require-ments of the Fire Safety Order within its area. It has been this author's experience that many employers are still unclear about what part the FRS play in the enforcement process. This author is currently unconvinced, some years after the Fire Safety Order came into force, that all employers and managers understand the massive shifts which have taken place. As already stated, the FRS cannot carry out the FRA. The FRS enforcement role is to select and prioritise those premises which they wish to monitor for compliance. Should such an inspection reveal shortfalls in the fire safety provisions, the FRS are empowered to serve one or more of three notices on the responsible person: the FRS can serve an 'enforcement notice', an 'alterations notice' or, in the case of the discovery of an excessive risk, a 'prohibition notice'. The latter can lead to the full or partial closure of a premise until the excessive fire risk is lowered. Responsible persons must be mindful that the fact that the FRS have not carried out an audit for self-compliance is no excuse for failure to ensure that all relevant requirements for general fire precautions have been complied with. FRS managers on front-line appliances are trained to recognise fire safety shortfalls and to alert their fire safety specialist counterparts of any defects. A failure by a responsible person to comply with the Order's requirements and which places any person at risk of death or serious injury can result in imprisonment for up to 2 years, or a maximum fine, or both a fine and imprisonment. A range of other offences and penalties exist within the Order (article 32).

Summary and conclusions

This chapter has highlighted the additional fire risks that are presented to care staff and managers in psychiatric care premises. It has identified the major change in UK fire safety legislation that places the onus of responsibility for preventing fire and for ensuring fire safety on the providers of those premises. Practical steps to ensure compliance with the Fire Safety Order have been presented. In conclusion, the Order, by placing an unconditional responsibility on the shoulders of those caught by the definitions in article 5(3), creates a very heavy burden indeed. These burdens are added to for responsible persons within psychiatric care premises, who have the additional challenges and responsibilities that working with this category of patient poses. However, a close adherence to the above pointers, augmented by the advice provided within the guidance literature mentioned, and by an unceasing vigilance on all aspects of occupant safety from fire, should mean that the law will have been complied with and, most importantly, that no occupant of psychiatric care and treatment premises should have been placed at risk of death or serious injury from fire.

References

Canter, D. (ed.) (1980) *Fires and Human Behaviour*. Wiley.

Department for Communities and Local Government (2006a) *Learning Lessons from Real Fires: Lessons from Fatal Fire Investigation Reports*. Arson Control Forum Research Bulletin no. 9. Department for Communities and Local Government. At http://www.arsoncontrolforum.gov.uk/download/628 (accessed 17 December 2010).

Department for Communities and Local Government (2006b) *Fire Safety Risk Assessment: Healthcare Premises*. Department for Communities and Local Government. At http://www.communities.gov.uk/documents/fire/pdf/152119.pdf (accessed 17 December 2010).

Department for Communities and Local Government (2009) *Fire Statistics United Kingdom 2007*. Department for Communities and Local Government. At http://www.communities.gov.uk/publications/corporate/statistics/firestatisticsuk2007 (accessed 17 December 2010).

Department of Health (2010) *Hospital Activity Statistics*. Department of Health. At http://www.performance.doh.gov.uk/hospitalactivity/data_requests/beds_open_overnight.htm (accessed 17 December 2010).

Geller, J. L., Fisher, W. H. & Moynihan, K. (1992) Adult lifetime prevalence of firesetting behaviours in a state hospital population. *Psychiatric Quarterly*, **63**, 129–142.

Grice, A. (2008) *Fire Risk: Fire Safety Law and Its Practical Application*. Thorogood.

Hansard (1968) Shelton Hospital (fire). *House of Commons Debates*, 26 February, 759, cc. 945–947. At http://hansard.millbanksystems.com/commons/1968/feb/26/shelton-hospital-fire (accessed 17 December 2010).

Office of the Deputy Prime Minister (2002) *A Consultation Document on the Reform of Fire Safety Legislation*. Office of the Deputy Prime Minister.

Rollin, H. (2003) One hundred years ago. Terrible fire at Colney Hatch Asylum. *British Journal of Psychiatry*, **182**, 553.

Index

Compiled by Judith Reading